Disease Ecology

Disease Ecology

Community structure and pathogen dynamics

EDITED BY

Sharon K. Collinge

and

Chris Ray
University of Colorado, USA

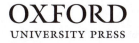

OXFORD
UNIVERSITY PRESS

OXFORD

UNIVERSITY PRESS

Great Clarendon Street, Oxford OX2 6DP

Oxford University Press is a department of the University of Oxford.
It furthers the University's objective of excellence in research, scholarship,
and education by publishing worldwide in

Oxford New York

Auckland Cape Town Dar es Salaam Hong Kong Karachi
Kuala Lumpur Madrid Melbourne Mexico City Nairobi
New Delhi Shanghai Taipei Toronto

With offices in

Argentina Austria Brazil Chile Czech Republic France Greece
Guatemala Hungary Italy Japan Poland Portugal Singapore
South Korea Switzerland Thailand Turkey Ukraine Vietnam

Oxford is a registered trade mark of Oxford University Press
in the UK and in certain other countries

Published in the United States
by Oxford University Press Inc., New York

British Library Cataloguing in Publication Data

Data available

Library of Congress Cataloging-in-Publication Data

Disease ecology / edited by Sharon K. Collinge and Chris Ray.
    p. cm.
    Includes bibliographical references.
    ISBN 0–19–856708–1 (alk. paper) — ISBN 0–19–856707–3 (alk. paper)
    1. Communicable diseases—Environmental aspects.   2. Host-parasite
relationships—Environmental aspects.   3. Communicable diseases in
animals—Environmental aspects.   I. Collinge, Sharon K.   II. Ray, Chris.
    [DNLM: 1. Communicable Diseases—epidemiology.   2. Ecology.
3. Host-Parasite Relations.   WA 110 D6113 2006]
RA643.D57 2006
614.5—dc22

                                                      2005020774

Typeset by Newgen Imaging Systems (P) Ltd., Chennai, India
Printed in Great Britain
on acid-free paper by
Antony Rowe, Chippenham, Wiltshire

ISBN 0–19–856707–3   978–0–19–856707–3
ISBN 0–19–856708–1 (Pbk.)   978–0–19–856708–0 (Pbk.)

10 9 8 7 6 5 4 3 2 1

To all the creatures that delight and inspire

Preface

Our research on disease ecology began several years ago when our collaborative research group was awarded funding from the NSF/NIH joint program, "Ecology of Infectious Diseases" to study landscape change and disease dynamics in prairie dogs. Many of the ideas and relationships that led to this book were generated through the annual PI network meetings for this program. We have learned volumes from the participants in this group and especially appreciate the support and vision of Joshua Rosenthal (NIH Fogarty Center) and Sam Scheiner (NSF) in fostering collaborative interactions among a diverse group of scientists interested in ecology and infectious disease dynamics.

The idea for this book arose at the 2002 meeting of the Ecological Society of America, where we were inspired by the growing number of presentations on disease ecology. We followed up on this trend by organizing a symposium explicitly focused on community ecology and epidemiology for the 2003 ESA meeting in Savannah. As two ecologists with experience in population, community, and landscape ecology, we sought to gather the collective expertise of ecologists working at the interface of disease ecology and epidemiology. The symposium in Savannah was highly successful (despite the delays incurred because participants had to catch a ferry to reach our 8 a.m. symposium!) and we were encouraged by Ian Sherman's enthusiasm for a related book project through Oxford University Press. We contacted additional contributors to add to the breadth of topics covered, and began soliciting the chapters that you see in this volume.

We especially thank our prairie dog disease research group for stimulating our thoughts and engaging discussions regarding disease ecology, including Jack Cully, Ken Gage, Whit Johnson, Michael Kosoy, Andrew Martin, and Bai Ying, as well as the graduate students in the group, Ellen Bean, Jory Brinkerhoff, David Conlin, Tammi Johnson, Ryan Jones, Kimberly Kosmenko, Amy Markeson, Sue Rodriguez-Pastor, and Bala Thiagarajan. We would have made little progress without the enthusiastic work of numerous field assistants over the past 3 years, and we sincerely thank them all.

This book benefited greatly from careful review and discussion of chapters by an informal "Disease ecology discussion group" at the University of Colorado-Boulder, including Ellen Bean, Jory Brinkerhoff, David Conlin, Ryan Jones, Matthew Kern, Amy Markeson, Andrew Martin, Susan Perkins, and Jamie Voyles. We are grateful for their contributions and are happy to report that many of the comments and insights made by this group found their way into the final versions of these chapters.

No serious project is completed without the understanding and endless patience of those people close to us. So a million thank-yous to Joan and Jeff for the emotional support, for being there with the Chipotle burritos, and for putting up with the late nights and early mornings.

Finally, we are sincerely grateful to Ian Sherman at Oxford for his continued patience, encouragement, and support of this project, and to Kerstin Demata, Abbie Headon and Anita Petrie for expert answers to our seemingly endless supply of questions.

Contents

List of contributors

Nicole Achee, Department of Preventive Medicine and Biometrics, USUHS, 4301 Jones Bridge Rd., Bethesda, MD 20814, USA. E-mail: nachee@usuhs.mil

Susan R. Bolden, School of Forestry & Environmental Studies, Yale University, New Haven, CT 06511, USA. E-mail: susan.bolden@yale.edu

Julia M. Butzler, Department of Biological Sciences, Dartmouth College, Hanover, NH 03755, USA. E-mail: Julia.M.Butzler@dartmouth.edu

James E. Childs, Department of Epidemiology, Yale School of Medicine, Yale University, New Haven, CT 06510, USA. E-mail: jamesechilds@comcast.net

Keith Clay, Department of Biology, Indiana University, Bloomington, IN 47405, USA. E-mail: clay@indiana.edu

Sharon K. Collinge, Department of Ecology and Evolutionary Biology and Environmental Studies Program, University of Colorado, Boulder, CO 80309-0334, USA. E-mail: Sharon.Collinge@colorado.edu

Kathryn L. Cottingham, Department of Biological Sciences, Dartmouth College, Hanover, NH 03755, USA. E-mail: Kathryn.Cottingham@dartmouth.edu

Andrew A. Cunningham, Institute of Zoology, Zoological Society of London, Regent's Park, London NW1 4RY, U.K. E-mail: a.cunningham@ioz.ac.uk

Eddie W. Cupp, Department of Entomology and Plant Pathology, Auburn University, Auburn, AL 36849, USA. E-mail: ecupp@ag.auburn.edu

Peter Daszak, Consortium for Conservation Medicine, 460 West 34th Street, New York, NY 10001, USA. E-mail: Daszak@conservationmedicine.org

Andrew P. Dobson, Department of Ecology and Evolutionary Biology, Princeton University, Princeton, NJ 08544, USA. E-mail: dobber@princeton.edu

Jon H. Epstein, Consortium for Conservation Medicine, 460 West 34th Street, New York, NY 10001, USA. E-mail: Epstein@conservationmedicine.org

Hume E. Field, Animal Research Institute, Dept. of Primary Industries, LMB 4, Moorooka 4105, Brisbane, Queensland, Australia. E-mail: Hume.Field@dpi.qld.gov.au

L. Kealoha Freidenburg, School of Forestry & Environmental Studies, Yale University, New Haven, CT 06511, USA. E-mail: kealoha.freidenburg@yale.edu

Nicole A. Freidenfelds, Department of Natural Resources, University of New Hampshire, Durham, NH 03824, USA. E-mail: naf5@cisunix.unh.edu

Clay Fuqua, Department of Biology, Indiana University, Bloomington, IN 47405, USA. E-mail: cfuqua@bio.indiana.edu

John Grieco, Department of Preventive Medicine and Biometrics, USUHS, 4301 Jones Bridge Rd., Bethesda, MD 20814, USA. E-mail: jgrieco@usuhs.mil

Kim Halpin, CSIRO, Livestock Industries, Australian Animal Health Laboratory, Private Bag 24, Geelong, Victoria 3220, Australia. E-mail: kim.halpin@csiro.au

Ryan F. Hechinger, Department of Ecology, Evolution and Marine Biology, University of California, Santa Barbara, CA 93106, USA. E-mail: Hechige@lifesci.ucsb.edu

Richard M. Higashi, Environmental Chemistry Group, Crocker Nuclear Laboratory, University of California, Davis, CA 95616, USA. E-mail: rmhigashi@ucdavis.edu

Manja P. Holland, School of Forestry & Environmental Studies, Yale University, New Haven, CT 06511, USA. E-mail: manja.holland@yale.edu

Robert D. Holt, Department of Zoology, University of Florida, Gainesville, FL 32611-8525, USA. E-mail: rdholt@zoo.ufl.edu

Alex D. Hyatt, CSIRO, Livestock Industries, Australian Animal Health Laboratory, Private Bag 24, Geelong, Victoria 3220, Australia. E-mail: Alex.Hyatt@csiro.au

Abdul Aziz bin Jamaluddin, Deputy Director General, Department of Veterinary Services, Ministry of Agriculture, 8th & 9th Floor, Wisma Chase Perdana, Off Jalan Semantan, Damansara Heights, 50630 Kuala Lumpur, Malaysia. E-mail: aziz@jph.gov.my

Felicia Keesing, Biology Department, Bard College, Annandale-on-Hudson, NY 12504, USA. E-mail: keesing@bard.edu

Armand M. Kuris, Department of Ecology, Evolution and Marine Biology and Marine Science Institute, University of California, Santa Barbara, CA 93106, USA. E-mail: kuris@lifesci.ucsb.edu

Kevin D. Lafferty, USGS Western Ecological Research Center and Marine Science Institute, University of California, Santa Barbara, CA 93106, USA. E-mail: klafferty@usgs.gov

Curt Lively, Department of Biology, Indiana University, Bloomington, IN 47405, USA. E-mail: clively@bio.indiana.edu

Kathleen LoGiudice, Biology Department, Union College, Schenectady, NY 12308, USA. E-mail: logiudik@union.edu

Stephen Luby, Programme on Infectious Diseases and Vaccine Sciences, ICDDR,B, Centre for Health and Population Research, GPO Box 128, Mohakhali, Dhaka 1212, Bangladesh. E-mail: sluby@icddrb.org

Trent R. Malcolm, School of Forestry & Environmental Studies, Yale University, New Haven, CT 06511, USA. E-mail: trent.malcolm@aya.yale.edu

Penny Masuoka, Department of Preventive Medicine and Biometrics, USUHS, 4301 Jones Bridge Rd., Bethesda, MD 20814, USA. E-mail: penny@ltpmail.gsfc.nasa.gov

Charles E. Mitchell, Department of Biology and Curriculum in Ecology, University of North Carolina, Chapel Hill, NC 27599, USA. E-mail: mitchell@bio.unc.edu

Kevin J. Olival, Center for Environmental Research and Conservation and Department of Ecology, Evolution, and Environmental Biology, Columbia University, New York, NY 10027, USA. E-mail: kjo2002@columbia.edu

Richard S. Ostfeld, Institute of Ecosystem Studies, Millbrook, NY 12545, USA. E-mail: ostfeldr@ecostudies.org

Raina K. Plowright, University of California, Davis, One Shields Avenue, Davis, CA 95616, USA. E-mail: rkplowright@ucdavis.edu

Kevin Pope, Geo Eco Arc Research, Aquasco, MD 20608, USA. E-mail: kpope@starband.net

Mary F. Poteet, Section of Integrative Biology, The University of Texas at Austin, Austin, TX 78712-0183, USA. E-mail: mpoteet@mail.utexas.edu

Alison G. Power, Dept. of Ecology and Evolutionary Biology, Cornell University, Ithaca, NY 14853-2701, USA. E-mail: agp4@cornell.edu

Juliet Pulliam, Dept. of Ecology & Evolutionary Biology, Princeton University, Princeton, NJ 08544, USA. E-mail: pulliam@princeton.edu

Sohayati Abdul Rahman, Virology Section, Veterinary Research Institute, No 59, Jalan Sultan Azlan Shah, 31400 Ipoh, Perak Darul Ridzuan, Malaysia. E-mail: sohayati@jphvri.po.my

Chris Ray, Department of Ecology and Evolutionary Biology, University of Colorado, Boulder, CO 80309-0334, USA. E-mail: cray@colorado.edu

Leslie A. Real, Department of Biology, Center for Disease Ecology, Emory University, Atlanta, GA 30322, USA. E-mail: lreal@emory.edu

Eliška Rejmánková, Department of Environmental Science and Policy, University of California, Davis, CA 95616, USA. E-mail: erejmankova@ucdavis.edu

Donald Roberts, Department of Preventive Medicine and Biometrics, USUHS, 4301 Jones Bridge Rd., Bethesda, MD 20814, USA. E-mail: droberts@usuhs.mil

Syed Hassan Sharifah, Veterinary Research Institute, No 59, Jalan Sultan Azlan Shah, 31400 Ipoh, Perak Darul Ridzuan, Malaysia. E-mail: sharifas@jphvri.po.my

Jenny C. Shaw, Department of Ecology, Evolution and Marine Biology, University of California, Santa Barbara, CA 93106, USA. E-mail: Shaw@lifesci.ucsb.edu

David K. Skelly, School of Forestry & Environmental Studies and Department of Ecology & Evolutionary Biology, Yale University, New Haven, CT 06511, USA. E-mail: david.skelly@yale.edu

Craig S. Smith, Dept. of Primary Industries, LMB 4, Moorooka 4105, Brisbane, Queensland, Australia. E-mail: craig.s.smith@dpi.qld.gov.au

Robert S. Unnasch, Sound Science LLC, Boise, ID 83702, USA. E-mail: bunnasch@tnc.org

Thomas R. Unnasch, Division of Geographic Medicine, University of Alabama at Birmingham, Birmingham, AL, 35294-2170, USA. E-mail: tunnasch@uab.edu

Michael J. Wade, Department of Biology, Indiana University, Bloomington, IN 47405, USA. E-mail: mjwade@bio.indiana.edu

Kathleen Whitney, Department of Ecology, Evolution and Marine Biology, University of California, Santa Barbara, CA 93106, USA. E-mail: whitney@lifesci.ucsb.edu

CHAPTER 1

Community epidemiology

Sharon K. Collinge and Chris Ray

1.1 The *raison d'être* of this book

Many infectious diseases of recent concern have emerged from complex ecological communities, involving multiple hosts and associated parasites. Several of these diseases appear to be affected by anthropogenic impacts at trophic levels below or above the host community, which suggests that disease prevalence may be altered in unanticipated ways by changes in the structure of ecological communities. Predicting the epidemiological ramifications of such alteration in community composition should be a primary goal of community ecologists and provides a justification for strengthening the current union between community ecology and epidemiology. The purpose of this book is to highlight exciting recent advances in theoretical and empirical research toward understanding the importance of community structure in the emergence of infectious diseases. To that end, this book has one dominant message: studies of epidemiology can be approached from the perspective of community ecology, and students of community ecology can contribute to epidemiology.

To date, most research on host–parasite systems has explored a limited set of community interactions, including a community of host species infected by a single parasite species, or a community of parasites infecting a single host. Less effort has been devoted to addressing additional complications, such as multiple-host–multiple-parasite systems, sequential hosts interacting on different trophic levels, alternate hosts with spatially varying interactions, effects arising from trophic levels other than those of hosts and parasites, or stochastic effects resulting from small population size in at least one alternate host species. Many of these issues are addressed in this book, by studies that link community structure with pathogen transmission and disease dynamics.

This book follows several excellent recent volumes focused on aspects of disease ecology. Chief among these is *Ecology of Wildlife Diseases* (OUP, 2002), which emphasizes ecology and evolution of wildlife diseases, primarily at the scales of individuals and populations. *Parasites and the Behavior of Animals* (OUP, 2002) describes how parasitism may alter behavior of individual animals, with significant consequences for population and community dynamics. *Evolution of Infectious Disease* (OUP, 1994) forges links between evolutionary biology and medicine. *Conservation Medicine* (OUP, 2002) bridges gaps between ecosystem health, animal health, and human health. Our book on *Disease Ecology* is unique in its explicit emphasis on theory and empirical research in community ecology in relation to infectious diseases.

We believe that the timing of this book is ideal, as it corresponds with a new synthesis of theory in community ecology and epidemiology being developed by Robert Holt, Andrew Dobson, and their colleagues. Their exciting work illustrates epidemiological applications for many of the familiar theoretical tools of community ecology. These tools are opening inroads to the study of very complex host–pathogen communities. We begin the book (Chapter 2) with these new perspectives on community epidemiology and, wherever possible, illustrate how new analytical tools can be applied within the studies discussed in this book.

We expect that this book will engage a broad audience, including scholars active in the fields of community ecology and epidemiology, medical practitioners, and advanced undergraduates, post-graduates and land managers with some background in ecology or epidemiology. Each chapter relates to an area of theory in community ecology and illustrates how community-level processes operate in a particular study system to affect pathogen transmission and disease dynamics. Chapters explore several areas of theory in community ecology (e.g. predator–prey dynamics, keystone species effects, succession, disturbance, species invasions, diversity and stability). In order to foster consistency among chapters, we asked each contributor to consider the following three questions in preparing their chapter:

• What key concepts from community ecology are best illustrated in your study system?
• How do community interactions appear to contribute significantly to pathogen transmission and disease prevalence in your study system?
• What sorts of community complexity must be considered to effectively predict disease dynamics?

1.2 Some useful definitions

The chapters in this book should be accessible to most readers familiar with basic concepts in ecology and epidemiology. We provide here a brief glossary, in alphabetical order, of some commonly used terms to serve as introduction to the reader or just to refresh your memory.

Enzootic refers to an infectious disease that is present in a host population at all times, but having low incidence within the population.
Epizootic refers to an infectious disease outbreak in a population that affects a large number of animals simultaneously but does not persist.
An *infectious disease* refers to the change in the state of health of a host organism as a result of invasion of the body by pathogenic organisms. Note that the disease is the manifestation of the infection in a host organism, but infection can occur without causing disease. In this book, infectious agents include viruses, bacteria, fungi, protozoans, and multicellular endoparasites.

A *pathogen* is any disease-producing microorganism or material (e.g. prions are infectious proteins, but are not technically organisms).

A *parasite* is an organism that lives in (endoparasites) or on (ectoparasites) the living tissue of a host organism; the biological interaction between host and parasite is called parasitism. Microparasites, which include viruses and bacteria, reproduce within their hosts. Macroparasites, which include multicellular endo- and ectoparasites, generally spend some portion of the life cycle away from the primary host.

The basic or intrinsic reproductive rate, R_0, of a microparasite is usually defined as the number of infective hosts (secondary infections) resulting from a single infective host (primary infection). For microparasites, R_0 depends primarily on host–host or host–vector–host contacts. For macroparasites, R_0 is usually defined as the number of adult parasites produced by a single adult parasite. In both cases, R_0 applies only when parasites are rare. For $R_0 < 1$, the parasite does not increase when rare.

A *reservoir host* is an animal species that maintains a parasite life cycle and functions as the source of the infection for humans or other species.

SEIR models have been used in human epidemiology for decades, and more recently have been incorporated into wildlife disease models. These models describe disease dynamics within a population of *S*usceptible individuals, *E*xposed individuals, *I*nfectious individuals, and *R*ecovered (or resistant) individuals. Variations on this modeling framework include, for example, "SIS" models which apply to diseases with a rapid onset of the infectious period and no legacy of resistance.

A *zoonosis* is an infection or disease that can be shared between humans and wildlife. Many of the diseases discussed in these chapters are zoonoses.

1.3 How this book works

To emphasize our message that community ecology and epidemiology can be productively linked, each chapter contains two boxes that highlight key tools and concepts in community epidemiology. One box focuses on techniques that will be useful to other researchers studying community aspects of infectious diseases. The second box emphasizes aspects of disease transmission from the perspective of community structure. With these boxes, we intend to provide our readers with the theoretical framework and empirical tools necessary to design and evaluate studies that effectively address the community context of infectious diseases.

1.4 Chapter highlights and connections

Each of the chapters in this book provides a novel contribution to the understanding of disease dynamics within complex communities. Most chapters relate shifts in disease dynamics to alterations of community structure driven by anthropogenic activities, including intensive agriculture (Chapters 7 and 13), clear-cut forestry (Chapter 10), urbanization (Chapter 11), or habitat loss and fragmentation (Chapters 3 and 14). Although the authors' expertise spans a wide range of study systems, from microbial communities inside ticks to the continental spread of rabid omnivores, all emphasize the reciprocal interactions between host communities and disease emergence. Most of the chapters involve ecological field studies of diseases just emerging in the United States. This focus on emergent diseases and their community ecology is clearly applicable to disease dynamics worldwide.

To begin, Holt and Dobson (Chapter 2) note that most emerging diseases involve more than one host, and many involve fairly complex host–pathogen communities. Understanding these diseases requires a framework in which to examine the dynamics of pathogens that infect two or more host species. These authors explore epidemiology of host–pathogen communities through analysis of "community modules," or small sets of interacting species. They adapt familiar tools from community ecology to analyze pathogen transmission dynamics in several types of communities, and develop a series of simple models to elucidate the dynamics of parasite coexistence. Holt and Dobson's chapter provides a very useful conceptual foundation and introduction to analytical tools that can be applied to many host–pathogen systems. One application is explored by Ray and Collinge (Chapter 14), who consider potential effects of a keystone species on the dynamics of plague in the United States.

The functional role of species richness in communities has been the subject of much recent research in ecology, and several chapters in this volume explore this topic in the context of disease dynamics. For example, Ostfeld *et al.* (Chapter 3) note that both mammal species richness and species composition are critical to prevalence of Lyme disease in northeastern US forests. The authors' detailed field studies and modeling efforts demonstrate that "species-specific functional roles can depend on the composition of the remaining community." This theme is considered again in Chapter 5 by Mitchell and Power in a very different study system involving plant pathogens, but the message that more diverse communities may have reduced pathogen loads is consistent. Both chapters also discuss the importance of pathogen "spillover," whereby high pathogen loads on one species within the community can result in higher pathogen prevalence in other species. The presence of this one species clearly can have dramatic effects on disease dynamics within the community. In the case of Lyme disease, it's the white-footed mouse, and in the case of barley yellow dwarf virus, it's wild oats.

Also relevant to the dynamics of Lyme disease, Clay *et al.* (Chapter 4) explore the intriguing possibility that microbial communities within ticks may influence expression of disease. These authors have found that microbes pathogenic to humans are often relatively rare within these communities, suggesting that the prevalence of human disease may be affected by community interactions between pathogenic and non-pathogenic microbes within the vectors themselves. Moreover, they draw from ecological theory on assembly rules to consider the abundance and distribution of microbes within ticks. These authors have discovered a surprising diversity of microbes within individual ticks, suggesting a great opportunity to use these (highly replicated) microbial communities to test several concepts in community ecology that have proven difficult to test in larger (less replicated) systems.

Several highly virulent, arthropod-borne viruses ("arboviruses") that cause serious human neurological diseases, such as West Nile encephalomyelitis and St Louis encephalomyelitis, are transmitted by mosquitoes that feed on both wildlife and human hosts. The recent emergence of these viruses has prompted investigation into those mosquito species and wild birds that are conspicuously involved in transmission cycles. Unnasch *et al.* (Chapter 6) describe an innovative molecular technique to identify the source of mosquito blood meals, which is proving to be quite useful in discerning the roles of particular vector and host species. One interesting result is their discovery that reptiles also host arboviruses and may play a critical role in maintaining these pathogens over the winter. They also use this molecular technique to determine the vectorial capacity of different mosquito species. Vectorial capacity is a term that takes into account the efficiency of the vector in transmitting the pathogen, the lifespan of the infectious hosts, and the degree of contact between the host and vector. Because species interactions are of prime importance in determining vectorial capacity, an understanding of community ecology is clearly essential for elucidating the epidemiology of vectored diseases.

Rejmánková *et al.* (Chapter 7) further discuss vectorial capacity in the context of malaria transmission in Belize. These authors describe how nutrient enrichment from intensive agricultural activities leads to dramatic shifts in wetland plant communities (to marshes dominated by cattails), which in turn cause changes in the abundance of particular mosquito species involved in malaria transmission. Their results show that the mosquito species most favored by these plant community changes is also the most capable vector of malaria in their study area. Moreover, a less capable vector, which was the more abundant mosquito species before nutrient enrichment, also survives well in cattail marshes. Thus, this shift in the marsh community may result in higher overall vector density, perhaps causing increased risk of malaria for humans.

Nutrient enrichment of aquatic systems can also promote conditions that favor growth of pathogenic microorganisms. For example, nutrient addition may directly increase the growth rate of *Vibrio cholerae*, the causative agent of cholera, or may enhance the growth of plankton that serve as attachment substrates for the bacteria (Cottingham and Butzler, Chapter 8). Until quite recently, there were no techniques available to examine the community ecology of microorganisms. Not surprisingly, little is known about how interactions among bacterial strains or species, for example, may affect relative abundance or expression of pathogenicity in infectious bacteria. Clearly, there is a great opportunity for research on the roles of key interspecific interactions, such as competition and predation, in affecting bacterial abundance, morphology, and possibly virulence. Cottingham and Butzler report on the current understanding of the environmental context in which *V. cholerae* dynamics unfold, and suggest that community ecology provides an excellent conceptual foundation for understanding both the pathogen and the disease it causes.

Aquatic ecosystems are often foci of disease caused by both microparasites (as in cholera, above) and macroparasites, because water is an excellent medium for survival and transmission of parasites, and because aquatic systems are often heavily modified by humans. Three chapters of this volume (Chapters 9–11) provide excellent examples of community influences on macroparasite transmission in three very different aquatic systems. Lafferty *et al.* (Chapter 9) extend a long history of food web studies in community ecology by adding parasites to an exceptionally detailed description of a salt-marsh food web. The authors show that including parasites in the food web changes considerably the metrics calculated for typical food webs. For example, food web "connectance" (the average proportion of other species with which each species interacts), increases dramatically in food webs where parasites are included, compared with where they are excluded. This finding has profound implications for our understanding of community structure and function.

Both Poteet (Chapter 10) and Skelly *et al.* (Chapter 11) examine how human modification of aquatic systems affects rates of macroparasitism. Poteet studied how forestry practices influence each host and parasite stage of a trematode parasite that infects giant salamanders in the northwestern United States. The complex life cycle of this macroparasite includes stoneflies, snails, and salamanders, which constitute key components of aquatic food webs in small streams. Completion of the parasite life cycle depends on predation of stoneflies by salamanders, and Poteet shows how the rate of transmission depends critically on the predator–prey functional response curve. Further, habitat disturbance due to clear-cut forestry alters the form of this functional response, with intriguing consequences for parasite transmission. On the opposite US coast, Skelly *et al.* (Chapter 11) examine how urbanization and associated habitat modification influence the prevalence of macroparasites in two common amphibian species, green frogs and spring peepers. Across two parasite taxa and these two host species, the authors detected no effect of urbanization on infection prevalence. However, they did find evidence of severe parasitism within three of the 16 wetlands studied; interestingly, these were the most heavily human-modified wetlands in the study and supported the highest densities of the snails that act as intermediate hosts for these parasites (echinostomes). Skelly *et al.* conclude that parasite infections are clearly context dependent, and suggest that it would be productive to examine a greater number of species in these communities to determine why emergence is likely in particular contexts.

Animal movement is notoriously difficult to study, yet is clearly a critical component of the dynamics of many diseases. Chapters 12 (Real and Childs) and 13 (Daszak *et al.*) incorporate animal movement explicitly into studies of viral transmission and spread. In their well-studied example, Real and Childs use spatially explicit models to show that movement of rabies across large geographic areas is impeded by landscape features such as rivers. This suggests that rivers may slow movement of raccoons and therefore provide barriers for movement of rabies. Very little is known about the impacts of rabies on vertebrate communities, or about how host species composition may affect transmission rates. Because vertebrate species composition varies spatially and temporally, it is likely that there are combinations of mammalian assemblages that create higher or lower rates of risk for rabies transmission to humans and domestic animals.

The emergence of Nipah virus in Malaysia (Chapter 13) involves interactions between domestic livestock (pigs), two native species of frugivorous flying foxes, and several species of fruiting trees. Satellite telemetry allowed Daszak *et al.* to reject the hypothesis that drought-related changes in flying-fox movement patterns led to the emergence of Nipah virus. On the contrary, their movement data suggest that Nipah virus is present continually in peninsular Malaysia, and was therefore likely to be available for introduction into pigs prior to the large drought that occurred in the mid-1990s. Additionally, their study of Nipah virus indicates that interspecific interactions affect viral prevalence. Fruiting trees planted next to hog containment facilities provide feeding and roosting sites for fruit-eating bats that harbor the virus. These sites provide opportunities for pathogen spillover from bats to pigs, and ultimately to humans. The authors' ability to link the presence of fruiting trees at hog farms to Nipah virus emergence has led to livestock management plans that specify buffer zones at pig farms where fruit trees are excluded.

As editors of this volume, we have had the opportunity to review the concepts covered in each chapter of this book, and to apply these concepts where possible to our own studies of disease. In the final chapter (Ray and Collinge, Chapter 14), we use this opportunity to discuss an old disease in several new ways. We discuss plague as an emergent disease of wildlife in the western US, noting the potential feedbacks between plague dynamics and community structure. Plague has caused much local extinction of the black-tailed prairie dog, which is arguably a keystone of prairie ecology. We suggest the added potential for key effects of the prairie dog on plague dynamics, using the models of Holt and Dobson (Chapter 2) to explore how prairie dogs may mediate both direct and apparent competition among alternate hosts of plague. The take-home message from our study is similar to that of most studies in this book: the key to understanding zoonoses is understanding interspecific transmission.

This should prove to be a useful book. Turn the page and start reading, because the world needs your contributions to community epidemiology.

CHAPTER 2

Extending the principles of community ecology to address the epidemiology of host–pathogen systems

Robert D. Holt and Andrew P. Dobson

2.1 Background

Community ecologists grapple with the structure and dynamics of ensembles of species that live in the same habitat, landscape, or region, and so potentially interact (Morin 1999; Lawton 2000). This concern with interspecific interactions has led to sustained interest in several questions. One is to understand how species within a single trophic level, competing for the same resources, manage to coexist (Chesson 2000a; Holt 2001). Other central concerns of community ecology go beyond coexistence within a trophic level to include topics such as understanding the structure and dynamics of food webs, and the relationship between diversity and ecosystem stability (e.g. McCann 2000). In addressing these issues, including the core issue of coexistence, parasites are increasingly recognized as "hidden" but vital constituents of natural communities (Morand and Arias-Gonzalez 1997; Thompson et al. 2001). In turn, there is a growing appreciation of the community dimensions of infectious disease epidemiology, as witnessed by the chapters of this volume.

In applied ecology, understanding the community context of infectious disease is critically important (e.g. zoonotic diseases, Ostfeld et al. 2001 and Chapter 3, this volume; invasive species, Mitchell and Power 2003; conservation, McCallum and Dobson 1995; Woodroffe 1999; Lafferty and Gerber 2002; Torchin et al. 2003). Such understanding can improve our ability to interpret and mitigate the emergence of novel infectious diseases (Daszak et al. 2000; Woolhouse 2002). Community structure can influence disease emergence in many ways. Parasites can infect multiple host species, and most hosts are vulnerable to infection by multiple parasite species (Dobson and Foufopoulos 2001, Morgan et al. 2004). Even specialist host–pathogen interactions are embedded in complex food webs, generating complex feedbacks. For instance, a generalist predator with a nonlinear functional response to a prey species that itself harbors a specialist parasite can lead to cyclic or chaotic patterns of disease prevalence (Hall et al. 2004; Holt, in press; Holt et al., in review). Maintenance of natural host–parasite dynamics may be crucial for maintaining species diversity and facilitating successional dynamics (Gilbert 2002); anthropogenic disruption (e.g. species introductions) can potentially lead to cascading shifts in host–parasite interactions, with devastating effects on community structure.

A key issue at the interface of community ecology and infectious disease epidemiology is how the interdependence of hosts and parasites affects species coexistence. Many processes can influence coexistence, often in idiosyncratic ways, yet coexistence is most broadly understood as arising from the interplay of three factors (Chesson 2000a; Holt 2001): (1) the inherent properties of the species themselves (e.g. feeding specializations), (2) properties of the extrinsic environment (e.g. abundance of food resources), and (3) the dynamic impacts each species in turn has upon the environment (e.g. influence of feeding on future food resources). Trade-offs between species are usually required for coexistence (Kneitel and Chase 2004). For instance, consider two consumer species competing via exploitation for two discrete, renewable food resources (see, for example, Chase and Leibold 2003). For stable competitive coexistence, where each species can increase when rare, the two species have to differ in terms of their responses to resource availability—an example of niche differentiation. Moreover, the two resources in turn need to respond differently to the two consuming species, such that the two consumer species experience distinct feedback effects arising from their impacts upon the resource supply. Finally, the abundance and renewal rates of the resources cannot be too different; otherwise, despite the existence of niche differences, one species will be able to exclude the other.

When analyzing coexistence, it is often insufficient to consider just pairs of species and their required resources in a local environment over short timescales. Interactions with other trophic levels can permit coexistence (as in keystone predation on competing species, Holt *et al.* 1994), or preclude it (as in apparent competition between prey species, Holt 1977; Holt and Lawton 1994). Noncompetitive interactions such as facilitation can moderate the impact of competition. Spatial flows of resources and species are often central to maintaining species coexistence at broader spatial scales (e.g. Holt 1993; Leibold and Miller 2004), as is temporal variation in resource availability or environmental conditions, when species have different responses to such variation (Chesson 2000a). Increasing the temporal, spatial, and trophic scales of inquiry broadens the range of trade-offs, environments, and feedbacks that can permit (or preclude) coexistence (Chesson 2000a; Holt 2001).

All of these questions in community ecology bear on the issue of understanding the persistence of multispecies assemblages of parasites and their hosts. This is a broad and rapidly evolving topic (see prior syntheses in Grenfell and Dobson 1995; Hudson *et al.* 2002). Because of the large numbers of species in communities, and the complexity and fluidity of the interaction webs that link these species, understanding community dynamics is a substantial challenge, even ignoring parasites and infectious disease! One fruitful approach to unraveling the dynamics of complex food webs is the analysis of "community modules" (Holt 1997a; Persson 1999). A community module is a carefully

chosen multispecies extension of pairwise interactions, chosen because the configuration of interactions is found in a wide range of species assemblages. Several familiar modules at the heart of community ecology are shown in Fig. 2.1. Figure 2.2 displays similar community modules involving infectious diseases. The community modules that have received greatest attention are those elucidating the coexistence of species competing for resources. Because hosts provide resources, habitats, and dispersal mechanisms for parasites, models from classical community ecology can be used to elucidate controls on parasite community structure. Toward this end, we will consider here several models based on simple epidemiological modules that address coexistence. We first focus on coexistence of parasites, then turn to the issue of how parasites influence host coexistence.

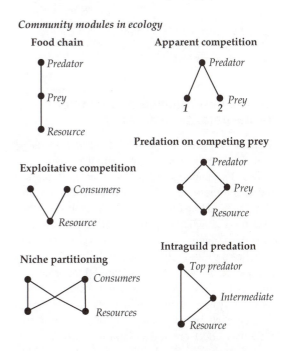

Community modules in ecology

Figure 2.1 Multispecies assemblages involving a relatively small number of species interacting in a defined way provide a useful conceptual waystation between pairwise interactions and highly complex food webs (after Holt 1997a). Note that some of these community modules may go by different names depending on the outcome of interactions; for example, predation on competing prey may be referred to as "keystone predation" if it facilitates prey coexistence, or "predator-mediated competition" if it excludes one prey species (resulting in a "food chain").

Community modules in epidemiology

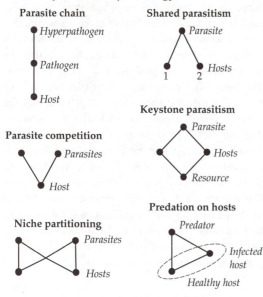

Figure 2.2 Many problems at the interface between community ecology and infectious disease epidemiology can be viewed as modules analogous to those in Fig. 2.1.

2.2 The host community: a templet for the parasite community

A theme of growing interest (and the focus of several chapters in this book) is that parasites can be key determinants of host population dynamics and community organization (e.g. Anderson and May 1978; Hudson *et al.* 1998; Dobson 1999; Hudson *et al.* 2002). For many ecologists (including ourselves), the dramatic impacts of parasites upon their hosts provide the principal *"raison d'être"* for studies of parasite–host ecology. However, for some purposes it may be useful to consider the host community as an arena in which parasite dynamics and interactions play out, without a significant reciprocal affect on host community structure. In the felicitous phrase of Jaenike and Perlman (2002), at times parasites are only a kind of "trophic garnish" on the food web.

The "trophic garnish" perspective on parasites may approximate reality in many cases. Human hosts, for instance, harbor large numbers (at least thousands) of microbial species, mostly bacteria (B. Bohannan and M. McFall-Ngai, personal communication). Some bacteria are always pathogenic,

and others can be pathogenic in particular circumstances (e.g. due to wounding or stress), but it is surely true that many of these potential parasites usually have only a negligible impact on their human hosts, in effect being commensals that do not impact host fitness (Levin and Antia 2001). Similarly, nematodes in *Drosophila* may have negligible effects on host fecundity (Perlman and Jaenike 2003). Competitive interactions within individual hosts (e.g. chemically mediated interference among nematodes) can provide density dependence that regulates parasites, even if host fecundity and mortality are not affected (Jaenike 1998; Poulin 1998). Density-dependent resource competition or facultative host defenses may reduce parasite survival or reproduction, without altering host demography (Shostak and Scott 1993; Jaenike 1996). An assumption of fixed host numbers is often made in classical human epidemiology, such as the Kermack–McKendrick (1927) model; such models in effect assume that the combined determinants of host abundance are effectively independent of pathogen impacts. Even harmful pathogens may fail to influence host population size if host population growth is density-dependent. For instance, "damping disease" may reduce seedling survival in a plant cohort (Augspurger 1983), but if the number of survivors exceeds the number of adult plants that can be sustained on a site, the overall course of plant population dynamics may be unchanged. Finally, many parasites that can in principle regulate host numbers do so only in certain contexts (e.g. where hosts experience stressful conditions, Brown *et al.* 2003; Lafferty and Holt 2003).

By assuming that total host numbers are fixed, independent of parasite load, one can identify key mechanisms of coexistence acting primarily on the parasites. Once understood, these mechanisms provide a useful yardstick for interpreting the consequences of relaxing the assumption of fixed host abundances. Given that the host community provides a templet for parasite dynamics, one can then ask how the properties of this templet influence patterns of parasite community organization and richness. This broad question is the focus of much work in classical parasitology (reviewed in Price 1980; Poulin 1998), but we suggest it would be useful to revisit this question more specifically using the conceptual framework provided by contemporary community ecology. Here we sketch some potentially fruitful applications of community ecology, using simple, illustrative models.

As noted above, a fundamental concern of community ecology is to understand how the strength and pattern of interspecific interactions influence species coexistence. Classical community ecology focused on equilibrial properties of species interactions in closed ecosystems in stable environments. If each of a set of consumer species is limited by the abundance of a single, depletable, limiting factor (as in the "exploitative competition" module of

Fig. 2.1), then at equilibrium at most one species is expected to persist (Levin 1970). For instance, in a well-mixed chemostat where algae compete for a single nutrient, theory predicts (and experiments confirm) that a single species of algae dominates, driving inferior competitors to extinction (Tilman 1982; Grover 1997). If multiple species stably coexist, one or more of the conditions required for competitive exclusion must be violated (Chesson 2000a; Holt 2001). We can categorize mechanisms of coexistence in terms of how they differ from this simple limiting case. Box 2.1 provides one typology of coexistence mechanisms.

Box 2.1 A précis of mechanisms of coexistence

Several key mechanisms of coexistence have been identified by community ecologists. These mechanisms depend generally on differences in how species exploit resources, and how the environment responds to such exploitation (Chesson 2000a; Holt 2001). In practice, these mechanisms are neither sharply defined nor mutually exclusive. See the text for further exploration of several scenarios of coexistence among competing parasites.

A. Coexistence in closed, equilibrial communities

Some systems (e.g. terrestrial communities on remote islands) are essentially closed to immigration, and may experience little temporal variation. Much of classical community theory assumes such closed, equilibrial communities.

Classical niche partitioning. In a stable environment with populations at equilibrium, species coexistence requires niche partitioning (e.g. Schoener 1989). Models of niche partitioning assume: (1) the environment is heterogeneous, with multiple potential limiting factors (e.g. a heterogeneous resource base), and (2) species have different requirements (e.g. due to trade-offs in exploitative ability for distinct resources). Such niche differences are necessary but not sufficient for coexistence; species must also be similar in how they respond to general abiotic factors (the "equalizing" conditions of Chesson 2000a), and have differential impacts upon the limiting factors themselves (Chase and Leibold 2003). Often, local coexistence is permitted by subtle variation in microhabitats and in the selection of microhabitats by individuals (e.g. Kotler and Brown 1999).

Localized interactions between individuals. Even in spatially homogeneous communities, dispersal following reproduction can be spatially circumscribed. This increases the impact of intraspecific competition relative to interspecific competition, potentially facilitating coexistence at local scales (Bolker and Pacala 1999).

Food-web effects. Frequency-dependent consumption by natural enemies (e.g. due to predator switching) can promote competitive coexistence. If superior competitors for resources are more vulnerable to predation, coexistence can occur (see the keystone predation module in Fig. 2.1; Holt et al. 1994; Leibold 1996; Chase and Leibold 2003). If an inferior resource competitor can directly prey upon the superior competitor, coexistence may be permitted (see the intraguild predation module; Holt and Polis 1997).

Nontrophic mechanisms of population regulation. Many biological mechanisms can influence population regulation, and thus interactions among species. For instance, if superior exploiters also experience strong intraspecific interference, this can permit the continued existence of inferior competitors (Schoener 1976).

B. Closed, nonequilibrial communities

Although much of theoretical community ecology assumes that the environment is constant, many natural systems in fact experience substantial temporal variation in abiotic conditions and resource supply rates. Moreover, populations may have intrinsically unstable dynamics, leading to cycles or chaotic dynamics even in constant environments. Given temporal variability, other mechanisms of coexistence can operate.

continues

Box 2.1 *continued*

Temporal niche partitioning (storage effects). In variable environments, coexistence may reflect temporal variation in the performance of different species on the same resource. This mechanism requires devices to slow the rate of population decline during bad times, such as seed banks or long-lived adult classes (Chesson 2000a). High recruitment into the seed bank or adult classes during better times can permit the population to persist through poor times. If different species are superior at different times, a large number of species with demographic storage effects can potentially coexist on a shared resource.

Nonlinear dynamics. Often, population growth rates are highly nonlinear functions of the magnitude of limiting factors (e.g. resource availability), leading to unstable dynamics. If competing species have different nonlinear responses to shared limiting factors, nonequilibrial coexistence may occur (Grover 1997; Huisman and Weissing 1999; Chesson 2000a; Abrams and Holt 2002). More subtle mechanisms of coexistence involving nonlinear dynamics reflect shifts between different dynamical regimes in systems with cyclical or chaotic dynamics (e.g. Harrison *et al.* 2001).

C. Open communities

Many natural communities are open, coupled to an external landscape or regional species pool via dispersal

(Polis *et al.* 2004; Holyoak *et al.* 2005). This permits the operation of a broad range of coexistence mechanisms involving species movement patterns in response to spatial and temporal variation (Holt 1993; Chesson 2000b).

Migration and habitat selection. Some species (e.g. migratory birds) may circumvent (and exploit) temporal variation by migration or seasonal habitat selection. If different species are regulated at different seasons and/or in different habitats, they can potentially coexist. Moreover, species that disperse at different rates in effect average over spatial variation in different ways; this subtle effect can at times permit coexistence (McPeek and Holt 1992; Debinski *et al.* 2001).

Metapopulation processes. Coexistence may occur if inferior competitors can rapidly colonize and establish populations following disturbance, permitting the exploitation of transient habitats, whereas superior competitors disperse more sluggishly. This mechanism requires recurrent loss of the superior competitor from local sites (e.g. through disturbance).

Source-sink dynamics. An inferior competitor may persist in one community if it is a superior competitor in a nearby community. Dispersal from "source" habitats then permits sustained presence in what would otherwise be "sink" habitats for the inferior competitor (Holt 1993; Leibold and Miller 2004).

2.3 Mechanisms of coexistence in parasite assemblages

We think it is fair to assert that the relative importance of each potential coexistence mechanism (Box 2.1) is not well understood for *any* natural community; parasite communities are certainly no exception. However, there are hints in the literature that many of these mechanisms may influence the structure of parasite assemblages. One basic question is the degree to which parasite species richness reflects processes acting within individual hosts (dubbed the "infracommunity" in parasitology; Holmes 1973, Holmes and Price 1986; Goater *et al.* 1987, Poulin 1998), versus processes acting at the level of entire host populations and communities. Here we focus on the latter.

2.3.1 Simple models for microparasite competition and coexistence

Parasites compete for susceptible hosts and the resources those hosts contain. In principle, analogues of any mechanism in Box 2.1 could help explain parasite coexistence. There is considerable room for developing theory that formalizes these mechanisms in a manner specifically tailored to host–parasite systems. We sketch here several models for microparasites (e.g. viruses, bacteria), illustrating different modes of coexistence.

Parasites abstractly compete at two levels of organization: within individual hosts and between hosts. Microparasites establish populations within individual hosts. Because hosts provide resources that can be consumed, this permits exploitative competition between multiple species that co-occur within a "patch" (individual host). For the moment, assume that only a single parasite species can persist in an individual host, and that whichever species initially colonizes that host excludes other species; that is, there is no coinfection by multiple species leading to either within-host coexistence or superinfection (where one parasite can supplant another). The absence of coinfection is assumed in many theoretical studies (e.g. Dushoff and Dwyer 2001). (We will relax this assumption below.)

Even if coinfection can at times occur, one can safely ignore it in a number of plausible circumstances. Consider a system in which two parasite species with similar birth and death rates use the same tissues within a host that does not exhibit species-specific immune responses (Iwasa *et al.* 2004). If infective propagules are small and infrequent, then whichever species first colonizes (infects) an individual host is likely to exclude the other species. After the first species has achieved an equilibrium between births and deaths within its host, small and infrequent propagules of a second species cannot invade unless its birth or death rates are relatively favorable. Species with similar birth and death rates will generally be distributed in a checkerboard pattern, with each host infected by just one of these similar parasite species. This outcome of parasite competition for host tissues within an individual parallels that of competition for host individuals within a population, as modeled in Equation (2.1) below. In other systems, assuming no coinfection can be viewed as a simple limiting case of a more complex epidemiological model. For instance, if coinfection rapidly leads to host mortality, few host individuals will in practice be coinfected. Alternatively, if encounter rates are low, hosts infected by any single parasite species are likely to recover or die before encountering a host infected with another parasite. Finally, for our purposes, assuming no coinfection is conceptually useful, because it permits us to identify various mechanisms operating at the host level to influence parasite coexistence.

Assuming two parasite species and no coinfection, we can divide a host population into one uninfected class and two, nonoverlapping classes of individuals infected with either parasite 1 or

parasite 2. Recall that for the moment we are assuming the host is regulated at its carrying capacity, *K*, by factors other than parasitism. A simple "SI" model describing "susceptible" and "infected" hosts and the exploitative competition between two species of microparasite spread by density-dependent transmission includes the following terms for the dynamics of each parasite:

$$\frac{dI_i}{dt} = (\beta_i S - d_i)I_i, \quad i = 1,2$$
$$K = S + I_1 + I_2 \tag{2.1}$$

Here, S is the density of susceptible hosts, I_i the density of hosts infected with parasite species i, β_i the transmission rate for parasite species i, and d_i the rate of parasite loss from the host population (including death and recovery of infected hosts). The second equation states that total host numbers are fixed at carrying capacity by factors other than parasitism.

When parasite i occurs alone, the first equation in model (2.1) reveals that the equilibrial density of susceptible hosts is $S^* = d_i/\beta_i$. Parasite j can invade if $dI_j/dt > 0$; that is, if $\beta_j S^* - d_j > 0$ or $d_i/\beta_i > d_j/\beta_j$. If this is true, when parasite j is alone at equilibrium, parasite i cannot invade. Thus, model (2.1) predicts competitive exclusion, and the winning parasite is the one that can persist at the lowest density of susceptible hosts. This model parallels in its essential features standard resource–consumer models (Grover 1997), which formalize the idea that, at equilibrium, a single species will dominate any single limiting resource. Here, the resource is the susceptible host subpopulation. See Allen *et al.* (2004) for more complex epidemiological models of this type.

If we substitute $S = K - I_1 - I_2$ into the first equation in (2.1), and do this for each of the two parasite species, we generate a competition model of Lotka–Volterra form, with nonintersecting zero-growth isoclines, corresponding to competitive exclusion. This very simple model predicting competitive exclusion provides a springboard for more complex models that illuminate how different aspects of host population and community properties influence parasite coexistence. Next, we sketch some plausible scenarios corresponding to the coexistence mechanisms of Box 2.1. Due to limitations in space and in the current state of theory, we consider some potential mechanisms in more detail than others; these mechanisms are not necessarily more important in natural communities.

2.3.1.1 Classical niche partitioning

In a multispecies host community, if each parasite species is specialized to a different host species, and the hosts do not themselves compete, parasite coexistence is trivial, as it is determined entirely by the independent responses each parasite has to its own host (e.g. each respective host should exceed the threshold density for its parasite). In effect, this scenario assumes a rigid niche partitioning among parasites. But in many natural systems, parasites are shared by multiple host species (Cleaveland *et al.* 2001; Dobson 2004; Woolhouse 2002; Woolhouse *et al.* 2001), and hosts harbor multiple parasites. In a species-rich host assemblage, heterogeneity among parasites in how they use different host species can in principle permit the sustained coexistence of multiple species of parasites.

There is now a rich theoretical literature on the dynamics of multi-host, one-pathogen systems (e.g. Holt and Pickering 1985; Bowers and Begon 1991; Begon *et al.* 1992; Begon and Bowers 1995; Bowers and Turner 1997; Greenman and Hudson 2000; Dobson 2004). Understanding cross-species transmission can be of great importance for addressing applied issues, and ignoring such transmission can lead to erroneous conclusions. For instance, Hess (1994) provocatively argued that increasing connectivity in a metapopulation might not always be a helpful conservation strategy, because connectivity also facilitates movement of pathogens. Several authors have noted that this result may be moot if transmission is generally facilitated by alternative, "reservoir" hosts (Gog *et al.* 2002; McCallum and Dobson 2002).

A simple listing of known hosts does not quantify the dynamical importance of multiple host species for parasite dynamics and coexistence. Compilations of parasite "host range" conflate several alternative dynamical scenarios. First, cross-species transmission may be only of historical or biogeographic importance. For HIV, contact with the original source host (presumably an African primate) was historically crucial but is now irrelevant

in determining the subsequent dynamics of the disease in humans. Many emerging diseases of economically important plants involve single introductions, not recurrent infection within a single community (Anderson *et al.* 2004). Second, in the case of recurrent cross-species transmission, the incidence of the disease in a focal host can be influenced by the presence, abundance, and epidemiological properties of alternative hosts. In this case, it is useful to distinguish several alternative scenarios (elaborating on a suggestion by Antonovics *et al.* 2002; see also May *et al.* 2001):

1. The focal host species may be a permanent demographic sink for the parasite, in that each primary infection in the focal host generates less than one secondary infection within its own population ($R_0 < 1$). Under this scenario, focal host infections are generally due to "spillover" of the parasite from a source host. Reciprocal transmission back to the source host (Antonovics *et al.* 2002) may alter prevalence in both source and sink hosts. This scenario is particularly likely when no host species alone is sufficiently dense to sustain the infection.
2. The focal host species may be able to sustain the parasite entirely on its own ($R_0 > 1$), but recurrent infection from alternative hosts may nonetheless significantly perturb dynamics within the focal host population.
3. As an intermediate case, the focal host may be an intermittent sink, such that R_0 varies through time. Alternative hosts may then be particularly important for ensuring parasite persistence through times of low R_0 in the focal host. In some ways, this scenario is reminiscent of the "migration and habitat selection" mechanism in Box 2.1.

Density-dependent disease transmission implies a threshold host population size, below which $R_0 < 1$. A host may be a sink for a parasite not because of the poor physiological suitability of the host, but because of ecological factors influencing host abundance or background mortality rates, such as microhabitat or resource availability, predation, or competition with other species. In model (2.1) above, the rate at which an uninfected individual becomes infected is proportional to the density of infectives in the host population. In some sexually transmitted or vector-transmitted diseases, however, the rate of infection depends upon the frequency of infection in the host population (i.e. the fraction of individuals infected). With pure frequency-dependent disease transmission, there is not a threshold host population density. But more realistic models of frequency-dependent transmission suggest that density-dependence often emerges at sufficiently low host numbers (Antonovics *et al.* 1995). So, it is likely that a threshold host density describes a wide range of infectious disease systems.

With recurrent cross-species infection, determining the criterion for microparasite invasion ($R_0 > 1$) requires a more complex approach than considering R_0 in each host alone (Dobson and Fofopoulos 2001; Holt *et al.* 2003; Dobson 2004). Here we exemplify one approach, and extend it to consider competition and effective niche partitioning among parasite species.

We can generalize model (2.1) to include two parasite and two host species, as follows:

$$\frac{dI_1}{dt} = \beta_{11}S_1I_1 + \beta_{12}S_1I_2 - \Gamma_1I_1$$

$$\frac{dI_2}{dt} = \beta_{22}S_2I_2 + \beta_{21}S_2I_1 - \Gamma_2I_2$$

$$\frac{dI_1'}{dt} = \beta_{11}'S_1I_1' + \beta_{12}'S_1I_2' - \Gamma_1'I_1'$$

$$\frac{dI_2'}{dt} = \beta_{22}'S_2I_2' + \beta_{21}'S_2I_1' - \Gamma_2'I_2'$$

$$(2.2)$$

The first two equations describe dynamics of parasite 1 in host species 1 and 2; the second two equations (with primes) describe parasite 2. The quantity β_{ij} denotes transmission of infection from infected individuals of species j to susceptible individuals of species i; Γ_i scales loss rates (mortality plus clearance or recovery) of infected individuals of host species i.

To complete the model, we must describe dynamics of the rest of the host populations. As before, we assume each host is regulated by strong density dependence (e.g. territoriality) independent of parasitism, so $K_i = S_i + I_i + I_i'$, $i = 1,2$. [Note that with this assumption about host regulation, we preclude apparent competition (Holt 1977; Holt and Pickering 1985; Hudson and Greenman 1998; Bowers 1999). We turn to such indirect interactions between hosts below.] Alternative models include

exponential or logistic growth of hosts, regulated at least in part by parasitism. For example, Begon *et al.* (1992) assume $dN_i/dt = r_iN_i(1 - N_i/K_i) - \alpha_iI_i$, $i = 1,2$, for each of two host species; the first term is logistic growth experienced by all individuals in species i, and the second denotes additional mortality experienced by infected individuals. In Box 2.2, we describe how a model with fixed host density (2.2) leads to isoclines that describe qualitatively the conditions for invasion of each parasite species; these isoclines can then be used to characterize some necessary conditions for parasite coexistence.

The zero-growth isoclines depicted in Box 2.2 characterize, for a system of two fixed-density host species, the densities of susceptible hosts that permit shared parasites to increase when rare. With this graphical tool in hand, we can now address some aspects of competitive coexistence without wallowing in complex algebra. Each parasite has its own zero-growth isocline. By jointly plotting each species' isocline, one can qualitatively characterize necessary conditions for coexistence of a pair of parasite species competing for susceptible individuals of two host species. If the isocline for parasite i lies entirely inside the isocline for parasite j, then i can invade the system and depress susceptible host density enough to keep j out. Thus, a necessary condition for parasite coexistence is that the two isoclines cross. (To characterize sufficient conditions, one must also consider host properties, such as the degree of regulation of hosts by parasitism.)

Parasites can coexist through different types of niche partitioning. Coexistence may be related either to the capacity each parasite has for using individual hosts, or to the pattern of transmission within and among host species. If parasite transmission is similar within and among host species, the zero-growth isoclines are straight lines. In this case, for these isoclines to cross, each parasite species must experience a lower loss rate in a different host species (Fig. 2.3 (a) and (b)). For example, parasites may coexist if each can better resist clearance from a different host. Such niche differentiation may be due to differential tolerance of induced or constitutive host defenses. Alternatively, if parasites have equivalent loss rates in both host species, they can coexist only if each has its highest transmission rate in a

Box 2.2 A graphical model for parasite invasion: zero-growth isoclines

Before addressing coexistence in the community represented by model (2.2), we need to characterize persistence conditions for each parasite species alone. If we assume host abundance is fixed (e.g. each host is at its respective carrying capacity), we can ask whether a given parasite (say species 1) can invade the host community. To determine the answer analytically, it is useful to rewrite the equations for parasite 1 (shown in main text) in the form

$$\frac{d}{dt}\begin{bmatrix} I_1 \\ I_2 \end{bmatrix} = \begin{bmatrix} (\beta_{11}S_1 - \Gamma_1) & \beta_{12}S_1 \\ \beta_{21}S_2 & (\beta_{22}S_2 - \Gamma_2) \end{bmatrix}\begin{bmatrix} I_1 \\ I_2 \end{bmatrix}$$

from which it is clear that the growth rate of the parasite is represented by the matrix. In fact, the asymptotic growth rate of the parasite is equivalent to the dominant eigenvalue of this matrix. The dominant eigenvalue equals zero (i.e. $R_0 = 1$) when the determinant of this matrix (det[]) is zero, resulting in the following condition for zero parasite growth:

$$\det \begin{bmatrix} (\beta_{11}S_1 - \Gamma_1) & \beta_{12}S_1 \\ \beta_{21}S_2 & (\beta_{22}S_2 - \Gamma_2) \end{bmatrix}$$
$$= (\beta_{11}S_1 - \Gamma_1)(\beta_{22}S_2 - \Gamma_2) - \beta_{12}S_1\beta_{21}S_2 = 0$$

When this condition is plotted in relation to the densities of susceptible hosts (S_1 and S_2, as in Fig. 2.3), it describes the "zero-growth isocline" for the parasite. If the combination of susceptible host densities lies outside the isocline, then the parasite can invade; conversely, if susceptible host densities are between the isocline and the origin, the parasite will decline toward extinction. The shape of the zero-growth isocline reflects the pattern of parasite transmission resulting from the type of interaction among host species (see Holt et al. 2003, and main text). In this particular model, host-specific loss rates, Γ_i, influence the intercepts, but not the curvature of the parasite's zero-growth isocline.

There is a subtle distinction between the zero-growth isoclines in Fig. 2.3 and the more familiar isoclines of resource–consumer theory (Grover 1997). In a typical resource–consumer model, the current growth rate of the consumer is simply a function of current resource abundance, with no explicit effect of time. In a host–parasite system, susceptible host abundance is indeed a "resource" for the parasite. But the growth rate in question here is the *asymptotic* growth rate for the parasite, after enough time has passed following invasion for the parasite to settle into its stable pattern of distribution across the host species.

The zero-growth isoclines derived above and depicted in Fig. 2.3 generalize the concept of a minimum host density to two host populations, and encapsulate graphically the minimal host community configurations permitting parasite invasion. One can also plot additional isoclines of constant R_0 as a function of susceptible host densities (Fig. 2.4). The zero-growth isocline is that set of susceptible host densities for which $R_0 = 1$; that is, although total host densities are fixed in model (2.2), parasites may regulate susceptible host densities. At equilibrium with a given parasite, the density of susceptible hosts will be depressed to levels somewhere on the zero-growth isocline for that parasite. This equilibrium then determines the initial array of susceptible host densities that a second parasite species will face when it attempts to invade the host community. By plotting isoclines for each parasite simultaneously, we can begin to characterize conditions for exclusion, versus coexistence. With similar parasite transmission rates within and among host species, the isoclines are straight lines (Fig. 2.3(b)). If most transmission is within host species, the isoclines instead bow out from the origin (Fig. 2.3(d)). Begon et al. (1999) analyzed transmission dynamics of the cowpox virus in mixed populations of bank voles and wood mice, and showed that despite their close co-occurrence, transmission between host species was negligible, so convex isoclines are quite plausible in this system, and doubtless many others as well.

In Fig. 2.3 and in model (2.2) in the text, both zero-growth isoclines have negative slope; this is not necessarily the case for systems with frequency-dependent transmission, vector-mediated transmission, or free-living infectious stages (Holt et al. 2003; J. Antonovics, personal communication). Figure 2.4 compares the isoclines describing contours of constant R_0 as a function of host density for several frequency-dependent systems, each with two host species. With multiple hosts, frequency-dependent transmission can buffer disease outbreaks, leading to the "dilution" effect described by Ostfeld and Keesing (2000), while density-dependent transmission usually leads to enhanced potential for parasite establishment and outbreak. When the frequency-dependent case is expanded to explicitly consider transmission vectors for the parasite, then the "height" of each R_0 contour varies approximately with the square root of vector abundance (Dobson 2004). So increasing vector density increases the potential for an epidemic. This effect helps explain why vector control has been so effective in controlling diseases such as malaria and yellow fever.

continues

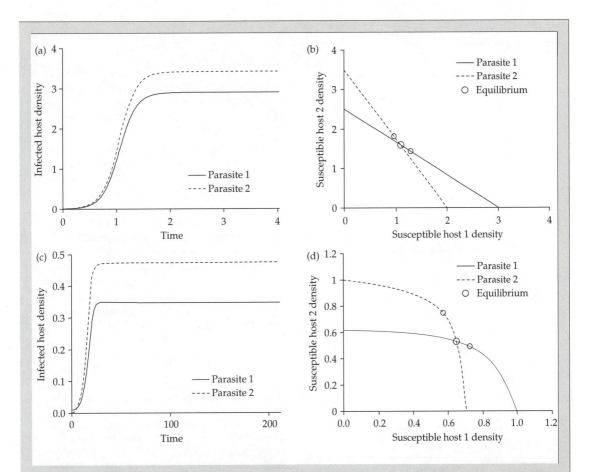

Figure 2.3 Examples of isocline shapes and coexistence for two parasite species competing for susceptible individuals of two (fixed-density) host species. In (a) and (b), transmission is similar within and between host species, but each parasite persists longer in a different host. In (c) and (d), parasite loss rates are similar between species, but there is more intra- than interspecific transmission. The time plots (a) and (c) are numerical simulations demonstrating that the parasites can coexist. In the isocline plots (b) and (d), the smaller dots indicate equilibrial densities of susceptible hosts when each parasite occurs alone; in these examples, the equilibria shift so as to facilitate invasion by the other parasite. The specific parameters are as follows: (a) Total number of hosts infected by each parasite, starting with host 1 infected by each parasite at a density of 0.001. $\beta_{11} = \beta_{12} = \beta_{21} = \beta_{22} = \beta_{11}' = \beta_{12}' = \beta_{21}' = \beta_{22}' = 1$, $\Gamma_1 = 3$, $\Gamma_2 = 2.5$, $\Gamma_1' = 2$, $\Gamma_2' = 3.5$, $K_1 = 4$, $K_2 = 5$. (b). Isoclines for parameters in (a). When both parasites are present, the system approaches the point at which the isoclines cross. (c and d). Same as (a) and (b), but $\beta_{11} = 0.5$, $\beta_{12} = 0.1$, $\beta_{21} = 0.4$, $\beta_{22} = 0.8$, $\beta_{11}' = 0.7$, $\beta_{12}' = 0.3$, $\beta_{21}' = 0.1$, $\beta_{22}' = 0.5$, $\Gamma_1 = \Gamma_2 = \Gamma_1' = \Gamma_2' = 0.5$, $K_1 = K_2 = 1$.

An important subtlety arises with pathogens that use ticks as vectors. The abundance of ticks may be tightly coupled to the abundance of their hosts—hosts that also harbor the pathogens that ticks transmit. In this case, increases in host abundance may lead to both increased vector abundance and enhanced amplification of disease transmission. If factors other than host availability can regulate vector numbers when hosts are common, nonlinear isoclines can readily occur.

In systems where vector transmission is by mosquitoes or tsetse flies, whose abundance is independent of host abundance, an increase in host numbers may dilute the per capita vector attacks and the per capita production of fresh infections from any given infected host (R_0). Models that

continues

Box 2.2 *continued*

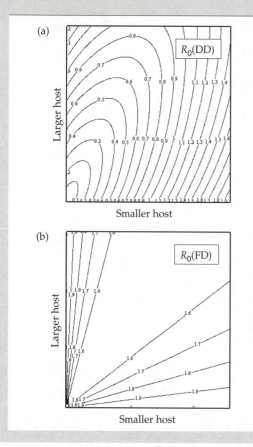

include a free-living pool of pathogens can generate isoclines with positive slope (Holt *et al.* 2003). If different pathogens have very different isoclines in these two-host systems, the interactions between them may not resemble familiar competition isoclines at all.

The isocline approach to analyzing coexistence of parasites in host communities provides useful insights, but it may be difficult to apply to particular empirical systems. In natural systems it can even be difficult to show that threshold densities exist (Begon *et al.* 2003). Detailed case studies seem to reveal that parasite persistence is not governed so much by average host density, as by the detailed spatial structuring of infection processes (e.g. Keeling and Gilligan 2000). An important task for future work is to articulate the impact of alternative forms for transmission dynamics, and the spatial structuring of transmission, on the coexistence conditions for parasites potentially competing for the same suite of host species.

Figure 2.4 Zero-growth isoclines resulting from density-dependent (a) or frequency-dependent (b) transmission. These isoclines with nonlinear or positive slopes depict contours of constant R_0 for a single parasite species infecting two hosts (see Dobson 2004). Were one to simultaneously plot isoclines for two parasite species infecting these two hosts, it is clear that the resulting figures would not match those of classical competition theory (details not shown).

different host, corresponding to nonlinear isoclines (Fig. 2.3 (c) and (d)). Transmission rates can differ in this way for a variety of reasons. Each parasite species may increase contact behavior in a different host species, or each may be specialized to exploit contacts in a different host.

Crossing isoclines are necessary but not sufficient for parasite coexistence. For coexistence, host carrying capacities cannot differ too greatly. A parasite that is better at exploiting a host with a low carrying capacity is vulnerable to exclusion by a parasite that is better at exploiting a host with a higher carrying capacity. This effect arises in model (2.5) below, which is a limiting case of model (2.2).

It should be noted that in model (2.2), we assume that hosts that are susceptible to infection by one parasite species in general are also

susceptible to the other parasite. If hosts have specialized immune responses, then host individuals that recover and become immune to one parasite species may still be available for infection by a second parasite species. This leads to a kind of niche partitioning within a single host species, which can facilitate the coexistence of competing parasites (Pej Rohani, personal communication).

2.3.1.2 *Spatially localized competition*
Roberts and Dobson (1995; see also Dobson 1985) explored a model for competing macroparasites that are characteristically aggregated within the host population. This model incorporates both exploitative competition for hosts, and direct interference. Parasite aggregation can facilitate coexistence,

particularly given negative cross-species correlations in the parasite distributions. The model of Roberts and Dobson (1995) assumed that hosts are solely regulated by the parasites (which increased host mortality). If, as in model (2.1), we instead assume that host density is constant and regulated by factors other than parasitism, the macroparasite equations presented in Roberts and Dobson (1995, p. 194) can be re-written as the familiar Lotka–Volterra competition equations, with parameters such as the competition coefficient expressed as a function of epidemiologically relevant quantities such as parasite fecundity and aggregation strength (details not shown). This simplification of the model reveals that the coexistence of competing macroparasites requires that they not be too dissimilar in their inherent ability to use the host. For example, macroparasites with similar rates of growth when rare may coexist via this "equalizing mechanism" (*sensu* Chesson 2000a). This simplification of the model also reveals that competing macroparasites must differ in their patterns of aggregation. If aggregation patterns ensure that intraspecific interference exceeds interspecific interference, then macroparasites may coexist via this "stabilizing mechanism" (*sensu* Chesson 2000a).

We are not aware of parallel theoretical studies directly pertinent to microparasites. However, we note that the degree of aggregation created in any host macroparasite system reflects the interplay between heterogeneities in host susceptibility (immunological, spatial, and genetic) and parasite virulence. In general, parasites that are more virulent will exhibit lower levels of aggregation and thus will be less likely to coexist with other species (Shaw and Dabson 1998) (barring spatial heterogeneities in parasite transmission efficiency, which would tend to promote parasite coexistence).

2.3.1.3 *Frequency-dependent mortality*

As in community ecology in general, food-web interactions may influence which parasite dominates and whether there will be exclusion or coexistence, depending upon the detailed structure of the trophic interactions (see Chapter 9, this volume, for further treatment of parasites in food webs). In model (2.1), the loss rate of infected hosts implicitly incorporates losses due to predation. In that case,

predation can potentially influence parasite community structure if different parasite strains lead to different (fixed) predation rates for infected hosts; for example, by affecting host behavior.

In models that allow the death rate of infected hosts to increase with the density of infected hosts, coexistence may be promoted (Pugliese 2002). Assume that parasite species 1 has higher transmission rates and also causes its host to attract generalist predators, who respond facultatively to the abundance of the infected prey. We can modify model (2.1) to account for this effect by allowing infected host deaths to increase directly with their own abundance:

$$\frac{dI_1}{dt} = (\beta_1 S - d_1(I_1))I_1 \tag{2.3}$$

Now assume that parasite 2 has lower transmission rates and does not affect host predation rates, so that host dynamics follow model (2.1). For simplicity, assume the death rate of hosts with parasite 1 is a linear function of their density, $d_1(I_1) = d_1 + d'I_1$, whereas hosts with parasite 2 have a fixed death rate; moreover, assume that each parasite can invade when alone with the host. The condition for parasite coexistence is:

$$\frac{\beta_1}{d_1} > \frac{\beta_2}{d_2} > \frac{\beta_1 + d'}{Kd' + d_1}$$

The left-hand inequality describes when parasite 1 can invade, given that parasite 2 is present and at equilibrium. The right-hand inequality describes when parasite 2 can invade, given that parasite 1 is present and at equilibrium. The full condition reveals that coexistence is more likely with larger host carrying capacity and larger effects of parasite 1 on host predation rates.

Packer *et al.* (2003) and Ostfeld and Holt (2004), building upon earlier work by Dobson (1988) and Lafferty (1992), have recently emphasized the importance of predation as a factor governing host–parasite dynamics, even if predators act simply as density-independent mortality agents upon various classes of prey. There are many reasons to focus on systems combining predation and parasitism. When predators attack both healthy and infected prey individuals, the full relationship corresponds to intraguild predation (Holt and Polis 1997; see Fig. 2.1), because predators both compete with parasites for healthy hosts and inflict mortality upon parasitized hosts. Generalist top predators in many communities seem particularly at risk to anthropogenic impacts. If disruption of natural predator–prey interactions reduces prey mortality rates, one indirect consequence could be the unleashing of host–pathogen interactions present in lower trophic levels. This could involve both increases in disease incidence in species that are already sustaining the pathogen, and spread to novel hosts (Packer *et al.* 2003; Ostfeld and Holt 2004; Hethcote *et al.* 2004; Hall *et al.* 2005; Holt, in press). If selective predation promotes parasite coexistence, as in model (2.3), predator removal may also bring certain parasites to dominance.

An interesting example comes from studies by Hudson and colleagues on the interplay between gamekeepers, predators, grouse, and a parasitic nematode (Hudson *et al.* 1992, 1998). Predators selectively attack heavily infected grouse. The job of a gamekeeper is to reduce predator numbers, in order to increase the game available for hunters. Across sites, Hudson found that the percentage of grouse heavily infected with worms actually *increases* with the density of gamekeepers! This suggests that although there may indeed be more grouse where gamekeepers are doing their job, those grouse on average are wormier. This effect should be expected whether or not predators differentially prey upon wormier grouse; with fewer predators, parasite-infested prey can simply live longer and generate more secondary infections.

We should caution that the impacts of predator removal upon disease dynamics may differ dramatically from the descriptions above. For instance, predators may themselves be hosts, or be transmission agents for the parasite (as is true in many complex life cycles, Parker *et al.* 2003; see also Lafferty 1992 and Chapters 9 and 10, this volume). Predator removal may then disrupt transmission dynamics and reduce disease incidence among the remaining hosts. Moreover, prey behavioral responses to predation can alter transmission dynamics directly (Dobson 1988; Lafferty 1992). If prey tend to be less mobile in the presence of predators, a reduction in predation may lead to an increase in prey contacts and disease transmission. If reduced predation leads to higher prey densities and more competition, prey may become more vulnerable to infection (Keesing *et al.*, in preparation). Caveats aside, we suggest that the elimination of top predators can often lead to an upsurge in the abundance of infected prey and the potential for disease transmission across host species.

2.3.1.4 Storage effects
Temporal fluctuations in the environment can promote parasite species coexistence via the storage effect if, for instance, competing parasite species have different abiotic optima for reproduction, and are able to produce long-lived resting stages. Baciloviruses with a long-lived resting stage may coexist via this storage effect. We are unaware of any formal theory addressing storage-effect mechanisms for parasite species coexistence.

2.3.1.5 Temporal fluctuations and nonlinearities
If transmission rates do not vary with host abundance or quality, then (using time-averaging techniques, Holt 1997a) it can be shown for model (2.1) that coexistence cannot be facilitated by temporal fluctuations in the host. However, there is growing evidence in many systems that transmission rates can be nonlinear functions of host density (Hochberg 1993; McCallum *et al.* 2001). If one parasite transmits better at low host densities, and the other transmits better at high host densities, it is conceivable that fluctuations in host density could promote parasite coexistence.

2.3.1.6 Alternating habitats
Many macroparasites have complex life cycles, making coexistence feasible if different species are regulated at different stages of life history (e.g. see Chapters 9–11, this volume). A complication here is that one must also characterize how the different hosts are themselves regulated, and if this regulation depends upon parasitism. This scenario is ripe for theoretical development.

2.3.1.7 Competition–colonization trade-offs
In model (1), we assumed that there is no coinfection. If individual hosts can harbor multiple

parasite species then coexistence may occur even if there is just a single host species. As a simple example, consider the following modification of model (2.1):

$$\frac{dI_1}{dt} = (\beta_1 S - \beta_2 p I_2 - d_1)I_1,$$
$$\frac{dI_2}{dt} = (\beta_2(S + p I_1) - d_2)I_2, \qquad (2.4)$$
$$K = S + I_1 + I_2$$

Here, the parameter p describes the rate of super-infection of hosts by parasite 2, or the ability of parasite 2 to infect individuals already infected with parasite 1 (relative to susceptibles). Model (2.4) in effect ignores coinfection by assuming that parasite 2 quickly supplants parasite 1 in any hosts that become jointly occupied.

With this modification in transmission dynamics, coexistence can now occur, if parasite 1 can persist at a lower host density than can parasite 2. Model (2.4) is similar in form to familiar models of competition–colonization trade-offs in metapopulations. This scenario is also in a sense a form of intraguild predation; both parasites compete for healthy hosts, and in addition the superior within-host parasite "preys" upon the other parasite. Hochberg and Holt (1990) explore a version of this model in which the host is regulated by parasites. That model can also be viewed as a variant of intraguild predation; in general, if a predator consumes the required resource of its prey, that prey species must be superior in exploitative competition for it to persist (Holt and Polis 1997).

2.3.1.8 Spatial subsidies

A simple mechanism for enriching local communities of parasites inhabiting a given host species in one location is "spillover" from other locations or other species. Model (2.1) can be modified to illustrate such spillover effects, as follows:

$$\frac{dI_1}{dt} = (\beta_1 S - d_1)I_1$$
$$\frac{dI_2}{dt} = (\beta_2 S - d_2)I_2 + S\beta'I' \qquad (2.5)$$
$$K = S + I_1 + I_2$$

Here $\beta'I'$ is the net force of infection of susceptible hosts occurring from external sources ("spillover"). Note that we have assumed that parasite species 1 is maintained solely by local dynamics, and there is just one host species available.

If parasite species 2 is locally inferior (i.e. $d_2/\beta_2 > d_1/\beta_1$), then it will surely be excluded in a closed community. In an open community with spillover, it will persist and equilibrate at

$$I_2^* = \frac{I'\beta'(d_1/\beta_1)}{d_2 - d_1(\beta_2/\beta_1)}$$

This equilibrium follows from examination of the first and second equations in model (2.5), which give us $S^* = d_1/\beta_1$ and $I_2^* = S^*I'\beta'/(d_2 - S^*\beta_2)$, respectively. Because we have assumed fixed host abundance, we can express the abundance of the resident parasite as $I_1^* = K - I_2^* - S^*$. Because I_1^* declines with I_2^*, and I_2^* is directly proportional to $I'\beta'$, the equilibrial abundance of parasite 1 declines linearly with the force of spillover infection from the alternative host for parasite 2.

At low spillover rates, one will observe coexistence. The coexistence mechanism in this case reflects habitat partitioning at a broader spatial scale; parasite 1 is locally superior, but parasite 2 can persist elsewhere and so be maintained locally in the focal community. However, if spillover is too great, the locally superior parasite can be excluded. This is particularly likely for host species with low K. Host–parasite models with density-dependent transmission predict minimum host population sizes, below which specialist parasites are likely to disappear. Spillover infections can amplify this trend, by permitting inferior generalists (maintained in large measure outside the focal host) to supplant specialist parasites in hosts that are low in abundance.

2.4 Back to parasite-driven host dynamics

We have explored some ways in which the standard repertoire of coexistence mechanisms that are of such enduring interest in community ecology may pertain to parasite species coexistence, and sketched simple models illustrating several mechanisms. We deliberately made the simplifying assumption that the abundance of each host species was set by ecological factors, independent of parasitism itself. But one reason for the increasing attention to parasites is that they can drive host population and community dynamics. Relaxing the assumption that hosts are regulated independently of parasitism increases the degrees of freedom that must be considered in analyzing community dynamics. Host species may themselves go extinct, and so one must ascertain the conditions for the joint maintenance of diversity in hosts as well as in their parasites. Moreover, unstable dynamics become more likely, permitting nonequilibrial influences on species exclusion and coexistence to arise.

Each of the modules shown in Fig. 2.2 warrants considerable treatment, well beyond the space limits of this chapter, and examples are beginning to appear in the literature (Hochberg and Holt 1990; Grenfell 1992; Holt and Hochberg 1998; Taylor *et al.* 1998, Dwyer *et al.* 2004). Here we highlight just a few simple points about regulation by parasites.

Consider again the basic model (2.1) of exploitative competition between parasites for a single host species, but now allow the parasite-free host population to grow in an unlimited fashion, following $dS/dt = rS - \beta_1 I_1 S - \beta_2 I_2 S + e_1 I_1 + e_2 I_2$. The last two terms describe contributions to susceptibles due to recovery or reproduction by infected individuals. The winning parasite species is still the one persisting at the lowest value of $S^* = d_i/\beta_i$. But the equilibrium may not exist; adding the equations for infected hosts, one finds that a condition for host population regulation is that $d_i < e_i$; that is, the death rate of infected hosts must exceed their combined rates of recovery and reproduction (Holt and Pickering 1985). Moreover, there is now a tendency for dynamic instability; for example, the lower the reproductive rate of infected hosts, the longer one observes damped oscillations when the system is perturbed.

2.4.1 Apparent competition

As noted above, one plausible mechanism for the coexistence of parasites is niche partitioning among host species. But if parasites influence host dynamics, a rich array of outcomes become possible. Embedded within the niche partitioning module (Fig. 2.2) is the module of shared parasitism. If a parasite can limit the numbers of each of several host species, apparent competition between hosts may occur, leading to reduced host abundance or even elimination of some host species from the community (Holt and Lawton 1994; Hudson and Greenman 1998). Shared parasitism could play important roles in community structure and biodiversity, and in the emergence of disease. For instance, Power and Mitchell (2004) experimentally demonstrated that wild oats facilitated spillover of the yellow dwarf virus onto several other host species, reducing their abundance through apparent competition (see also Chapter 5, this volume).

Holt and Pickering (1985) provided a formal treatment of apparent competition due to shared parasitism for a standard susceptible-infected (SI) model in which hosts are not regulated independently of parasitism, and in which disease transmission was density-dependent within and between host species. By examining conditions for each species to increase when rare, they identified conditions that led to exclusion of one host species, and conditions permitting coexistence. These conditions combine intrinsic host properties, impacts of disease on host fitness, and patterns of transmission. Host species with low intrinsic growth rates are vulnerable to exclusion; for robust coexistence, such that each host species can increase when rare, within-species disease transmission must exceed between-species transmission.

The potential for indirect exclusion via shared parasitism arises in almost any model in which parasites can regulate host numbers. For instance, Bowers and Begon (1991) examined a model for two hosts interacting via a pathogen with a free-living infectious stage. The single-host case can lead to a stable equilibrium or limit cycles. Despite the seeming potential for nonequilibrial coexistence, coexistence did not occur. At equilibrium, the host contributing most to the free-living pool of pathogens won out. This result parallels that of predator-mediated competition models in which the winning competitor is often the one that can sustain more predators (Holt *et al.* 1994). Begon and Bowers (1995) showed again in a model of multiple host species that one species would exclude all others if both transmission and density-dependent host growth were in proportion to total host density. In general, host coexistence in the face of a single, shared parasite seems to require the classical niche partitioning suggested by Holt and Pickering (1985); that is, stronger intraspecific than interspecific disease transmission.

Bowers and Begon (1991) also observed that nonequilibrial dynamics may occur, allowing the winner of competition between hosts to depend on the starting conditions. Since then, further evidence has mounted that even simple one-pathogen, two-host models can display a rich diversity of dynamical outcomes. Greenman and Hudson (1997) demonstrated that the Holt–Pickering model could generate alternative equilibria; under the same parameter values, one host species could exclude the other or, if the second host were introduced in sufficient numbers, both hosts could persist in a stable limit cycle. Similar phenomena can arise even with direct intraspecific density dependence in host dynamics (as in Begon *et al.* 1992; Begon and Bowers 1995). However, if such intraspecific density dependence is sufficiently strong, the system settles into a stable equilibrium. Intraspecific density dependence depresses host productivity, reduces the equilibrial level of infection, and weakens the indirect interaction between host species.

There are often substantial differences among host species in transmission rates and other key parameters reflecting body size, diet, and other important ecological dimensions. Figure 2.5 illustrates the long-term transient dynamics of a system of four host species when rates of interspecific transmission vary across four orders of magnitude (after Dobson 2004). In this system we have scaled the dynamics of the host species by their body sizes; these allometric rescalings allow numerical examination of more complex systems for realistic ranges of parameter values (DeLeo and Dobson 1996). When interspecific transmission is low, each host species exhibits persistent epidemic cycles of a frequency determined by the demographic speed

with which the pool of susceptible hosts recovers; host species with small body size exhibit faster epidemic cycles (Fig. 2.5(a)). As interspecific transmission increases, outbreaks are dominated by the dynamics of smaller species until the system stabilizes and each species reaches a constant abundance. Eventually, interspecific transmission is sufficiently high to allow the smaller (least susceptible) to drive the larger (more susceptible) species to local extinction (Fig. 2.5(b)).

The theoretical studies discussed above focus on microparasites. Comparable phenomena arise in macroparasite models (Dobson 1990; Dobson and Pacala 1992; Greenman and Hudson 2000). Although such models are relatively complex and difficult to analyze, qualitatively similar messages emerge. In a wide range of circumstances, apparent competition mediated by macroparasites can lead to host exclusion. Adding direct competition exacerbates this trend, as suggested by data on the decline of the partridge in the United Kingdom (Tompkins *et al.* 1999, 2000, 2001).

2.4.2 Keystone parasitism

When there is competition among host species, parasites may facilitate coexistence—a "keystone parasitism" effect. For a parasite to play this role, the host species that is superior in competition must also be more vulnerable to parasitism. This situation can emerge if competitive dominance translates into high population size, and specialist parasites are more likely to evolve on abundant hosts. A specialist parasite can regulate the abundance of a superior competitor below the level set by resources, thus freeing resources for inferior competitors that can escape parasitism (e.g., Packer and Clay 2000). One suggestive line of evidence for the potential ubiquity of keystone parasitism comes from invasion biology. Introduced species often carry fewer parasites than inflict them in their native ranges, which may permit them to explode to high abundances in their new ranges, reducing the abundances of competing native species (Mitchell and Power 2003; Torchin *et al.* 2003). If invasive species suffer more parasitism and occur at lower densities within their native ranges than

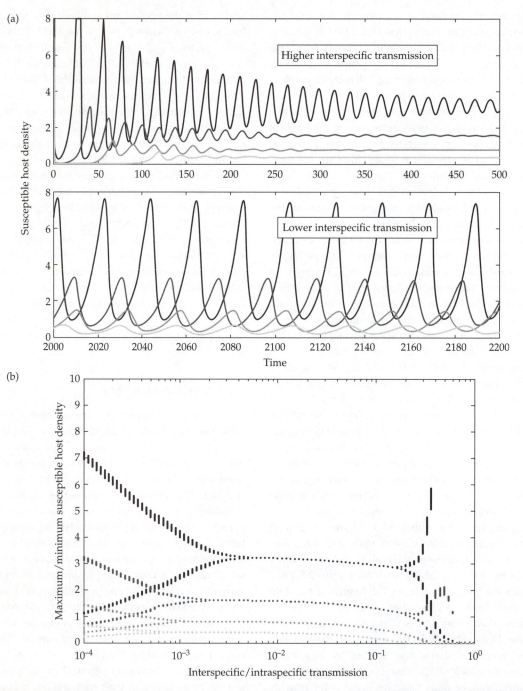

Figure 2.5 Examples of transient dynamics, coexistence, and exclusion in hosts sharing parasites. The examples shown are based on parameter values arising from the allometric scaling relationships noted by DeLeo and Dobson (1996). (a) An increase in interspecific transmission from low to intermediate rates may stabilize dynamics. (b) Further increases in transmission can lead to exclusion of hosts with low intrinsic growth rates (e.g. hosts with large body sizes).

within their introduced ranges, then keystone parasitism may be keeping these competitive dominants in check within their native ranges.

2.5 Future directions

Ultimately, everything described above suggests that ecologists need to reconsider the role that parasites play in communities (Marcogliese and Gone1997; Dobson *et al.* 2005). In Chapter 9 of this volume, Lafferty *et al.* quantify the abundance of parasites in a salt marsh community. This work reinforces earlier studies by Memmott *et al.* (2000) and others suggesting that consideration of parasites increases the diversity of species in a community by between 50% and 100%, often quadrupling the number of links in a food web. The methods described here illustrate how we can illuminate aspects of these complex systems by breaking them into individual modules of multiple interacting species. Quantifying the relative importance of the different types of modules in different communities remains an important task for the future of parasite-host community ecology.

Acknowledgments

RDH thanks Mike Barfield and Erin Taylor for their assistance with manuscript preparation, the University of Florida Foundation and NIH for financial support, and the editors for their patience.

References

Abrams, P. A. and R. D. Holt. (2002). The impact of consumer-resource cycles on the coexistence of competing consumers. *Theoretical Population Biology* **62**:281–296.

Allen, L. J. S., N. Kirupaharan, and S. M. Wilson. (2004). SIS epidemic models with multiple pathogen strains. *Journal of Difference Equations and Applications* **10**:53–75.

Anderson, P. K., A. A. Cunningham, N. G. Patel, F. J. Morales, P. R. Epstein, and P. Daszak. (2004). Emerging infectious diseases of plants: pathogen pollution, climate change and agrotechnology drivers. *Trends in Ecology and Evolution* **19**:535–544.

Anderson, R. M. and R. M. May. (1978). Regulation and stability of host-parasite population interactions. I. Regulatory processes. *Journal of Animal Ecology* **47**:219–247.

Antonovics, J., Y. Iwasa, and M. P. Hassell. (1995). A generalized model of parasitoid, venereal, and vector-based transmission processes. *American Naturalist* **145**:661–675.

Antonovics, J., M. Hood, and J. Partain. (2002). The ecology and genetics of a host shift: *Microbotryum* as a model system. *American Naturalist* **160**:S40–S53.

Augspurger, C. K. (1983). Seed dispersal by the tropical tree, *Platypodium elegans*, and the escape of its seedlings from fungal pathogens. *Journal of Ecology* **71**:759–771.

Begon, M. and R. G. Bowers. (1995). Beyond host-pathogen dynamics. In B. T. Grenfell and A. P. Dobson, eds. *Ecology of Infectious Diseases in Natural Populations*, pp. 478–509. Cambridge University Press, Cambridge, UK.

Begon, M., R. G. Bowers, N. Kadianakis, and D. E. Hodgkinson. (1992). Disease and community structure: the importance of host self-regulation in a host-host-pathogen model. *American Naturalist* **139**: 1131–1150.

Begon, M., S. M. Hazel, D. Baxby, K. Bown, R. Cavanagh, J. Chantrey, T. Jones, and M. Bennett. (1999). Transmission dynamics of a zoonotic pathogen within and between wildlife host species. *Proceedings of the Royal Society of London B* **266**:1939–1945.

Begon, M., S. M. Hazel, S. Telfer, K. Bown, D. Carslake, R. Cavanagh, J. Chantrey, T. Jones, and M. Bennett. (2003). Rodents, cowpox virus and islands: densities, numbers and thresholds. *Journal of Animal Ecology* **72**:343–355.

Bolker, B. and S. Pacala. (1999). Spatial moment equations for plant competition: understanding spatial strategies and the advantages of short dispersal. *American Naturalist* **153**:575–602.

Bowers, R. G. (1999). A baseline model for the apparent competition between many host strains: the evolution of host resistance to microparasites. *Journal of Theoretical Biology* **200**:65–75.

Bowers, R. G. and M. Begon. (1991). A host–host–pathogen model with free-living infective stages, applicable to microbial pest control. *Journal of Theoretical Biology* **148**:305–329.

Bowers, R. G. and J. Turner. (1997). Community structure and the interplay between interspecific infection and competition. *Journal of Theoretical Biology* **187**:95–109.

Brown, S. P., F. Renaud, J. F. Guegan, and Fl Thomas. (2001). Evolution of trophic transmission in parasites: the need to reach a mating place? *Journal of Evolutionary Biology* **14**:815–820.

Chase, J. M. and M. A. Leibold. (2003). Ecological niches: linking classical and contemporary approaches. University of Chicago Press, Chicago, IL.

Chesson, P. (2000a). Mechanisms of maintenance of species diversity. *Annual Review of Ecology and Systematics* **31**:343–366.

Chesson, P. (2000b). General theory of competitive coexistence in spatially-varying environments. *Theoretical Population Biology* **58**:211–237.

Cleaveland, S., M. K. Laurenson, and L. H. Taylor. (2001). Diseases of humans and their domestic mammals: pathogen characteristics, host range and the risk of emergence. *Philosophical Transactions of the Royal Society of London B* **356**:991–999.

Daszak, P., A. A. Cunningham, and A.D. Hyatt. (2000). Emerging infectious diseases of wildlife – threats to biodiversity and human health. *Science* **287**:443–453.

Debinski, D. M., Ray, C., and E. H. Saveraid. (2001). Species diversity and the scale of the landscape mosaic: do scales of movement and patch size affect diversity? *Biological Conservation* **98**:179–190.

DeLeo, G. A. and A. P. Dobson. (1996). Allometry and simple epidemic models for microparasites. *Nature* **379**:720–722.

Dobson, A. P. (1985). The population dynamics of competition between parasites. *Parasitology* **91**:317–347.

Dobson, A. P. (1988). The population biology of parasite-induced changes in host behavior. *Quarterly Review of Biology* **63**:139–165.

Dobson, A. P. (1990). Models for multi-species parasite-host communities. In G. Esch, C.R. Kennedy, and J. Aho, eds. *The Structure of Parasite Communities*, pp. 261–288. Chapman and Hall, London.

Dobson, A. P. (1999). The role of parasites in ecological systems. In A. Farina, ed. *Perspectives in Ecology. A Glance from the VII International Congress of Ecology (Florence, 19–25 July 1998)*, pp. 51–64. Backhuys Publishers, Leiden, NL.

Dobson, A. P. (2004). Population dynamics of pathogens with multiple host species. *American Naturalist* **164** (Suppl.):S64–S78.

Dobson, A. and J. Foufopoulos. (2001). Emerging infectious pathogens of wildlife. *Philosophical Transactions of the Royal Society of London B* **356**:1001–1012.

Dobson, A. P. and S. W. Pacala. (1992). The parasites of *Anolis* lizards in the northern Lesser Antilles. 2. The structure of the parasite community. *Oecologia* **91**:118–125.

Dobson, A. P., K. D. Lafferty, A. M. Kuris, and C. Packer. (2005). Parasites and food webs. In M. Pascual and J. Dunne, eds. *Ecological Networks*. Oxford University Press, Oxford.

Dushoff, J. and G. Dwyer. (2001). Evaluating the risks of engineered viruses: modeling pathogen competition. *Ecological Applications* **11**:1602–1609.

Dwyer, G., J. Dushoff, and S. H. Yee. (2004). The combined effects of pathogens and predators on insect outbreaks. *Nature* **430**:341–345.

Gilbert, G. S. (2002). Evolutionary ecology of plant diseases in natural ecosystems. *Annual Review of Phytopathology* **40**:13–43.

Goater, T. M., G. W. Esch, and A. O. Bush. (1987). Helminth parasites of sympatric salamanders: ecological concepts at infracommunity, component, and compound community levels. *American Midland Naturalist* **118**:289–300.

Gog, J., R. Woodroffe, and J. Swinton. (2000). Disease in endangered metapopulations: the importance of alternative hosts. *Proceedings of the Royal Society of London B* **269**:671–676.

Greenman, J. V. and P. J. Hudson. (1997). Infected coexistence instability with and without density-dependent regulation. *Journal of Theoretical Biology* **185**:345–356.

Greenman, J. V. and P. J. Hudson. (2000). Parasite-mediated and direct competition in a two-host shared macroparasite system. *Theoretical Population Biology* **57**: 13–34.

Grenfell, B. T. (1992). Parasitism and the dynamics of ungulate grazing systems. *American Naturalist* **139**: 907–929.

Grenfell, B. T. and A. P. Dobson, eds. (1995). *Ecology of Infectious Diseases*. Cambridge University Press. Cambridge, UK.

Grover, J. P. (1997). *Resource Competition*. Chapman and Hall.

Hall, S. R., M. A. Duffy, and C.E. Caceres (2005). Selective predation and productivity jointly drive complex behavior in host-parasite systems. *American Naturalist* **165**:70–81.

Harrison, M. A., Y. C. Lai, and R. D. Holt. (2001). Dynamical mechanism for coexistence of dispersing species. *Journal of Theoretical Biology* **213**:53–72.

Harvell, D. *et al.* (2004). The rising tide of ocean diseases: unsolved problems and research priorities. *Frontiers in Ecology and the Environment* **2**:375–382.

Hess, G. R. (1994). Conservation corridors and contagious disease: a cautionary note. *Conservation Biology* **8**:256–262.

Hethcote, H. W., W. Wang, L. Han, and Z. Ma. (2004). A predator-prey model with infected prey. *Theoretical Population Biology* **66**:259–268.

Hochberg, M. E. (1993). Nonlinear transmission rates and the dynamics of infectious diseases. *Journal of Theoretical Biology* **153**:301–321.

Hochberg, M. E. and R. D. Holt. (1990). The coexistence of competing parasites. I. The role of cross-species infection. *American Naturalist* **136**:517–541.

Holmes, J. C. (1973). Site selection by parasitic helminths: interspecific interactions, site segregation, and their importance to the development of helminth communities. *Canadian Journal of Zoology* **51**:333–347.

Holmes, J. C. and P. W. Price. (1986). Communities of parasites. In J. Kikkawa and D. J. Anderson, eds. *Community Ecology: Patterns and Processes*, pp. 187–213. Blackwell, London.

Holt, R. D. (1977). Predation, apparent competition, and the structure of prey communities. *Theoretical Population Biology* **12**:197–229.

Holt, R. D. (1993). Ecology at the mesoscale: the influence of regional processes on local communities. In R.E. Ricklefs and D. Schluter, eds. *Species Diversity in Ecological Communities*, pp. 77–88. University of Chicago Press, Chicago, IL.

Holt, R. D. (1997a). Community modules. In A.C. Gange and V. K. Brown, eds. *Multitrophic Interactions in Terrestrial Ecosystems*, pp. 333–349. Blackwell, Oxford.

Holt, R. D. (1997b). From metapopulation dynamics to community structure: some consequences of spatial heterogeneity. In I. Hanski and M. Gilpin, eds. *Metapopulation Biology*, pp. 149–164. Academic Press, New York.

Holt, R. D. (2001). Coexistence of species. *The Encyclopedia of Biodiversity* (S. Levin, ed.) **5**:413–426.

Holt, R. D. The community context of disease emergence: could changes in predation be a key driver? In R. Ostfeld, F. Keesing, and V. Eviner, eds. *The Ecology of Infectious Diseases*. Princeton University Press, Princeton, NJ.

Holt, R. D. and M. E. Hochberg. (1998). The coexistence of competing parasites. II. Hyperparasitism and food chain dynamics. *Journal of Theoretical Biology* **193**:485–495.

Holt, R. D. and J. H. Lawton. (1994). The ecological consequences of shared natural enemies. *Annual Review of Ecology and Systematics* **25**:495–520.

Holt, R. D. and J. Pickering. (1985). Infectious disease and species coexistence: a model of Lotka-Volterra form. *American Naturalist* **126**:196–211.

Holt, R. D., A. P. Dobson, M. Begon, R. G. Bowers, and E. Schauber. (2003). Parasite establishment and persistence in multi-host-species systems. *Ecology Letters* **6**:837–842.

Holt, R. D., J. Grover, and D. Tilman. (1994). Simple rules for interspecific dominance in systems with exploitative and apparent competition. *American Naturalist* **144**:741–777.

Holt, R. D. and G. A. Polis. (1997). A theoretical framework for intraguild predation. *American Naturalist* **149**:745–764.

Holt, R. D., M. Roy, and M. Barfield. Predation and disease dynamics: effects of host immunity and regulation (in review).

Holyoak, M., M. A. Leibold, and R. D. Holt, eds (2005). *Metacommunities: Spatial Dynamics and Ecological Communities*. University of Chicago Press, Chicago, IL (2005).

Hudson, P. J. and J. Greenman. (1998). Competition mediated by parasites: biological and theoretical progress. *Trends in Ecology and Evolution* **13**:387–390.

Hudson, P. J., A. P. Dobson, and D. Newborn. (1992). Do parasites make prey vulnerable to predation? Red grouse and parasites. *Journal of Animal Ecology* **61**:681–692.

Hudson, P. J., A. P. Dobson, and D. Newborn. (1998). Prevention of population cycles by parasite removal. *Science* **282**:2256–2258.

Hudson, P. J., A. Rizzoli, B. T. Grenfell, H. Heesterbeek, A. P. Dobson, eds. (2002). *The Ecology of Wildlife Diseases*. Oxford University Press, Oxford.

Huisman, J. and F. J. Weissing. (1999). Biodiversity of plankton by species oscillations and chaos. *Nature* **402**:407–410.

Iwasa, Y., F. Michor and M. Nowan (2004). Some basic properties of immune selection. *Journal of Theoretical Biology* **229**:179–188.

Jaenike, J. (1996). Population-level consequences of parasite aggregation. *Oikos* **76**:155–160.

Jaenike, J. (1998). On the capacity of macroparasites to control insect populations. *American Naturalist* **155**:84–96.

Jaenike, J. and S. J. Perlman. (2002). Ecology and evolution of host-parasite associations: mycophagous *Drosophila* and their parasitic nematodes. *American Naturalist* **160**:S23–S39.

Keeling, M. J. and C. A. Gilligan. (2000). Bubonic plague: a metapopulation model of a zoonosis. *Proceedings of the Royal Society of London B* **267**:2219–2230.

Keesing, F., R. D. Holt, and R. S. Ostfeld. Effects of species diversity on disease risk. (in preparation).

Kermack, W. O. and A. G. McKendrick. (1927). Contributions to the mathematical theory of epidemics, part I. *Proceedings of the Royal Society of London A* **115**:700–721.

Kneitel, J. M. and J. M. Chase. (2004). Trade-offs in community ecology: linking spatial scales and species coexistence. *Ecology Letters* **7**:69–80.

Kotler, B. P. and J. S. Brown. (1999). Mechanisms of coexistence of optimal foragers as determinants of local abundances and distributions of desert granivores. *Journal of Mammalogy* **80**:361–374.

Lafferty, K. D. (1992). Foraging on prey that are modified by parasites. *American Naturalist* **140**:854–867.

Lafferty, K. D. and L. R. Gerber. (2002). Good medicine for conservation biology: the intersection of epidemiology and conservation theory. *Conservation Biology* **16**:593–604.

Lafferty, K. D. and R. D. Holt. (2003). How does environmental stress affect the population dynamics of disease? *Ecology Letters* **6**:654–664.

Lawton, J. H. (2000). *Community Ecology in a Changing World*. Ecology Institute, Oldendorf/Luhe, Germany.

Leibold, M. A. (1996). A graphical model of keystone predators in food webs: trophic regulation of abundance, incidence and diversity patterns in communities. *American Naturalist* **147**:784–812.

Leibold, M. A. and T. E. Miller. (2004). From metapopulations to metacommunities. In I. Hanski and O. E. Gaggiotti, eds. *Ecology, Genetics and Evolution of Metapopulations*, pp. 133–150. Elsevier/Academic Press, London, UK.

Levin, B. R. and R. Antia. (2001). Why we don't get sick: the within-host population dynamics of bacterial infections. *Science* **292**:1112–1115.

Levin, S. A. (1970). Community equilibria and stability, and an extension of the competitive exclusion principle. *American Naturalist* **104**:413–423.

Marcogliese, D. J. and D. K. Cone. (1997). Food webs: a plea for parasites. *Trends in Ecology and Evolution* **12**:320–325.

May, R. M., S. Gupta, and A. R. McLean. (2001). Infectious disease dynamics: what characterizes a successful invader? *Philosophical Transactions of the Royal Society of London B* **356**:901–910.

McCallum, H. and A. Dobson. (1995). Detecting disease and parasite threats to endangered species and ecosystems. *Trends in Ecology and Evolution* **10**:190–194.

McCallum, H. and A. Dobson. (2002). Disease, habitat fragmentation and conservation. *Proceedings of the Royal Society of London B* **269**:2041–2049.

McCallum, H., N. Barlow, and J. Hone. (2001). How should parasite transmission be modelled? *Trends in Ecology and Evolution* **16**:295–300.

McCann, K. S. (2000). The diversity-stability debate. *Nature* **405**:228–233.

McPeek, M. A. and R. D. Holt. (1992). The evolution of dispersal in spatially and temporally varying environments. *American Naturalist* **140**:1010–1027.

Memmott, J., N. D. Martinez, and J. E.Cohen. (2000). Predators, parasitoids, and pathogens: species richness, trophic generality, and body sizes in a natural food web. *Journal of Animal Ecology* **69**:1–15.

Mitchell, C. E. and A. G. Power. (2003). Release of invasive plants from fungal and viral pathogens. *Nature* **421**:625–627.

Morand, S. and E. Arias-Gonzalez. (1997). Is parasitism a missing ingredient in model ecosystems? *Ecological Modelling* **95**:61–74.

Morgan, E. R., E. J. Milner-Gulland, P. R. Torgerson, and G. F. Medley. (2004). Ruminating on complexity: macroparasites of wildlife and livestock. *Trends in Ecology and Evolution* **19**:181–188.

Morin, P. J. (1999). *Community Ecology*. Blackwell, Oxford.

Myers, J. H. and D. R. Bazely. (2003). *Ecology and Control of Introduced Plants*. Cambridge University Press, Cambridge, UK.

Norman, R., R. G. Bowers, M. Begon, and P. J. Hudson. (1999). Persistence of tick-borne virus in the presence of multiple host species: tick reservoirs and parasite mediated competition. *Journal of Theoretical Biology* **200**:111–118.

Ostfeld, R. S. and F. Keesing. (2000). The function of biodiversity in the ecology of vector-borne zoonotic diseases. *Canadian Journal of Zoology* **78**:2061–2078.

Ostfeld, R. S. and R. D. Holt. (2004). Are predators good for your health? Evaluating evidence for top down regulation of zoonotic reservoirs. *Frontiers in Ecology and the Environment* **2**:13–20.

Ostfeld, R. D., E. M. Schauber, C. D. Canham, F. Keesing, C. G. Jones, and J. O. Wolff. (2001). Effects of acorn production and mouse abundance on abundance and *Borrelia burgdorferi* infection prevalence of nymphal *Ixodes scapularis* ticks. *Vector-Borne and Zoonotic Diseases* **1**:55–63.

Packer, A. and K. Clay. (2000). Soil pathogens and spatial patterns of seedling mortality in a temperate tree. *Nature* **404**:278–285.

Packer, C., R. D. Holt, A. Dobson, and P. Hudson. (2003). Keeping the herds healthy and alert: impacts of predation upon prey with specialist pathogens. *Ecology Letters* **6**:797–802.

Parker, G. A., J. C. Chub, M. A. Ball, and G. N. Roberts. (2003). Evolution of complex life cycles in helminth parasites. *Nature* **425**:480–484.

Perlman, S. J. and J. Jaenike. (2003). Infection success in novel hosts: an experimental and phylogenetic study of *Drosophila*-oarasutuc benatides. *Evolution* **57**:544–557.

Persson, L. (1999). Trophic cascades: abiding heterogeneity and the trophic level concept at the end of the road. *Oikos* **85**:385–397.

Polis, G. A., M. Power, and G. R. Huxel, eds. (2004). *Food Webs at the Landscape Level*. University of Chicago Press, Chicago, IL.

Poulin, R. (1998). *Evolutionary Ecology of Parasites: From Individuals to Communities*. Chapman and Hall, London.

Power, A. G. and C. E. Mitchell. (2004). Pathogen spillover in disease epidemics. *American Naturalist* **164**:S79–S89.

Price, P. W. (1980). *Evolutionary Biology of Parasites*. Princeton University Press, Princeton, NJ.

Pugliese, A. (2002). On the evolutionary coexistence of parasite strains. *Mathematical Biosciences* **177**:355–375.

Roberts, M. G. and A. P. Dobson. (1995). The population dynamics of communities of parasitic helminths. *Mathematical Biosciences* **126**:191–214.

Schoener, T. W. (1976). Alternatives to Lotka-Volterra competition: models of intermediate complexity. *Theoretical Population Biology* **10**:309–333.

Schoener, T. W. (1989). The ecological niche. In J.M. Cherrett, ed. *Ecological Concepts*, pp. 79–113. Blackwell, Oxford.

Shaw, D. J. and A. P. Dobson (1998). Patterns of macroparasite aggregation in wildlife populations. *Parasitology* **117**:597–610.

Shostak, A. W. and M. E. Scott. (1993). Detection of density-dependent growth and fecundity of helminths in natural infections. *Parasitology* **107**:527–539.

Taylor, D. R., A. M. Jarosz, R. E. Lenski, and D. W. Fulbright. (1998). The acquisition of hypovirulence in host-pathogen systems with three trophic levels. *American Naturalist* **151**:343–355.

Thompson, J. N., O. J. Reichman, P. J. Morin, G. A. Polis, M. E. Power, R. W. Sterner, *et al.* (2001). Frontiers of ecology. *Bioscience* **51**:15–24.

Tilman, D. (1982). *Resource Competition and Community Structure*. Princeton University Press, Princeton, NJ.

Tompkins, D. M., G. Dickson, and P. J. Hudson. (1999). Parasite-mediated competition between pheasant and grey partridge: a preliminary investigation. *Oecologia* **119**:378–382.

Tompkins, D. M., J. V. Greenman, P. A. Robertson, and P. J. Hudson. (2000). The role of shared parasites in the exclusion of wildlife hosts: *Heterakis gallinarum* in the ring-necked pheasant and the grey partridge. *Journal of Animal Ecology* **69**:829–840.

Tompkins, D. M., J. V. Greenman, and P. J. Hudson. (2001). Differential impact of a shared nematode parasite on two gamebird hosts: implications for apparent competition. *Parasitology* **122**:187–193.

Torchin, M. E., K. D. Lafferty, A. P. Dobson, V. J. McKenzie, and A. M. Kuris. (2003). Introduced species and their missing parasites. *Nature* **421**:628–630.

Woodroffe, R. (1999). Managing disease threats to wild mammals. *Animal Conservation* **2**:185–193.

Woolhouse, M. E. J., L. H. Taylor, and D. T. Haydon. (2001). Population biology of multihost pathogens. *Science* **292**:1109–1112.

Woolhouse, M. E. J. (2002). Population biology of emerging and re-emerging pathogens. *Trends in Microbiology* **10** (Suppl.):S3–S7.

CHAPTER 3

Community ecology meets epidemiology: the case of Lyme disease

Richard S. Ostfeld, Felicia Keesing, and Kathleen LoGiudice

3.1 Background

Any vector-borne zoonotic disease involves *at least* four species: the human victim, the pathogen, the vector, and the wildlife reservoir. Typically, though, the pathogen (usually viral or bacterial) can infect multiple species of wildlife hosts, and the vector (usually an arthropod) can feed from many wildlife species in addition to the human and wildlife reservoir. In addition, population density of the reservoir (usually a mammal or bird) and vector might be controlled or regulated by natural enemies or resources. To fully understand disease risk, scientists therefore might need to study interactions among a formidable number of species, and potentially between each species and its abiotic environment. Thus, although epidemiology appears to have primacy as the science devoted to analysis of variation in human disease risk and incidence, a key role for community ecology also seems fundamental.

The crucial importance of community ecology in understanding disease risk is best explored by considering a particular disease system whose ecological components are relatively well understood. Lyme disease (LD) is a tick-borne zoonosis caused by the bacterium *Borrelia burgdorferi*. LD was first described in the mid-1970s in the US state of Connecticut, but it is now known from Eurasia, Africa, and Australia in addition to North America (Barbour and Fish 1993). In some temperate regions, LD is the most commonly reported vector-borne disease (CDC 2003). Ticks in the *Ixodes ricinus* complex are the primary vectors; in the United States, the most important vector is the blacklegged tick, *I. scapularis*. In the enzootic cycle, *B. burgdorferi*

is reciprocally transmitted between ticks and wildlife reservoir hosts; LD exists because humans can serve as hosts for both the tick and the pathogen and thus can become an accidental part of this cycle. The *Ixodes* tick life cycle includes four stages: egg, larva, nymph, and adult. Larvae, nymphs, and adults each take a single blood meal, lasting from several days to a week, from a vertebrate host before dropping off and molting into the next stage (in the case of larvae and nymphs) or before reproducing and dying (in the case of adults). Larvae and nymphs are highly generalized in their choice of hosts and are known to parasitize dozens of species of mammals, birds, and lizards. Adults tend to be restricted to larger mammals, particularly white-tailed deer, *Odocoileus virginianus*. Two years are required for the life cycle to be completed (Barbour and Fish 1993; Ostfeld 1997).

3.2 Vertebrate communities and Lyme-disease risk

Larval ticks, which hatch from eggs uninfected, can acquire a *B. burgdorferi* infection if they feed on an infected vertebrate host. Those that acquire infection during the larval meal then molt into infected nymphs capable of transmitting the disease agent during the nymphal blood meal. The probability that a larval tick will become infected during its larval blood meal is largely a function of the species of host on which it feeds. The white-footed mouse, *Peromyscus leucopus*, is considered the principal natural reservoir for *B. burgdorferi* infection in North America; recent research shows that 92% of larvae feeding from free-ranging white-footed mice acquire infection and molt into infected nymphs (LoGiudice *et al.* 2003). A few other competent reservoirs exist, principally eastern chipmunks (*Tamias striatus*) and short-tailed shrews (*Blarina brevicauda*), but most vertebrate species have low capacity to infect feeding ticks.

Most cases of LD are transmitted by nymphs. Nymphs are tiny and therefore hard to detect and they have a potentially high probability of being infected with *B. burgdorferi*. Nymphs are also active in summer, which increases their contact rates with humans. Adult ticks have an even higher probability of being infected, but are much more conspicuous and are most active in mid-to-late autumn when encounters with humans are less likely. Nymphal infection prevalence (NIP), the proportion of host-seeking nymphs infected with the disease agent, is considered an important measure of human risk of exposure to LD (Ostfeld *et al.* 2001; LoGiudice *et al.* 2003), because it reflects the probability that a tick bite will result in a case of LD. In the United States, LD incidence is high in the northeastern and upper midwestern regions. In this "hyperendemic" zone, NIP tends to be above 15%. In contrast, LD incidence is quite low despite abundant populations of blacklegged ticks in southeastern and lower midwestern states, where NIP tends to be <5% (Ostfeld and LoGiudice 2003). Therefore, NIP would appear to be an epidemiologically relevant measure of disease risk at both small and large scales.

Nymphal infection prevalence is determined by the distribution of larval meals among members of the vertebrate community, which differ strongly in reservoir competence—the probability that they will infect ticks that feed on them. A vertebrate community dominated by highly competent reservoirs should produce a nymphal cohort having high NIP, whereas a community with many incompetent reservoirs should produce lower NIP. Natural variation in species composition within the community of hosts from which ticks feed, which is essentially the entire community of grounddwelling mammals, birds, and lizards, should be accompanied by variation in NIP. As vertebrate species composition changes due to anthropogenic or natural causes, it might be possible to predict the consequent changes in disease risk.

3.3 Modeling community disassembly

Habitat destruction, fragmentation, and conversion are responsible for changing both diversity and species composition of vertebrate communities worldwide (Hilton-Taylor 2000). Frequently, species diversity declines and species composition shifts towards domination by species most resistant to, or even favored by, these habitat changes. Therefore, a strong potential exists for habitat fragmentation to influence risk of human exposure to LD via its impacts on both diversity and species composition within the community of grounddwelling terrestrial vertebrates. To predict how habitat loss and fragmentation will change LD risk, precise knowledge of three factors is essential: (1) what functional role is played by each potentially important host species in contributing to overall NIP; (2) which species are most likely to be lost from (or severely reduced within) remaining tick habitat as the landscape is fragmented; and (3) how the loss of species changes the abundance or functional role of the remaining species. We address each of these fundamental issues next.

3.3.1 Species-specific contributions to NIP

Nymphal infection prevalence in any given year is equal to the proportion of the prior year's larval cohort that acquired infection, adjusted by any difference in survival (from fed larva to questing nymph) between infected and uninfected ticks. Because no evidence suggests that infection with *B. burgdorferi* reduces survival probability of larval *I. scapularis*, NIP can be considered equivalent to the proportion of larvae acquiring infection in the previous year. Within endemic zones for LD, virtually every terrestrial mammal and ground-dwelling bird species acts as a host for larval *I. scapularis*. These species vary strongly, however, in the fraction of the larval cohort they feed and in the fraction of feeding larvae they infect. To account for speciesspecific contributions to overall NIP, LoGiudice *et al.* (2003; see also Ostfeld and LoGiudice 2003) constructed a simple model with the following parameters: Density (number ha^{-1}) of host species $i = N_i$; species-specific body burdens (mean larval ticks host^{-1}) $= B_i$; and species-specific reservoir competence (proportion of larvae acquiring infection) = C_i. Therefore, $m_i = N_i\, B_i$, where m_i is the number of larval meals taken from species i, and $I_i = m_i\, C_i$, where I_i is the number of nymphs infected from their larval meal on species i; and the total number of nymphs infected from their larval meal is $I_T = \sum m_i\, C_i$. The number of nymphs not infected in their larval meal on species i is given by $U_i = m_i \times (1 - C_i)$, and the total number of nymphs not infected is $U_T = \sum m_i (1 - C_i)$. Thus, the total nymphal infection prevalence is $\text{NIP}_T = I_T / (I_T + U_T)$.

To validate this model, LoGiudice *et al.* (2003) exhaustively live-captured mammals and birds within a hyperendemic zone for LD in Dutchess County, New York State (US), and directly estimated N_i, B_i, and C_i. For some species, estimates of N_i had to be drawn from published studies conducted in similar oak-mixed hardwood habitats. Because long-term studies of white-footed mice and eastern chipmunks reveal dramatic inter-annual variation in population density (Ostfeld

et al. 1996; 2001; Schmidt and Ostfeld 2001), LoGiudice *et al.* (2003) allowed N_i values for these species to vary within the bounds of observed variation. The model provided predicted values of NIP for a fully intact host community with varying densities of mice and chipmunks (Fig. 3.1). Empirical data on NIP as a function of the previous year's rodent density closely matches the model's predictions (Fig. 3.1), which suggests that: (1) important hosts for ticks were not missed in the field sampling; (2) estimates of parameter values for each host species are reasonably accurate; and (3) a combination of high species richness and low mouse density reduces NIP and therefore LD risk.

3.3.2 Species loss with habitat fragmentation

Habitat fragmentation and destruction are considered the primary causes of declines in abundance and local extirpation of many species (e.g. Hilton-Taylor 2000). However, some species appear relatively insensitive to habitat fragmentation and others clearly benefit. Intrinsic traits of species that influence their sensitivity to habitat fragmentation are known in only a few cases (e.g. Kirkland and Ostfeld 1999; Davies *et al.* 2000; Crooks 2002; Pereira *et al.* 2004), and the importance of these traits appears to vary taxonomically and geographically. At present, for mammals and birds in the northeastern United States (within the LD hyperendemic zone), little is known concerning either which species are most vulnerable to habitat fragmentation or which intrinsic traits most strongly influence vulnerability.

In contrast, intensive study of the mammalian fauna in agricultural landscapes of the midwestern United States, suggests that: (1) species richness declines log-linearly with decreasing forest fragment size (i.e. there is a strong species–area relationship; Rosenblatt *et al.* 1999); (2) carnivorous and some granivorous species occur only in relatively large fragments (Rosenblatt *et al.* 1999); and (3) white-footed mice occur in fragments of all sizes, but their density is highest in the smallest forest patches (Nupp and Swihart 1996, 2000; Krohne and Hoch 1999).

Whether responses to habitat fragmentation are idiosyncratic or predictable on the basis of

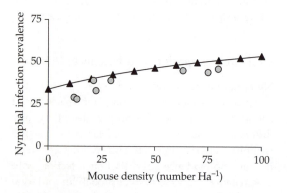

Figure 3.1 Change in LD risk, as measured by nymphal infection prevalence (NIP=percentage of nymphs infected with *B. burgdorferi*) with changing density of white-footed mice. Dark triangles and line represent model predictions based on a complete host community consisting of ca. 12 species of mammals and 4 species of birds, with each species except mice fixed at their long-term average densities. Less diverse communities show higher values of NIP at all mouse densities (LoGiudice *et al.* 2003). Gray circles represent empirical values of NIP in year t and mouse density in year $t-1$ averaged over three 2.25-ha forest plots on which ticks and small mammals have been monitored for the past 10 years (updated from LoGiudice *et al.* 2003). The good fit between predicted and observed NIP as mouse density varies suggests relatively complete accounting of host species, an appropriate model, and accurate parameter values (empirically determined) of host abundance, tick burdens, and reservoir competence.

species-specific traits is unknown. Assessing the importance of species-specific traits, such as body size, trophic level, degree of trophic, or habitat specialization, dispersal ability, intrinsic rate of increase, variability in population size, etc., is fraught with difficulties. A key obstacle is the covariation in many of these traits within and among species (Davies *et al.* 2000). For instance, large-bodied animals typically have low intrinsic rates of increase and need extensive habitat areas (which would increase their vulnerability to extirpation with habitat fragmentation), but also tend to be highly mobile and have relatively constant population densities (which would decrease vulnerability to fragmentation-caused extirpation). Consequently, no strong empirical basis exists for posing "disassembly rules" (Ostfeld and LoGiudice 2003) for the mammalian and avian faunas in fragmented forest landscapes of the northeastern United States.

Our strategy, therefore, is to pose a plausible set of disassembly rules, and ask whether different rules result in different predictions concerning the way that LD risk changes with changing species richness and composition (Ostfeld and LoGiudice 2003). Our rules allow us to construct virtual communities with different richness levels and species composition, and our model (see Section 3.3.1) allows us to predict the value of NIP that arises from each community. We next describe a set of plausible rules for community disassembly and assess their consequences for NIP by applying each rule to determine the sequence of species lost from a fully intact community.

Nihilism

For the nihilism "rule" (actually, an anti-rule), species respond entirely idiosyncratically to habitat fragmentation, such that no intrinsic trait is a good predictor. This rule is simulated by selecting species for removal entirely at random. Note that this is the rule often used for assessing the impact of species diversity on ecosystem functions in experimental field or microcosm approaches (Loreau *et al.* 2001; Tilman *et al.* 1997).

Quasi-nihilism

For this rule, we rely on strong empirical evidence that white-footed mice do not decline or disappear

from small forest fragments (reviewed above). We assume that mice are present in all communities, but randomly select all other species for removal.

Body size/home-range size

Here we assume that larger-bodied (higher mass) species are most sensitive to habitat fragmentation, owing to the scaling of habitat size to body size. Because home-range size scales with body size for the mammals of northeastern United States (Ostfeld and LoGiudice 2003), rules involving body size and home range are equivalent. For this and the remaining disassembly rules, we assume that white-footed mice and white-tailed deer are necessary for the tick life cycle to be completed, and therefore are present in all communities.

Trophic level

For this rule, we assume that the most carnivorous species are most sensitive to habitat fragmentation, owing to their need for greater habitat area to meet dietary requirements (Pimm and Lawton 1977; Holt 1996). Herbivores and omnivores are expected to be least sensitive, and insectivores of intermediate sensitivity.

Midwestern United States

For this "rule" we simply apply empirical observations by Rosenblatt *et al.* (1999) and Nupp and Swihart (2000) regarding the sequence of mammalian species loss with decreasing habitat area in the midwestern United States. A few species found at our sites are not included in the communities studied in the Midwest; for those species, we apply the trophic level rule.

The consequences of applying different disassembly rules to changes in NIP are dramatic (Figs 3.2 and 3.3). Under the Nihilism "rule," declining species richness results in declining NIP because the probability of mice being included in the community is reduced as richness becomes lower. In contrast, including mice in all communities under the Quasi-nihilism "rule" causes NIP to soar with declining richness as larger and larger proportions of the larval cohort feed on mice (Fig. 3.2). NIP is constrained between ca. 40% at

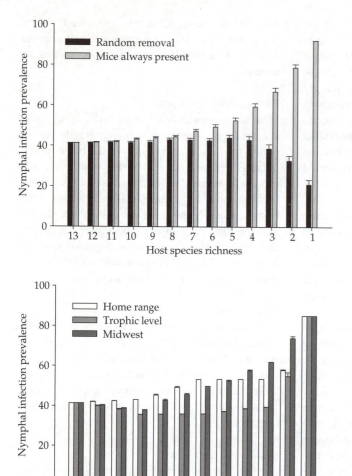

Figure 3.2 Results of a simulation model in which nymphal infection prevalence (defined in Fig. 3.1) changes as species richness in the host community varies. Two community disassembly rules are represented: the nihilism "rule," in which species are removed in random sequence; and the quasi-nihilism rule, in which mice are assumed to be present in all communities and all other species are removed in random sequence. Bars represent means with standard errors from 100 simulations at each level of species richness. See Ostfeld and LoGiudice (2003) for more details. Redrawn and updated from Ostfeld and LoGiudice (2003).

Figure 3.3 Results of a simulation model in which nymphal infection prevalence (defined in Fig. 3.1) changes under three nonrandom disassembly rules: the body size/home-range size rule, in which species with larger bodies/home ranges are lost first; the trophic level rule, in which the most carnivorous species are lost first; and the Midwest "rule," in which species are lost in roughly the order observed in fragmented landscapes in midwestern United States (see text).

maximal species richness and ca. 85% when only white-footed mice and white-tailed deer remain (Fig. 3.3). Nevertheless, at intermediate levels of species richness, different disassembly rules create different patterns of change in NIP. For example, under the home-range rule, species loss from 13 to 7 elicits a gradual increase in NIP, followed by a plateau until the final two species are lost at which point NIP soars (Fig. 3.3). The Midwest "rule" gives rise to a more gradual increase in NIP throughout the entire range of species loss. In marked contrast, the trophic level rule results in a *decrease* in NIP from high to intermediate levels of species richness. Only when the final two species are lost does NIP skyrocket to the maximal level.

Differences among the disassembly rules in the relationship between species richness and NIP are affected both by the species lost and by the composition of the remaining community. In other words, whether the loss of a particular species results in an increase or decrease in NIP, and the magnitude of that effect, depends on the aggregate effects of the remaining species on NIP. To exemplify this concept, first consider a high-diversity community that consequently has a low NIP. If shrews (*Sorex* and *Blarina* spp.) are lost from this community, the result will be a decrease in NIP, because shrews have a moderately high reservoir competence and feed a large number of larval ticks (Fig. 3.4). This early loss of shrews under the

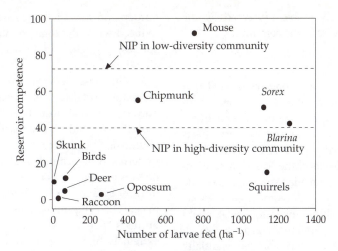

Figure 3.4 Position of host species in phase space, defined as the combination of realized reservoir competence (measured proportion of larvae that acquire infection through feeding from a particular host species; Schauber and Ostfeld 2002) and number of larvae fed by that host species per hectare. The "Reservoir competence" axis can be viewed as a measure of the direction of species-specific effects on total NIP, and the "number of larvae fed" axis can be viewed to represent the magnitude of species-specific effects on total NIP. In a fully intact community at our field sites, NIP values range between 35% and 40% (lower dashed line), whereas in species-poor communities, NIP is much higher (upper dashed line, see Allan et al. 2003). In a species-poor community, with high NIP, loss of species such as *Sorex* and *Blarina* shrews and chipmunks would have the effect of increasing NIP even further. But in a species-rich community, with lower NIP, loss of these same species would reduce NIP even further. This situation illustrates the contingent nature of the net effects of species loss on this particular ecosystem function.

trophic level rule appears responsible for the general reduction in NIP with species loss at high and intermediate levels of species richness (Fig. 3.3). However, if shrews are lost from a low-diversity community that has a high NIP, the effect is to strongly elevate NIP even further. This effect of shrews is responsible for the patterns arising from the home-range and Midwest rules.

Host species can be arrayed in a phase diagram with the x-axis representing the total number of larvae fed by that species, and the y-axis representing reservoir competence (Fig. 3.4). Whether NIP increases or decreases following loss of species X depends on whether the reservoir competence of species X is below or above the NIP value for the current community (Fig. 3.4). This example illustrates a concept increasingly recognized by community ecologists—that species-specific functional roles can depend on the composition of the remaining community. It also reinforces the importance of knowing the sequence with which species are lost as habitat is degraded, in order to predict the consequences for ecosystem functioning (Wardle et al. 1999; Schwartz et al 2000; Ostfeld and LoGiudice 2003).

3.3.3 Impact of species loss on abundance or functional role of remaining species

So far, we have assumed that all host species interact only with ticks directly and not with one another, an assumption that is quite likely to be false. Many of the species in these host communities are likely to interact directly via predator–prey or competitive relationships. Moreover, indirect effects of each species on other members of the community could occur via trophic webs or "competition" for ticks.

Recall that species-specific effects on NIP are determined by population density, average tick burden per individual, and reservoir competence. Despite the convenient assumption that each of these parameters can be treated as a species-specific constant, we have every reason to expect that each parameter is influenced by the composition of the remaining community. Unfortunately, for lack of data, we cannot incorporate the net effect of each species on parameter values for all other species into our models. Nevertheless, it seems useful to describe qualitatively how the population density, mean tick burdens, and reservoir competence of a focal species are likely to be influenced by the presence of other species in the community.

Population density

Community ecologists have long recognized that species influence one another's abundance both through direct effects (predator–prey, competitive, and mutualistic interactions) and indirect effects mediated by third parties (reviewed by Pimm 1991; Lawton 2000). For instance, the loss of a carnivorous or omnivorous mammalian species (e.g. skunk, raccoon) that preys on omnivorous/granivorous rodents (e.g. mice, chipmunks, squirrels) could result in enhanced population growth of all rodent species. Or, if the carnivore preferentially fed on one of the species (e.g. mice), then the loss of the carnivore species may elicit disproportionate increases in population growth of mice, which may then suppress populations of the sciurid rodents with which they compete. The observed correlation between carnivore loss and increased abundance of white-footed mice in fragmented landscapes in Indiana and Illinois (Nupp and Swihart 1996, 2000; Krohne and Hoch 1998; Rosenblatt et al. 1999) suggests a direct trophic interaction, but the evidence is weak. To our knowledge, the existence of indirect interactions, such as apparent competition, between mice and sciurid rodents in these or similar landscapes has not been assessed. It might be necessary to construct interaction webs in which all pairwise interactions are quantified in order to predict net effect of species loss on abundance of the remaining species.

Average tick burdens

Ticks are weakly mobile and move at most a few meters by crawling, relying on vertebrate hosts for longer-distance movements. As such, their ability to actively pursue and select hosts is quite limited, and their host-finding strategy is largely sit-and-wait. The active host-seeking season for each tick stadium (larval, nymph, or adult stage) extends for only a few months (Fish 1993; Ostfeld et al. 1996a). The number of available, host-seeking ticks should be "depleted" rapidly when encounter rates with hosts are high, but might decline slowly when encounter rates are low. It follows that average tick

burdens on any given species of host should be reduced when the total abundance of hosts (of all species) is high, and increased when total host abundance is low.

Nevertheless, effects of the abundance of alternate hosts (or all hosts) on average tick burdens on focal hosts have been neglected until recently. A study of impacts of alternate host abundance on focal-host tick burdens was undertaken by Schmidt et al. (1999), who assessed how varying density of eastern chipmunks influenced average tick burdens on white-footed mice. When chipmunk density was low, larval tick burdens per mouse were variable and often extremely high, whereas when chipmunk density was high, larval burdens on mice were lower and less variable (Fig. 3.5). This relationship supports the contention that host-seeking ticks can be depleted by increasing availability of hosts, and that this can reduce tick burdens on individual host species. The data in Fig. 3.5 also support the assertion that average larval burdens on host species might be determined as much by host community composition as by species-specific characteristics.

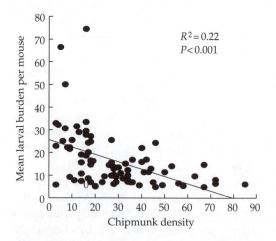

Figure 3.5 Effects of variation in the population density of chipmunks (number per 2.25-ha plot) and average larval tick burdens on the white-footed mice on that plot. Each data point represents a different plot-year covering our sites of long-term monitoring of rodents and ticks at the Institute for Ecosystem Studies in Millbrook, New York. The relationship demonstrates the strong potential for changes in the abundance of one host (in this case, chipmunks) to affect encounter rates between ticks and a focal host (white-footed mice).

Reservoir competence

Reservoir competence for any vector-borne pathogen is typically measured by determining the probability that an infected host will transmit an infection to a feeding vector. Generally, reservoir competence is high when the immune response by the host to the pathogen is insufficient to prevent high concentrations of pathogens in blood or other tissues, resulting in the acquisition of pathogens by the vector during its blood meal. For many host species, however, reservoir competence initially increases following the infection event (during the pathogen dissemination phase) and then declines as the immune system removes pathogens. Schauber and Ostfeld (2002) termed the latter "reservoir competence decay." In the case of LD, and probably for many other zoonoses, hosts become repeatedly inoculated during vector meals, and each new inoculation results in a temporary increase in reservoir competence as pathogen levels circulating in the host increase (reviewed in Schauber and Ostfeld 2002). Therefore, true reservoir competence values for a given host change dynamically with the rate of inoculation, and published values for particular host species almost certainly represent averages that hide these dynamics.

Schauber and Ostfeld (2002) found that, even if the shape of reservoir competence decay is a species-specific trait, the "realized" reservoir competence—which is the probability that a blood meal taken by a vector from a host under field conditions will result in infection of the vector—depends strongly on the composition of the host community. If the community is dominated by highly competent reservoirs (e.g. mice), then the infection prevalence in the tick population should be high. As a result, the inoculation rate of all hosts should be high, and hosts' realized reservoir competence should remain near the maximum of the competence decay curve. On the other hand, if the host community is dominated by incompetent reservoirs, tick infection prevalence should be lower, resulting in lower inoculation rates and realized reservoir competence values that are closer to their minimum under decay.

In conclusion, all three key parameters that determine any individual species' contribution to NIP are quite likely to be influenced by the presence and abundance of other species in the host community. Therefore, considering them to be species-specific traits, as we have done in our modeling, probably oversimplifies the LD system considerably. Determining the net effect of changes in species composition on population density, average tick burdens, and reservoir competence of all host species, however, is a major logistical and conceptual challenge. We suggest that a combination of experimental, modeling, and comparative studies will allow investigators to approach this important issue (Box 3.1).

Box 3.1 Approaches for assessing the role of indirect interactions in disease dynamics

Most studies of disease dynamics have focused on a relatively small set of species directly involved in transmission. Most studies of malaria, for example, have emphasized monitoring abundances of reservoir hosts and mosquito vectors, and determining the prevalence of the *Plasmodium* parasite in these animals. Once the appropriate values are obtained from these observations, they are used to model transmission dynamics.

If disease systems are seen as embedded within ecological communities, however, then studying them also requires investigating species and interactions only *indirectly* involved in disease transmission. For example, investigators interested in the abundance of different malaria vectors might consider bottom-up controls of vegetation on mosquito recruitment (for an example, see Chapter 7, this volume). In the context of LD, we might consider potential

top-down and bottom-up controls on the abundance of competent hosts. In eastern North America, white-footed mice (*P. leucopus*) were known to be the most competent reservoir for the bacterial agent of LD (*B. burgdorferi*), as early as 1984 (Anderson and Magnarelli 1984; Levine *et al.* 1985). But what regulated mouse populations was not understood until long-term monitoring showed correlations between mouse abundance and pulses of acorn production (mast) by oak trees (Elkinton *et al.* 1996; Ostfeld *et al.* 1996b; Wolff 1996). To determine if acorn production *caused* high mouse abundance, Jones *et al.* (1998) conducted a large-scale field experiment in which they added almost a million acorns to experimental plots. This experimental pulse of acorn production caused significant increases in mouse densities the following year (Jones *et al.* 1998).

continues

Box 3.1 *continued*

Sometimes, though, field experiments of the dynamics of complex communities are not possible. For example, LoGiudice *et al.* (2003) were interested in the individual roles played by each host species in infecting ticks with the Lyme bacterium. Removing each host species from large plots of forest was infeasible. However, through extensive fieldwork and literature reviews, they estimated the densities of each host species, and then estimated their tick burdens and reservoir competencies directly. (Reservoir competence was measured by bringing field-caught animals into the laboratory and placing them in cages suspended over pans of water. Embedded ticks dropped off after feeding and were collected from pans. Ticks were allowed to molt and were tested for *B. burgdorferi* using a direct immunofluoresence assay. For details, see Ostfeld *et al.* 2001). With these data, they built a simple model that accounted for each species' contribution to the proportion of ticks infected with the Lyme bacterium. They tested the model by comparing the proportion of ticks the model predicted would be infected with the proportion of ticks that actually were infected in their forest plots. With close agreement between these values, Ostfeld and LoGiudice (2003) used the model to simulate the removal of individual host species and the effect of these removals on tick infection.

Laboratory experiments can also be useful for understanding complex ecological interactions that are impractical or impossible to study in the field. Shaw *et al.* (2003) were interested in why field-caught white-footed mice were infested with on average twice as many larval

ticks as were eastern chipmunks (*T. striatus)*. In a carefully controlled laboratory experiment, they tested two alternative explanations for this effect. They found that ticks oriented towards white-footed mice twice as often as they oriented towards eastern chipmunks (*T. striatus*), but that mice partially counterbalanced this attraction by being more efficient groomers than chipmunks were.

This careful integration of monitoring, experimentation, and modeling has its limitations for elucidating the epidemiological consequences of species interactions in complex ecological communities. LoGiudice *et al.* (2003) sought to make their model for estimating tick infection more realistic by allowing the removal of a particular host species to affect parameter values for other species. For example, what would be the net effect of removing eastern chipmunks from a forest community if this removal increased tick burdens on white-footed mice, or increased mouse density by reducing competition, or reduced mouse density by increasing predation pressure on mice? Unfortunately, LoGiudice *et al.* (2003) were unable to adapt their model in this way because they found that there were simply no field data to use to parameterize such a model, nor could they develop a realistic field protocol to gather these data themselves. Developing mathematical and experimental or comparative techniques for grappling with complex ecological systems is the greatest challenge for the future of disease ecology; it is also the greatest challenge for other disciplines that investigate the behavior of intricate networks of interactions.

3.4 Discussion

Epidemiology is the scientific discipline devoted to understanding the incidence, distribution, and control of disease in a population. For infectious diseases, the simplest disease system is one with a single species each of pathogen and host, and a highly specialized relationship between the two. Under these conditions, the importance of community ecology to epidemiology might be limited to: (1) the reciprocal roles of the host and pathogen in regulating each other; and (2) the roles played by various other (non-host, non-pathogen) species in controlling abundance of the host species (Keesing *et al.*, in review, Box 3.2; see also Holt and

Dobson, Chapter 2, this volume). However, when the pathogen can infect more than one species of host (the situation for all zoonoses), community ecology becomes even more fundamental, because species composition and interspecific interactions can influence abundance of all host species and contact rates between each host and the pathogen. Finally, vector-borne diseases increase the importance of community ecology even further by adding vector-host and vector-pathogen interactions to the mix.

We have focused on the LD system because of its epidemiological importance and relevance as a model of other vector-borne zoonoses. The LD system involves several key features that are

Box 3.2 What causes the "dilution effect" in disease systems?

In several recent studies, vertebrate communities composed of a diversity of host species have been found to pose lower LD risk than communities composed of few host species. This phenomenon, termed the "dilution effect" (Ostfeld and Keesing 2000a), may occur in a number of vector-borne disease systems (Ostfeld and Keesing 2000b). Despite the potential generality of this effect, however, there is confusion about the mechanisms underlying its occurrence. Keesing et al. (in review) argue that dilution is in fact the net effect of a suite of potential mechanisms, and that these mechanisms may operate in both vector-borne and non-vector-borne disease systems.

The mechanisms through which dilution could occur can be elucidated by examination of a model of a simple disease system. Imagine a system in which a microparasite is specialized on a single host species, and is passed from host to host through direct contact. The dynamics of the host population can be described by a susceptible-infected (SI) model (after Anderson and May 1978):

$$\frac{dS}{dt} = (b-m)S - \alpha \delta SI + (\gamma + b')I \qquad (3.1)$$

$$\frac{dI}{dt} = \alpha \delta SI - (\gamma + m')I \qquad (3.2)$$

where b and b' are the birth rates of susceptible and infected individuals, respectively, and m and m' are their respective death rates. Susceptible individuals become infected based on a rate of encounter with infected individuals, α, and a probability of transmission given an encounter, δ. Infected individuals recover at a rate γ to become susceptible again.

One measure of disease risk in this system is the rate of change in the density of infected individuals, dI/dt (Equation (3.2)). If the host species is already present in the focal community, the addition of a non-host species could result in declining disease risk if the presence of that species:

- decreased encounter rates between susceptible and infected individuals (α)—"encounter dilution";
- decreased rates of transmission given an encounter (δ)—"transmission dilution";
- decreased the abundance of susceptible individuals (S)—"susceptible host regulation";
- increased the rate of recovery of infected individuals (γ)—"recovery dilution"; or
- increased the rate of mortality of infected individuals (m')—"infected host mortality".

The first of these modes of dilution, encounter dilution, could occur if an added species (e.g. a predator) affected space use of the host in a way that reduced its rate of contact with other hosts. The third mode, susceptible host regulation, could occur if a non-host species added to this system were a predator or competitor of the host. Examples of this type of regulation abound.

Now we consider more complex systems in which multiple host species can be infected with the pathogen. We identify the host species with the highest probability of transmission (δ) as the most competent reservoir (MCR). In this system, disease risk is a function of the total density of infected hosts, including the MCR and other host species. We begin with a focal community initially containing the MCR. Adding a non-host species to this community could lead to dilution through any of our original five modes; these would decrease the density of infected MCR individuals. Because of our measure of risk, however, adding a host species would only increase disease risk, unless its addition resulted in a concomitant reduction in the density of infected MCR individuals through one of our five original modes. With a vector-borne disease system, such as LD, we introduce one additional mode of dilution, vector regulation, which occurs when the addition of a species regulates the abundance of the vector.

In the LD system, many of these modes appear to operate simultaneously. In diverse communities in the northeastern United States, predators and competitors of white-footed mice (P. leucopus), the MCR, might regulate its abundance, decreasing disease risk through "susceptible host regulation" and "infected host mortality" (Rosenblatt et al. 1999; Nupp and Swihart 1996, 2000; Allan et al. 2003). These same species serve as hosts for ticks, and thus may also decrease contact rates between infected ticks and uninfected mice (see Fig. 3.5), a form of "encounter dilution." Immature ticks that attempt to feed on non-mouse hosts tend to be less likely to survive than are ticks that feed on mice (Wilson et al. 1990; Craig et al. 1996; Ostfeld and Lewis 1999), a type of "vector regulation." And "transmission dilution" occurs when the presence of alternate species increases the average reservoir competence decay (sensu Schauber and Ostfeld 2002; see main text), resulting in a lower average rate of transmission.

Whether the dilution effect occurs in a given disease system is determined by the net effect of this suite of mechanisms operating simultaneously. Of course, these modes can in principle operate in reverse, such that adding species to a disease system could increase disease risk through an "amplification effect." Only further studies of the community ecology of a diversity of disease systems will reveal the frequency of these patterns.

characteristic of many other vector-borne disease systems: reliance by the pathogen on acquisition by vectors from hosts (rather than purely vertical transmission), a generalist vector that parasitizes many host species, and strong variation among host species in average reservoir competence (Ostfeld and Keesing 2000a). These characteristics suggest that disease risk to humans, which is affected by both the proportion of vectors infected with the pathogen and the abundance of infected vectors, will be influenced by host community composition. In the LD system, the most competent reservoir (white-footed mouse) is also ubiquitous, abundant, and insensitive to human disturbance of natural habitats. Consequently, as host diversity is eroded, the impact of white-footed mice increases and so does risk of human exposure to the pathogen. Conversely, high diversity in the vertebrate host community will provide a strong "dilution effect" (Ostfeld and Keesing 2000a), which protects humans from disease risk.

However, prior empirical and modeling approaches to studying the effect of species diversity and composition on LD risk have largely been limited to determining the individual roles played by each species in feeding and infecting ticks, and then assessing how species presence or absence affects tick infection prevalence or abundance. We have argued that such an approach provides a good beginning, but is limited by the likely possibility that species-specific effects are not fixed, but rather are strongly influenced by the composition of the remaining host community. Our empirically based simulation models suggest that knowing the relative sensitivities of various host species to habitat loss and degradation can be important in predicting consequences for human health. But the results also suggest that basic knowledge of the community ecology of familiar host species is insufficient for making quantitative predictions. The next key step will be to determine how the presence/absence of species influences the abundance, tick burden, and reservoir competence of the remaining species.

Zoonotic disease systems involve a network of interacting species directly involved in disease transmission, and understanding the complexity of interactions among these species is crucial for understanding disease risk. But disease systems also involve a larger network of species that play *indirect* but potentially critical roles in determining disease risk (see Box 3.1). In the LD system in eastern North America, oak trees (*Quercus* species) determine much of the interannual variation in LD risk, despite the fact that they are not directly involved as hosts for either the pathogen or the vector of this disease. Instead, because they produce occasional hyperabundant crops of nutritious acorns (mast), oaks indirectly affect LD risk by influencing the abundance of key hosts for the pathogen, including the white-footed mouse (Ostfeld *et al.* 1996b; Jones *et al.* 1998). Clearly, the concepts, approaches, and tools of community ecology are fundamental to the epidemiology of zoonotic disease.

Acknowledgments

This work was supported by a grant from NIH to RO, FK, and KL, by a grant from NSF to RO, and by a grant from NSF (CAREER) to FK. The authors thank Bob Holt for his partnership in developing ideas about modes of dilution. This is a contribution to the program of the Institute of Ecosystem Studies.

References

Allan, B. F., F. Keesing, and R. S. Ostfeld. (2003). Effects of habitat fragmentation on Lyme disease risk. *Conservation Biology* **17**:267–272.

Anderson, J. F. and L. A. Magnarelli. (1984). Avian and mammalian hosts for spirochete-infected ticks and insects in a Lyme disease focus in Connecticut. *Yale Journal of Biology and Medicine* **57**:627–641.

Anderson, R. M. and R. M. May. (1978). Regulation and stability of host-parasite population interactions. I. Regulatory processes. *Journal of Animal Ecology* **47**: 219–247.

Barbour, A. G. and D. Fish. (1993). The biological and social phenomenon of Lyme disease. *Science* **260**: 1610–1616.

Centers for Disease Control and Prevention. (2003). *Morbidity and Mortality Weekly Report* **51**:1169.

Craig, L. E., D. E. Norris, M. L. Sanders, G. E. Glass, and B. S. Schwartz. (1996). Acquired resistance and antibody response of raccoons (*Procyon lotor*) to sequential feedings of *Ixodes scapularis* (Acari: Ixodidae). *Veterinary Parasitology* **63**:291–301.

Crooks, K. R. (2002). Relative sensitivities of mammalian carnivores to habitat fragmentation. *Conservation Biology* **16**:488–502.

Davies, K. E., C. R. Margules, and J. E. Lawrence. (2000). Which traits of species predict population declines in experimental forest fragments? *Ecology* **81**:1450–1461.

Elkinton, J. S., W. M. Healy, J. P. Buonaccorsi, A. M. Hazzard, *et al.* (1996). Interactions among gypsy moths, white-footed mice, and acorns. *Ecology* **77**:2332–2342.

Fish, D. (1993). Population ecology of *Ixodes dammini*. In H. S. Ginsberg, ed. *Ecology and Environmental Management of Lyme Disease*, pp. 25–42. Rutgers University Press, New Brunswick, NJ.

Hilton-Taylor, C. (2000). *IUCN Red List of Threatened Species*. International Union for the Conservation of Nature. Gland, Switzerland.

Holt, R. D. (1977). Predation, apparent competition, and the structure of prey communities. *Theoretical Population Biology* **12**:197–229.

Holt, R. D. (1996). Food webs in space: an island biogeographic perspective. In G. A. Polis and K. O. Winemiller, eds. *Food Webs: Integration of Patterns and Dynamics*, pp. 313–323. Chapman and Hall, New York.

Keesing, F., R. D. Holt, and R. S. Ostfeld. In review. Effects of species diversity on disease risk.

Kirkland, G. L., Jr. and R. S. Ostfeld. (1999). Factors influencing variation among states in the number of federally listed and candidate mammals in the United States. *Journal of Mammalogy* **80**:711–719.

Krohne, D. T. and G. A. Hoch. (1999). Demography of *Peromyscus leucopus* populations on habitat patches: the role of dispersal. *Canadian Journal of Zoology* **77**:1247–1253.

Jones, C. G., R. S. Ostfeld, E. M. Schauber, M. Richard, and J. O. Wolff. (1998). Chain reactions linking acorns to gypsy moth outbreaks and Lyme-disease risk. *Science* **279**:1023–1026.

Lawton, J. H. (2000). *Community Ecology in a Changing World*. Ecology Institute, Oldendorf/Luhe Germany.

Levine, J. R., M. W. Wilson, and A. Speilman. (1985). Mice as reservoirs of the Lyme disease spirochete. *American Journal of Tropical Medicine and Hygiene* **34**:355–360.

LoGiudice, K., R. S. Ostfeld, K. A. Schmidt, and F. Keesing. (2003). The ecology of infectious disease: effects of host diversity and community composition on Lyme disease risk. *Proceedings of the National Academy of Sciences* **100**:567–571.

Loreau, M., S. Naeem, P. Inchausti, J. Bengtsson, J. P. Grime, A. Hector, *et al.* (2001). Biodiversity and ecosystem functioning: current knowledge and future challenges. *Science* **294**:804–808.

Nupp, T. E. and R. K. Swihart. (1996). Effect of forest patch area on population attributes of white-footed mice (*Peromyscus leucopus*) in fragmented landscapes. *Canadian Journal of Zoology* **74**:467–472.

Nupp, T. E. and R. K. Swihart. (2000). Landscape-level correlates of small-mammal assemblages in forest fragments of farmland. *Journal of Mammalogy* **81**:512–526.

Ostfeld, R. S. (1997). The ecology of Lyme disease risk. *American Scientist* **85**:338–346.

Ostfeld, R. S. and F. Keesing. (2000a). Biodiversity and disease risk: the case of Lyme disease. *Conservation Biology* **14**:722–728.

Ostfeld, R. S. and F. Keesing. (2000b). The function of biodiversity in the ecology of vector-borne zoonotic diseases. *Canadian Journal of Zoology* **78**:2061–2078.

Ostfeld, R. S. and D. N. Lewis. (1999). Experimental studies of interactions between wild turkeys and blacklegged ticks. *Journal of Vector Ecology* **24**:182–186.

Ostfeld, R. S. and K. LoGiudice. (2003). Community disassembly, biodiversity loss, and the erosion of an ecosystem service. *Ecology* **84**:1421-1427.

Ostfeld, R. S., K. R. Hazler, and O. M. Cepeda. (1996a). Temporal and spatial dynamics of *Ixodes scapularis* (Acari: Ixodidae) in a rural landscape. *Journal of Medical Entomology* **33**:90–95.

Ostfeld, R. S., C. G. Jones, and J. O. Wolff. (1996b). Of mice and mast: ecological connections in eastern deciduous forests. *Bioscience* **46**:323–330.

Ostfeld, R. S., E. M. Schauber, C. D. Canham, F. Keesing, C. G. Jones, and J. O. Wolff. (2001). Effects of acorn production and mouse abundance on abundance and *Borrelia burgdorferi* infection prevalence of nymphal *Ixodes scapularis* ticks. *Vector Borne and Zoonotic Diseases* **1**:55-64.

Ostfeld, R. S., F. Keesing, E. M. Schauber, and K. A. Schmidt, (2002). The ecological context of infectious disease: diversity, habitat fragmentation, and Lyme disease risk in North America. In A. Aguirre, R. S. Ostfeld, C. A. House, G. Tabor, and M. Pearl, eds. *Conservation Medicine: Ecological Health in Practice*, pp. 207–219. Oxford University Press, New York.

Pereira, H. M., G. C. Daily, and J. Roughgarden. (2004). A framework for assessing the relative vulnerability of species to land-use change. *Ecological Applications* **14**:730–742.

Pimm, S. L. (1991). *The Balance of Nature?* University of Chicago Press, Chicago, IL.

Pimm, S. L. and J. H. Lawton. (1977). Number of trophic levels in ecological communities. *Nature* **268**:329–331.

Rosenblatt, D. L., E. J. Heske, S. L. Nelson, D. M. Barber, M. A. Miller, and B. MacAllister. (1999). Forest fragments in east-central Illinois: islands or habitat patches for mammals? *American Midland Naturalist* **141**:115–123.

Schauber, E. M. and R. S. Ostfeld. (2002). Modeling the effects of reservoir competence decay and demographic turnover in Lyme-disease ecology. *Ecological Applications* **12**:1142–1162.

Schmidt, K. A. and R. S. Ostfeld. (2001). Biodiversity and the dilution effect in disease ecology. *Ecology* **82**:609–619.

Schmidt, K. A., R. S. Ostfeld, and E. M. Schauber. (1999). Infestation of *Peromyscus leucopus* and *Tamias striatus* by *Ixodes scapularis* (Acari: Ixodidae) in relation to the abundance of hosts and parasites. *Journal of Medical Entomology* **36**:749–757.

Schwartz, M. W., C. A. Brigham, J. D. Hoeksema, K. G. Lyons, M. H. Mills, and P. J. van Mantgem. (2000). Linking biodiversity to ecosystem function: implications for conservation biology. *Oecologia* **122**:297–305.

Shaw, M. T., F. Keesing, R. McGrail, and R. S. Ostfeld. (2003). Factors influencing the distribution of larval blacklegged ticks on rodent hosts. *American Journal of Tropical Medicine and Hygiene* **68**:447–452.

Tilman, D., J. Knops, D. Wedin, P. B. Reich, M. E. Ritchie, and E. Siemann. (1997). The influence of functional diversity and composition on ecosystem processes. *Science* **277**:1300–1302.

Wardle, D. A., K. J. Bonner, G. M. Barker, G. W. Yeates, K. S. Nicholson, R. D. Bardgett *et al.* (1999). Plant removals in perennial grassland: vegetation dynamics, decomposers, soil biodiversity, and ecosystem properties. *Ecological Monographs* **69**:535–568.

Wilson, M. L., T. S. Litwin, T. A. Gavin, M. C. Capkanis, D. C. MacLean, and A. Spielman. (1990). Host-dependent differences in feeding and reproduction of *Ixodes dammini* (Acari: Ixodidae). *Journal of Medical Entomology* **27**:945–954.

Wolff, J. O. (1996). Population fluctuations of mast-eating rodents are correlated with production of acorns. *Journal of Mammalogy* **77**:850–858.

CHAPTER 4

Microbial community ecology of tick-borne human pathogens

Keith Clay, Clay Fuqua, Curt Lively, and Michael J. Wade

4.1 Background

Microbial interactions within disease vectors may influence pathogen prevalence. For example, competitive or facilitative interactions among pathogenic microbes within vectors may affect their transmission and ensuing disease. And, the presence of nonpathogenic bacterial symbionts and other benign bacteria within a vector may facilitate or interfere with the acquisition and/or transmission of pathogenic bacteria. The role of microbial interactions in the organization of microbial communities within vectors and hosts has not been critically examined, yet these interactions may have an equal or even greater impact than cross-immunity, where exposure to one microbe reduces the likelihood of infection by a second microbe through elevated immune function.

Ticks vector more human pathogens than any other arthropod, and are the primary source of vector-borne infectious disease in many areas of Europe, Asia, and North America. In addition, ticks harbor non-pathogenic or commensal microbes and vertically transmitted symbionts. Prior studies of the relationship among ticks, vertebrate hosts, and pathogens have given little consideration to this microbial community and its interspecific interactions. The use of molecular genetic, cultivation-independent methods facilitates testing the direction and strength of ecological interactions among microbes within vectors. Incorporation of microbial interactions into epidemiological theory may better predict pathogen prevalence and disease incidence. In addition, these microbial systems lend themselves to rigorous tests of theory in community ecology, because each tick harbors a "replicate" community. The focus of this chapter is to consider the ecology of infectious disease transmission in relation to the microbial community within ticks. Similar relationships may occur in a wider range of arthropod vectors such as mosquitoes, fleas, lice, and bugs.

The microbial communities within ticks vary in species richness and relative species abundance. Our studies and those of others suggest that virtually all ticks are infected by several vertically transmitted (VT) symbionts whose identities vary with host phylogeny. Vertical transmission occurs when the symbiotic microbe colonizes undeveloped eggs within female ticks and proliferates in newly hatched larvae. Ticks also may be infected by horizontally transmitted (HT) bacteria that are obtained from the environment or from blood meals. We wish to determine whether the identity and/or number of endosymbiont species affect pathogen prevalence in tick microbial communities. More generally, are there predictable patterns of community organization in ticks, or do tick-borne microbial communities represent random assemblages of microbes from the available species pool? Randomly assembled communities are used as null models by ecologists and biogeographers to examine patterns of co-occurrence and to detect the signature of species interactions (Gotelli 2000). The comparative analysis of tick microbial communities offers a unique opportunity for detecting even subtle deviations from null model expectations, because each tick can be treated as a more or less independent observation of a single community, offering a great deal of statistical power from the high degree of replication.

Research on the ecology of infectious disease calls for study of the interactions among parasites or pathogens (Smith *et al.* 1995). The exclusion or facilitation of one microbe by another could change the pathogen load of the vector and the pattern of host coinfection (host infection with multiple pathogen species introduced by the vector). Models investigating microbial interactions within ticks can address these issues. In particular, we wish to determine whether there is selection for VT symbionts to competitively inhibit more virulent HT microbes. Vertical transmission of microbes through eggs is common among ticks and other arthropods (Sonenshine 1991). Theory predicts an association between mode of transmission among hosts and pathogen virulence (Ewald 1987; Kover and Clay 1998). When VT microbes harm their host, they may ensure their own extinction unless there is also some level of horizontal transmission. Similarly, when two microbial species coexist in a single host, if one is strictly VT, it may gain a transmission advantage by reducing the establishment of any HT pathogen that harms the host. It is in the interest of VT microbes to exclude pathogens from the host because infection by virulent pathogens may cause that host lineage and its VT community to become extinct. We know that complex communities of microorganisms can coordinate activities within hosts or interfere with other microbes via cell–cell communication (Fuqua *et al.* 2001). Such mechanisms may be relevant to the interactions among microbes within ticks.

4.2 Ticks as vectors of human pathogens

Hard ticks (Class Arachnida, Order Acari, Family Ixodidae) are obligate ectoparasites of terrestrial vertebrates. They can harm their hosts both directly and indirectly. Tick-produced toxins can cause paralysis, bite wounds can become festering sores prone to infection, and heavily parasitized hosts can literally be drained of blood (exsanguinated). More commonly, ticks harm their hosts indirectly by transmitting pathogenic microbes (Sonenshine 1991; Sonenshine and Mather 1994). The tick lifecycle includes egg, larval, nymphal, and adult stages, with a blood meal required for molting and egg production. Adult females may ingest more

than 100 times their body weight in blood (Sauer *et al.* 1995), and lay 5–10,000 eggs. Ticks can acquire pathogens during blood meals, but transmission of pathogens to susceptible vertebrate hosts requires that ticks maintain pathogen infection during "transstadial" molts from larvae to nymphs and from nymphs to adults (Sonenshine 1991).

Ticks carry a remarkable diversity of pathogens, including bacteria, viruses, protists, and nematodes, and a single tick bite can co-transmit multiple pathogens (Levin and Fish 2000; Rolain *et al.* 2005). Our research efforts have focused on the eastern United States and most of the following discussion is based on ticks and microbes from that region, where there are several newly recognized or emerging diseases (Table 4.1) such as southern tick-associated rash illness (Armstrong *et al.* 1996) and bartonellosis (Chang *et al.* 2001). Tick-borne pathogens classified as "select agents" with potential use as biological weapons include *Coxiella burnetii* and *Francisella tularensis* (responsible for Q fever and tularemia, respectively) and the rare, but highly virulent, encephalitic viruses (Atlas 2002). Other tick-borne pathogens, such as the viral agent of Crimean–Congo hemorrhagic fever, could spread beyond their current geographic ranges (Hoogstraal 1979), and established pathogens can jump to new tick vectors.

Three of the most medically important genera of ticks in the United States are *Amblyomma*, *Dermacentor*, and *Ixodes*. They serve as vectors for many human disease agents (Table 4.1). *Rickettsia rickettsii* is an obligate intracellular parasite and the causative agent of Rocky Mountain spotted fever. Rocky Mountain spotted fever is the most frequently reported rickettsial disease in the United States, with mortality ranging from 4% (with treatment) to ~20% (without) (CDC 1998). The primary vector is the American dog tick, *Dermacentor variabilis* (Burgdorfer 1975). *Borrelia burgdorferi* is the causal agent of Lyme disease, a tick-borne, systemic bacterial infection involving multiple organ systems leading to dermatologic, cardiac, neurologic, and arthritic abnormalities (Steere *et al.* 1977). Lyme disease is transmitted to humans by the bite of *Ixodes scapularis* and *I. pacificus* and is the most frequent vector-borne disease in the United States (see also Chapter 3, this volume). More than

Table 4.1 Diseases spread by tick bites (with primary tick vectors). Data from the United States

Disease	Pathogen	Tick	Reference
Rocky Mountain spotted fever	*Rickettsia rickettsii*	Da,Dv	Gage *et al.* (1995)
Lyme disease	*Borrelia burgdorferi*	Is	Lane (1994)
Human monocytic ehrlichiosis (HME)	*Ehrlichia chaffeensis*	Aa	Anderson *et al.* (1993)
Human granulocytic ehrlichiosis (HGE)	*Anaplasma phagocytophila*	Is	Dumler and Walker (2001)
Southern tick-associated rash illness	*Borrelia lonestari*	Aa	Barbour *et al.* (1996)
Q fever	*Coxiella burnetii*	Aa	Gage *et al.* (1995)
Tularemia	*Francisella tularensis*	Aa	Parola and Didier (2001)
Bartonellosis	*Bartonella henselae*	Is	Chang *et al.* (2001)
Powassan fever	Flavivirus	Is,Ic	Karabatsos (1985)
Colorado tick fever	Coltivirus	Da	Karabatsos (1985)
Babesiosis	*Babesia microti*[a]	Is	Sonenshine and Mather (1994)

Abbreviations:
Da = *Dermacentor andersoni*, Dv = *Dermacentor variabilis*, Is = *Ixodes scapularis*, Aa = *Amblyomma americanum*, Ic = *Ixodes cookei*.
[a] Protozoan.

115,000 cases were reported during the period 1982–1998 (CDC 1998). *Amblyomma americanum* vectors *Ehrlichia chaffeensis*, the causal agent of human monocytic ehrlichiosis, a recently recognized tick-borne disease (Anderson *et al.* 1993). Infection results in a flu-like febrile illness characterized by symptoms such as fever, headache, malaise, myalgia, chills, and abnormal liver enzyme levels that are sometimes difficult to differentiate from Rocky Mountain spotted fever or acute Lyme disease (McDade 1990; Rikihisa 1991). White-tailed deer are a natural reservoir host for the bacterium (Lockhart *et al.* 1997). Another tick-borne pathogen of emerging concern is *Anaplasma* sp. (poss. *equi* or *phagocytophila*), the causal agent of human granulocytic ehrlichiosis (anaplasmosis), an illness characterized by headache, myalgia, malaise, thrombocytopenia, leukopenia, and elevated levels of hepatic transaminases. In addition to humans, horses and dogs also appear to be susceptible to this disease (Ewing *et al.* 1997). Human granulocytic ehrlichiosis has the same geographic range as *B. burgdorferi*, and shares the same tick vector (*I. scapularis*, Ostfeld 1997). Another pathogen sharing the same vector species and range (Hofmeister *et al.* 1998) is *Babesia microti*, an intracellular, malaria-like, protozoan parasite. *B. microti* is the most recognized cause of human babesiosis in the United States (Herwaldt *et al.* 1996).

4.3 Microbial interactions within ticks

Human health concerns have prompted much research into the ecological relationships among tick vectors, microbial pathogens, and their vertebrate hosts. In contrast, ecological interactions among microbial taxa inhabiting the same tick or tick species have rarely been considered (but see Burgdorfer *et al.* 1981; Niebylski *et al.* 1997a). Interspecific interactions within ticks may occur during extended periods from several months up to a year or more between blood meals. Competition plays a central role in the organization of many communities, including those of some parasites or pathogens (Esch *et al.* 1990; Kuris and Lafferty 1994; McKenzie and Bossert 1997). Alternatively, parasite and pathogen communities may be relatively unstructured with random species assemblages and weak interspecific interactions (Holmes and Price 1986; Poulin 1997). Null models are helpful in determining if microbial interactions affect tick-borne community structure (Lafferty *et al.* 1994; Gotelli 2000). For example, Gotelli and Rohde (2002) examined community structure of ectoparasites in 45 species of marine fish and reported that most analyses could not distinguish observed community structure from that expected, given random colonization and extinction. Hubbell (2001) in his *Unified Neutral Theory of Biodiversity and*

Biogeography further suggested that predictable patterns in community organization can arise from random colonization by the available species pool, extinction, and speciation, rather than from niche differentiation and competitive exclusion. However, an assumption of the neutral theory is that biological communities are saturated with individuals, creating a zero-sum game where the addition of one new individual requires the loss of another. Parasite and pathogen communities within individual hosts may frequently violate this assumption, and exhibit great variation in parasite load or intensity of infection (Poulin 1997).

Some evidence exists to support the hypothesis that ecological interactions among microbes could limit the distribution and prevalence of tick-borne pathogens. Burgdorfer *et al.* (1981) described non-pathogenic rickettsiae of *D. andersoni* in the Bitterroot Valley of Montana (north-central United States) and suggested that they could be a limiting factor for the distribution of pathogenic *R. rickettsii*. Rocky Mountain spotted fever occurs predominantly among residents of the west side of the valley despite abundant tick populations on both sides of the valley. Burgdorfer and colleagues discovered that a large percentage of female, east-side ticks were infected by rickettsiae found primarily in the ovary. This "east-side agent" was similar to pathogenic *R. rickettsii* ultrastructurally, but could be differentiated by flourescent-labeled antibodies. Experimental inoculations of meadow voles and guinea pigs with the east-side agent induced at most a limited pathogenic response. When nymphal ticks harboring the east-side agent (via vertical transmission) were fed on guinea pigs infected by *R. rickettsii*, the ticks became highly co-infected by the pathogen and the east-side agent. Most co-infected ticks transmitted only the east-side agent to eggs. Those few ticks that transmitted *R. rickettsii* either lacked the east-side agent entirely or were only mildly infected. Thus, it appears that the east-side agent can limit vertical transmission of *R. rickettsii*. Burgdorfer *et al.* (1981) suggested that the non-virulent, VT symbiont might thereby effectively exclude pathogenic agents from large parts of the tick's range. It is noteworthy that pathogenic *R. rickettsii* can be VT and has been shown to induce high mortality in tick vectors (Niebylski *et al.* 1999).

Subsequently, several species of rickettsiae (*R. rickettsii, R. rhipicephali, R. montana,* and *R. bellii*) have been recognized from the Bitterroot Valley of Montana based on distinct serotypes (Philip *et al.* 1976). Recently, Niebylski *et al.* (1997b) described Burgdorfer's east-side agent as a new species, *R. peacockii*. Experiments with other non-virulent rickettsiae (*R. montana* and *R. rhipicephali*) demonstrated that they also blocked vertical transmission of *R. rickettsii* (Burgdorfer *et al.* 1981; Lane 1994). Paralleling the situation in the Bitterroot Valley and *D. andersoni*, Philip *et al.* (1976) reported that the Pacific coast tick, *D. occidentalis* is a vector for *R. rickettsii* in California but only rarely in populations that have a high frequency of infection by *R. rhipicephali*.

Recent work based on DNA sequence variation suggests that another endosymbiont might also reduce pathogen prevalence. This endosymbiont of *D. andersoni*, which is unrelated to rickettsiae, is closely related to *F. tularensis* subsp. *tularensis*, the causal agent of tularemia. Tularemia, a bacterial disease resembling plague, can be contracted through contact with infected animals or contaminated water, and by bites by infected arthropods (Gage *et al.* 1995). The related endosymbiont occurs at very high frequencies in the Bitterroot Valley of Montana and is effectively spread by vertical transmission (Niebylski *et al.* 1997a). It is absent from salivary glands and there is no evidence that it can be spread via tick bite, unlike *F. tularensis* subsp. *tularensis*. Niebylski *et al.* (1997a) suggested that these *Francisella* endosymbionts may prevent or reduce vertical transmission of the tularemia agent by competitively inhibiting pathogens in ovaries and eggs or by indirect mechanisms. The co-occurrence of pathogenic species of *Coxiella, Francisella,* and *Rickettsia* with closely related VT symbionts (Niebylski *et al.* 1997a, b; Noda *et al.* 1997, Macaluso *et al.* 2002) emphasizes the evolutionary lability of virulent pathogens and benign or mutualistic symbionts.

Individual ticks are often infected by multiple pathogens, as well as by VT symbionts, providing the opportunity for microbial interactions during the extended periods between blood meals when no additional microbial colonization occurs. Many studies have reported frequencies of ticks carrying various disease agents, sometimes also reporting co-infection frequencies (e.g. Leutenegger *et al.* 1999). However, these data were not collected to evaluate patterns of pathogen co-occurrence and generally do not consider VT symbionts and other non-pathogenic microbes. For example, in *I. ricinus* ticks in the Netherlands, 70% of ticks infected with *Ehrlichia* also carried *Bartonella* and 13% were additionally infected by *B. burgdorferi* (Schouls *et al.* 1999). Similarly, in New Jersey (US), 10% of *I. scapularis* ticks were co-infected with either *B. burgdorferi*, *A. phagocytophila*, or *B. microti* (Varde *et al.* 1998). Studies of 492 *I. ricinus* ticks from Germany revealed that 1.6% were infected by granulocytic ehrlichiae and 36% by *B. burgdorferi* with four ticks infected by both pathogens (Fingerle *et al.* 1999). In some cases, pathogen occurrence in the same tick was clearly independent of the presence or absence of other pathogens. For example, Schauber *et al.* (1998) reported that infections of *I. scapularis* ticks by *B. burgdorferi* and the agent of human granulocytic ehrlichiosis were independent of each other in New York (US). Similarly, Levin and Fish (2000) found that *A. phagocytophila* and *B. burgdorferi* were acquired by mice regardless of their prior infection status by the opposite agent, and likewise were transmitted independently.

Simultaneous infections by multiple tick-borne pathogens occur frequently in mammalian hosts, including humans. In a North Carolina (US) kennel, 26 of 27 dogs tested were seroreactive to *Ehrlichia*, 25 to *Bartonella vinsonii* (the agent of canine endocarditis), 22 to *R. rickettsii*, and 16 to *Babesia canis* (Kordick *et al.* 1999). Further polymerase chain reaction (PCR) analyses indicated that 15 dogs were infected by *Ehrlichia canis*, nine with *E. chaffeensis*, 8 with *E. ewingii*, 8 with *E. platys*, and 3 with *E. equi*, in addition to the other pathogens. Similarly, five deer from Georgia (US) were tested for *Ehrlichia* infection using serologic, molecular, and culture techniques. One of five was infected with *E. chafeensis*, three of five with the human granulocytic ehrlichiosis agent and all five with another *Ehrlichia*-like organism (Little *et al.* 1998). Of 96 human patients in Wisconsin and Minnesota infected with *B. burgdorferi*, 5 were co-infected with *A. phagocytophila*, 2 with *B. microti* and 2 were infected by all three pathogens (Mitchell *et al.* 1996).

Ticks could become co-infected (in addition to VT symbionts) by consuming a single blood meal containing multiple pathogens. Alternatively, transfer of pathogens between cofeeding ticks (simultaneously feeding on the same animal host) may account for co-infections (Piesman and Happ 2001). Coinfection via sequential blood meals is less likely given that the hard tick life cycle includes only three blood meals well-separated in time. In contrast, coinfections of vertebrates by tick-borne pathogens could easily result from sequential and independent tick bites given that a large animal host could have a tick burden in the hundreds or thousands. Moreover, hosts may be bitten by ticks coinfected with multiple pathogens as described above.

In contrast to competitive exclusion or random associations, mutual facilitation within ticks, whereby one microbe enhances the likelihood of infection by another, may also occur. For example, Mather *et al.* (1987) suggested that the agents of Lyme disease and babesiosis occurred together in ticks more frequently than expected. Similarly, pathogens may be positively associated within vertebrate hosts. In New York (US), 60–90% of patients diagnosed with human granulocytic ehrlichiosis tested positive for *B. burgdorferi*, a higher than expected rate based on pathogen prevalence (Wormser *et al.* 1997, see also Mitchell *et al.* 1996). In the rodent *Neotoma mexicana*, 24% of samples contained *A. phagocytophila*, 66% contained *B. burgdorferi*, and 78% of the animals infected by *A. phagocytophila* were simultaneously infected with *B. burgdorferi*, a higher rate than expected for independent infection (Zeidner *et al.* 2000). Mutual facilitation increases the health risk of tick bites.

Overall, these studies demonstrate that ticks harbor a diversity of pathogens and symbionts, potentially allowing for ecological interactions among microbes within ticks. Microbial interactions could affect pathogen prevalence and transmission within tick populations. However, few studies have explicitly tested this possibility, and those studies have generally ignored VT symbionts of ticks.

4.4 Microbial diversity within ticks

Determinative microbiology has relied for over a century on the ability to cultivate microorganisms derived from natural environments. Although this approach remains one of the most commonly employed and useful means of identifying microbes, it excludes the detection of a potentially vast range of microorganisms. Estimates from soil environments suggest that greater than 99% of active microorganisms are not detectable by conventional cultivation methods (Hugenholz et al. 1998; Rondon et al. 2000). Powerful molecular probing techniques now enable the detection of a much wider range of microorganisms from a diversity of environments (Box 4.1). Noncultivated microbes can be identified and phylogenetically categorized, often to the level of genus and species, using nucleic acid or antibody probes directed towards highly conserved macromolecules (Clements 1991). Although a range of conserved proteins, fatty acids and nucleic acids have been used as targets for this purpose, small subunit ribosomal RNAs (SSUs) such as bacterial 16S rRNA, are the most generally applicable, and often the most informative (Stahl 1995). Molecular analysis has revealed diverse arthropod-associated microbes for a variety of systems (Brune and Friedrich 2000, van Borm et al. 2002). Many of these microbes have not yet been cultured and their identification would be virtually impossible without cultivation-independent methods. Likewise, the study of tick-borne pathogens increasingly relies on molecular detection approaches to identify, distinguish, and compare pathogens among different tick species and populations (Burkot et al. 2001; Sparagano et al. 1999; Sun et al. 2000; Schabereiter-Gurtner et al. 2003).

We have initiated studies to examine the microbial diversity of eastern North American ticks. Over 400 bacterial rDNA sequences have been obtained and then used to probe the DNA sequence databases (Table 4.2). Three species of questing ticks (D. variabilis, A. americanum, and I. scapularis) were collected in the midwestern United States by dragging cloth swaths of fixed size through vegetation in numerous sampling areas. Most of our sampling sites are in southern Indiana where distances between sites range from 1–5 km up to 200 km. We targeted general habitat types (open woodlands for A. americanum, woodland margins for D. variabilis, and closed-canopy woodland for I. scapularis) but have found that all three ticks can be found almost anywhere. Collection success is often more of a function of weather, temperature, and time of day than site-specific characteristics. Collected ticks were surface-sterilized, individually homogenized, and extracted for total nucleic acid. Bacterial 16S rDNA sequences were amplified using eubacterial-specific primers and then fused en masse into plasmid vectors.

We have identified several unique 16S rDNA phylotypes associated with D. variabilis, A. americanum, and I. scapularis (Table 4.2). These findings clearly indicate that ticks are host to a diverse microbial community where interspecific interactions could occur. Analysis of microbial rDNA sequences associated with D. variabilis revealed two phylotypes likely to be VT symbionts from the gamma-Proteobacterial group (Table 4.2 and Box 4.1). The most prevalent of these, a Francisella-like sequence (Dermacentor-associated symbiont, or DAS) has been reported for D. variabilis from Connecticut and D. andersoni from Montana (Niebylski et al. 1997a; Sun et al. 2000). The second type represents a new branch of the Arsenophonus-type bacteria, originally identified as the "son-killing" endosymbionts of the parasitoid wasp Nasonia vitripennis (Gherna et al. 1991; Grindle et al. 2003). The D. variabilis-associated Arsenophonus (DAA) type microbes were detected in many tick populations (Table 4.2). Furthermore, analysis of larval ticks derived from engorged D. variabilis females revealed a clonal population of the DAA microbe, suggesting that they are VT, as documented for the Nasonia symbiont (Gherna et al. 1991). This is the first report of an Arsenophonus-type microbe from a noninsect, arthropod host. We also detected the rickettsiae, R. bellii and R. montana, in our samples. In addition, 16S rDNA phylotypes representing the alpha- and beta-Proteobacteria, Bacteroidetes, and Actinomycetes groups were identified. The proteobacterial and actinobacterial groups are well known for stable associations with arthropods, but the Bacteroidetes group has not been previously recognized. Several of these microbial groups are abundant in soils and could conceivably be due to bacteria or spores not

Box 4.1 **Characterizing microbial communities using molecular genetics**

Powerful molecular probing techniques now enable the detection of a much wider range of microorganisms from a diversity of environments, including arthropod-associated microbes. Many of these microbes have not been cultured and their identification would be virtually impossible without cultivation-independent methods. A direct approach for examining microbial diversity of ticks or other arthropods involves extracting total nucleic acid from surface-sterilized samples, and performing PCR amplification using primers specific for eubacterial rDNA sequences (Marchesi *et al.* 1998) (Fig. 4.1). The PCR products, 16S-rDNA amplicons, are fused *en masse* with plasmid cloning vectors and introduced into *Escherichia coli*.

The rDNA inserts carried on these plasmids are sequenced to identify the microbe and subsequent phylogenetic analysis provides taxonomic affiliations. (Note: the alpha-numeric abbreviations in the radial cladogram below indicate microbial taxa identified in our own work). Specific PCR primers detect targeted rDNA sequences nested within eubacterial amplicons, or directly amplified from the tick extracts. Specific probes can be developed to visualize the internal location of microbes by *in situ* hybridization. Quantitative PCR and T-RFLP analyses also provide data on relative and absolute densities of different microbial species within single ticks.

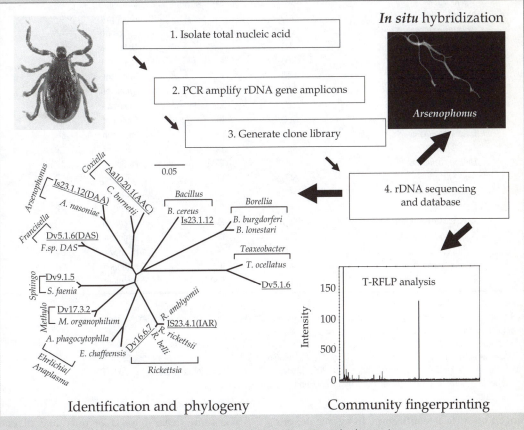

Figure 4.1 Sequence of steps involved in characterizing microbial communities using molecular genetics.

Table 4.2 Prokaryotes from ticks identified by DNA sequencing (SEQ) and/or direct probing (DP), their relative frequency, and association with ticks. All collection sites were in Indiana (US), including 16 *Dermacentor* sites and 5 sites each for *Amblyomma* and *Ixodes*

Tick[a]	Closest phylogenetic relative	Method[b]	Frequency[c]	Type	Group	N[d]
Dv	*Actinoplanes minutisporangius*	SEQ	R	Unknown	ACT	1,-
	Arsenophonus nasoniae	DP, SEQ	M-VF	Symbiont	GP	4,7
	Bradyrhizobium genosp. G	SEQ	R	Unknown	AP	1,-
	Corynebacterium genitalium	SEQ	R	Unknown	ACT	1,-
	Erwinia rhapontici	SEQ	R	Unknown	GP	1,-
	Francisella sp. DAS	DP, SEQ	VF	Symbiont	GP	4,8
	Friedmanniella antarctica	SEQ	R	Unknown	ACT	1,-
	Gordonia sp. SJS0289-JS1	SEQ	R	Unknown	ACT	1,-
	Methylobacterium organophilum	SEQ	R-IF	Unknown	AP	1,-
	Microlunatus phosphovorus	SEQ	R	Unknown	ACT	1,-
	Nocardioides jensenii	SEQ	R	Unknown	ACT	1,-
	Pseudomonas tolasii	SEQ	VF	Unknown	GP	1,-
	Rickettsiae	DP	M-VF	Variable	AP	2,8
	SFG Rickettsiae	DP	M	Variable	AP	-.1
	Rickettsia bellii	SEQ	R	Unknown	AP	1,-
	Rickettsia montana	SEQ	M	Symbiont	AP	1,-
	Sphingomonas faenia	SEQ	IF	Unknown	AP	2,-
	Taxeobacter ocellatus	SEQ	R	Unknown	BCT	1,-
Dv-L[e]	*Arsenophonus nasoniae*	SEQ	F	Symbiont	GP	1,-
	Francisella sp. DAS	DP, SEQ	VF	Symbiont	GP	1,-
	Pseudomonas sp. Gu5828	SEQ	M	Unknown	GP	1,-
Aa	*Arsenophonus nasoniae*	SEQ	M	Symbiont	GP	1,-
	Borrelia lonestari	DP	IF	Pathogen	SP	-,3
	Coxiella burnetii	SEQ	F-VF	Symbiont	GP	4,-
	Ehrlichia chaffeensis	DP	IF-M	Pathogen	AP	-,2
	Legionella sp.	SEQ	IF	Unknown	GP	1,-
	Rickettsia amblyommii	SEQ	IF	Pathogen	AP	1,-
	Sinorhizobium sp. FJ38 32-1-A	SEQ	R	Unknown	AP	1,-
Is	*Alcaligenes xylosoxidans*	SEQ	R	Unknown	BP	1,-
	Arsenophonus nasoniae	SEQ	IF	Symbiont	GP	1,-
	Bacillus cereus	SEQ	M	Unknown	BAC	1,-
	Borrelia burgdorferi	DP	IF-VF	Pathogen	SP	-,4
	Rickettsia sp. (I.s. symbiont)	SEQ	F-VF	Symbiont	AP	2,-

Abbreviations:

AP = Alphaproteobacteria, GP = Gammaproteobacteria, ACT = Actinobacteridae, BCT = Bacteroidetes, BAC = Bacillaceae, BP = Betaproteobacteria, SP = Spirochetes.

[a] Tick species as in Table 1.
[b] Prokaryotes identified by DNA sequencing (SEQ) or direct probing (DP).
[c] Very Frequent (VF) = 81–100%, Frequent (F) = 51–80%, Moderate (M) = 21–50%, Infrequent (IF) = 6–20%, Rare (R) = 1–5%.
[d] Number of sites where prokaryote identified by sequencing and/or by direct probing.
[e] Larval clutches.

removed by surface sterilization. In aggregate, our results expand considerably the diversity of microbes known from *D. variabilis*. It should be emphasized that it is unclear for many of these microbes whether they represent endosymbionts, commensals, or tick pathogens.

The same general trend of microbial diversity was observed in *A. americanum* and *I. scapularis*. Similar to the DAS-type microbe associated with *D. variabilis*, we have identified microbes likely to be dominant VT symbionts of each tick. Most of the microbes detected are specific to each tick species although the *Arsenophonus* species was found associated with all three ticks (Grindle *et al.* 2003; unpublished data). The abundance of these VT bacteria within each tick, based on the frequency of their identification in our clone libraries, appears to far exceed the pathogens as well as other commensal microbes associated with the ticks. For example, we find that the human pathogens are significantly underrepresented in our clone libraries, relative to the abundant non-pathogens. Therefore, the most prevalent microbial interaction within ticks may be with numerically dominant VT symbionts. But even those microbes maintained at low relative abundance within individual ticks could have

significant effects on microbial ecology and disease transmission.

The rDNA sequence library approach allows the identification of previously undiscovered microbial taxa but does not determine whether a particular microbe is absent in any given sample, nor does it provide a reliable measure of density. For this purpose, specific assays must be designed to identify microbial taxa of interest. Common assay formats employ PCR-based assays, fluorescent *in situ* hybridization, immunodetection, and traditional microscopy. We use a number of PCR assays for tick-borne microbes based upon signature sequences in the 16s rDNA sequences and in other target genes

---

Box 4.2 Effects of a VT microbe on the prevalence of pathogens in tick populations

Following the initial idea of Dobson (1985) that there could be competition among parasites within a single host, we consider microbial interactions within ticks (Lively *et al.* in preparation). In particular, we are exploring whether the co-occurrence of VT symbionts and HT pathogens within a vector leads to strong selection on VT symbionts to competitively inhibit the establishment or growth of more virulent HT pathogens. For a more general formulation and equations of interactions between microbes, see Lively *et al.* (2005). The tick-specific model describes the interaction between a HT pathogen that reduces vector survival and fecundity, and a VT pathogen that excludes the more virulent HT pathogen. The model assumes that nymphal and larval populations of ticks are limited by small mammal hosts (e.g. mice) but adult populations are limited by survival though the winter (see Van Buskirk and Ostfeld 1995).

In preliminary runs, tick populations were initiated without infection. After 100 generations, a single tick infected by the HT microbe was "introduced" by the simulation. After 100 additional tick generations, a single tick infected with the VT microbe was introduced. We followed the dynamics for an additional 400 generations. Key parameters for this baseline model were drawn from previous empirical work by Niebylski *et al.* (1999). High numbers of nymphs per mammalian host and high probabilities of vertical transmission for the VT microbe led to the near elimination of the HT microbe in tick populations (Fig. 4.2, upper panel) and relatively stable temporal dynamics, with the frequency of HT infection greatly reduced in small mammal host populations (Fig. 4.2, lower panel). In the absence of the

HT pathogen, the VT symbiont does not persist (not shown). These results show that microbial interactions can have dramatic effects on the frequency of pathogens in populations of ticks and their hosts, and correspond to our empirical findings of high prevalence of VT symbionts and low prevalence of HT pathogens in tick populations.

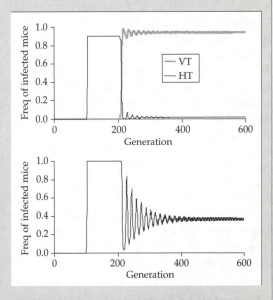

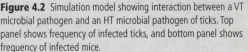
Figure 4.2 Simulation model showing interaction between a VT microbial pathogen and an HT microbial pathogen of ticks. Top panel shows frequency of infected ticks, and bottom panel shows frequency of infected mice.

such as those encoding glycolytic enzymes and bacterial flagella. Using these techniques we analyzed large numbers of samples collected over diverse geographies (Table 4.2). As reflected in the 16s-rDNA libraries we have found the abundant non-pathogens such as DAS in virtually 100% of ticks from every population that we have analyzed. Most other tick-associated microbes are less uniformly distributed. The pathogens, in particular, are variable in their distribution, with high infection rates in some sites, and other sites where no pathogens are detected. Such heterogeneous distribution predicts hotspots of potential transmission, as is often observed for tick-borne pathogens. The underlying causes are likely to be multifactorial, but we hypothesize that these include ecological interactions among the microbes harbored within the ticks.

In our initial analyses of the *D. variabilis* libraries, the *Arsenophonus*-type sequences (DAA) were not isolated from ticks that had *Francisella*-type sequences (DAS). As suggested by studies of the non-pathogenic rickettsiae in Montana's Bitterroot Valley (Burgdorfer *et al.* 1981), these VT microbes could conceivably act to exclude pathogenic bacteria (Box 4.2). It was essential to establish methods for directly detecting these microbes from individual ticks. Therefore, we designed and tested DAA-specific and DAS-specific 16S-rDNA PCR primers. All but one population carried DAA and DAS amplicons. Given the ubiquity of the DAS microbe it would not explain the presence or absence of the DAA microbe, which occurs at less than 100% frequency within tick populations. These tests do not however reveal relative abundances of co-occurring microbes, and thus we may not detect incomplete exclusion where the presence of DAA could restrict the abundance of DAS. Techniques that allow relative abundances to be determined within a single sample, such as quantitative PCR and T-RFLP (terminal restriction fragment length polymorphisms) can be used to measure the relative abundances of microbial rDNA within the individual ticks (Marsh 1999; Brunk *et al.* 2002).

4.5 Analysis of co-occurrence patterns of tick-borne microbes

Classic ecological theory has assumed that competition plays a pervasive role in the organization of ecological communities. In other words, biological interactions structure communities of organisms physiologically capable of growing in a given environment. More closely related species, which have similar physiological requirements and which utilize similar resources, are expected to compete more strongly than more distantly related species. Within a community, the co-occurrence of animal species that differ in a regular fashion in body size, morphology, or food preferences (character displacement) has been taken as evidence for interspecific competition and niche displacement. For example, negative correlations between the abundances of ecologically similar bird species on south Pacific islands have been interpreted as evidence that competition structures these avian communities (Diamond 1975).

The interpretations of patterns seen as consistent with competition have been questioned with the counterargument that patterns of co-occurrence can be explained as purely random assemblages of communities. This has led to a call for comparing observed patterns with purely random associations (e.g. Ricklefs and Travis 1980). Strong *et al.* (1979) reexamined the distribution of species of Darwin's finches among the Galapagos Islands, often cited as a classic case of niche displacement, and found that species composition among islands was not statistically different than random assemblages. In contrast, Schoener (1984) found evidence supporting the role of competition structuring hawk communities.

With respect to ticks, null models of community structure provide a useful approach to determine whether competitive interactions (interference) or mutual facilitation are important determinants of microbial community structure. In the simplest sense, one can ask whether two taxa occur together more or less frequently than expected purely by chance. As discussed above, evidence from *Dermacentor* ticks from Montana is consistent with the idea of mutual interference. East-side ticks have high levels of infection by nonpathogenic rickettsiae and low levels of pathogenic *R. rickettsii*, whereas west-side ticks exhibit the opposite pattern. Alternatively, this pattern could reflect founder effects where each microbe colonized tick populations on different sides of the valley. There is also evidence consistent with facilitation among microbial agents where two taxa co-occur more frequently than expected by chance, as in the case of *Ixodes* ticks simultaneously carrying *B. burgdorferi* and *Babsesia* (Mather *et al.* 1987; Wormser *et al.* 1997).

Microbial diversity data can be subjected to statistical tests to evaluate the hypothesis of microbial community interactions, that is, whether species co-occur more or less frequently than expected (i.e. facilitation or inhibition). Molecular data on the presence or absence of particular microbes can be used to form a matrix consisting of +s and 0s, where rows correspond to microbial taxa and columns to individual ticks. Diamond (1975) reasoned that the checkerboard distribution of bird species on islands (where two species are never found on a single island) was strong evidence that the assembly of communities reflected interspecific competition. Null models of community structure provide a useful approach to determine whether competitive or facilitative interactions within ticks are important determinants of microbial community structure. Gotelli (2000) provided a detailed analysis of the strength of different null model algorithms and indices summarizing co-occurrence patterns (see also Gotelli & Rohde 2002).

probability that the observed value does not exceed the expected value from a random assemblage are: A. 9.14 ($P < 0.0001$), B. 4.04 ($P < 0.30$), C. 4.93 ($P < 0.002$). This index and algorithm are generally robust with low probability of Type-I (false positive) error (Gotelli 2000). In the simple case of two microbial taxa, the data collapse to a 2 x 2 contingency table of the sort analyzed by McKenzie and Bossert (1999) with *G*-test statistics, using the resampling algorithim in the EcoSim computer package (Gotelli and Entsminger 2003).

Statistical power is an issue with respect to the frequency of microbial taxa and the number of tick samples that can be characterized. A power analysis (using the PASS sample size software from NCSS, Inc.) suggests that the minimal sample size for detecting mutual exclusion or facilitation of two microbes each occurring at 50% frequency is only $N = 11$. For two microbes at 1% frequency the minimum N is over 50,000. For two microbes at 50% and 10% frequency, respectively, the minimum N is 101. If there is less than 100% perfect exclusion, sample sizes need to be larger. Thus, there is little statistical power for evaluating interactions of microbes that occur at very low frequencies but good statistical power for evaluating interactions between

	Tick sample		
	A.	B.	C.
Microbial taxa	+ + + + 0 0 0 0	+ 0 0 + + + + 0	+ + 0 0 + + 0 0
	+ + + + 0 0 0 0	0 0 0 + + + + 0	+ + 0 0 + + 0 0
	+ + + + 0 0 0 0	+ + + + + + 0 0	0 0 + + 0 0 + +
	+ + + + 0 0 0 0	+ 0 + 0 0 + + 0	0 0 + + 0 0 + +
	0 0 0 0 + + + +	0 0 + 0 + 0 + 0	0 0 + 0 + 0 + 0
	0 0 0 0 + + + +	0 + + 0 0 0 0 0	0 + 0 0 0 0 0 0
	0 0 0 0 + + + +	0 + 0 + + 0 0 +	0 + 0 + + 0 + +
	0 0 0 0 + + + +	+ + + + + 0 0 +	+ 0 + + + 0 0 +

Three examples are shown here where microbial taxa (rows) are distributed among individual ticks (columns). Case A is highly structured where taxa 1–4 always co-occur but never with taxa 5–8. Case B is a totally random community. Case C is intermediate with some structure (taxa 1 & 2 and 3 & 4 co-occur but are mutually exclusive with the opposite pair, taxa 5–8 are randomly distributed). The C-score, which quantifies the average co-occurrence of all unique pairs of species (125), and

VT microbes at moderate prevalence (~50%) and less common (~10%) pathogens (Table 4.2).

The presence or absence of microbial taxa in individual ticks is analogous to the presence or absence of bird species on Pacific islands (Diamond 1975). However, given the small size of individual bacterial cells and their potentially enormous populations within a single tick, a quantitative measure of bacterial populations may be more informative. Hubbell (2001) has provided a framework for testing null models of community composition, as opposed to competition-based models, based on quantitative data on relative species abundances. With quantitative PCR and T-RFLP analyses it is possible to obtain data on relative and absolute densities of different microbial species within single ticks. This offers another approach to examine microbial interactions manifested as correlated population densities rather than presence/absence.

With quantitative data on relative species abundance it is possible to estimate reciprocal effects of interacting microbes. In particular, regression analysis can reveal whether population density of one species is correlated (positively or negatively) with population density of the other species within single ticks, and whether observed community composition is effectively neutral with respect to interspecific interactions. Hubbell's (2001) theory predicts a negative correlation between species abundances under the assumption of constant density per unit area. This assumption may apply if there is an upper limit to the number of microbial cells that can be supported by a single tick, such that an increase in density of one microbe must be balanced by a decrease in another. A key distinction between the predictions of Hubbell's neutral model and competition-based models would concern whether the identity of the dominant VT symbiont is consistent across ticks and independent of the likelihood of colonization via vertical or horizontal transmission.

4.6 Modeling microbial interactions

Epidemiological models have provided useful tools for examining risk factors involved in the transmission of a focal pathogen species among hosts. However, individual hosts or vectors may be co-infected with multiple, interacting pathogen or parasite species (Holmes and Price 1986; Esch et al. 1990; Kuris and Lafferty 1994; Petney and Andrews 1998). Despite abundant empirical data on co-occurrence, there are few models of interactions among pathogens. Existing multiple-pathogen models focus on the distribution of macroparasites across hosts or on host co-immunity, wherein immunity to one parasite confers partial protection

against others. For example, Dobson (1985) showed that, when one species of parasite was highly aggregated on individual hosts and had intermediate pathogenicity, it reduced niche overlap with competing parasite species and limited competitor density (see also Dobson and Roberts 1994). Mosquitoes accumulate multiple *Plasmodium* species (McKenzie and Bossert 1997), whereas human studies show a deficit of mixed-species infections (Richie 1988). Competition between *Plasmodium* species, which depends on their specific identity, could affect their coexistence and transmission (Richie 1988; McKenzie and Bossert 1999). In addition, cross-immunity may be a determinant of many mixed-pathogen communities (Feng and Velasco-Hernandez 1997; Tanaka et al. 1999).

Smith et al. (1995) identified several needs for more realistic epidemiological models, including examination of interactions among parasites. Since this call to action, however, little work has been done. The exclusion or co-facilitation of one microbe by another changes the parasite load of the disease vector, the pattern of coinfection of vertebrate hosts, and possibly the degree of cross-species acquired immunity. Thus, ecological interactions among microbes within the vector, and the antigenic interactions within the vertebrate host, interact with one another to affect the epidemiology of disease. We have begun to address these issues in models designed to investigate interactions within the microbial communities of ticks, including pathogens, symbionts, and commensals. In particular, we are exploring whether VT symbionts and HT pathogens that co-occur in the same disease vector lead to strong selection on VT microbes to competitively inhibit the establishment or growth of more virulent, HT microbes (see also Price 1953).

Host–pathogen coevolutionary theory predicts an association between mode of transmission among hosts (vertical or horizontal) and pathogen virulence (Ewald 1987; Lipsitch et al. 1996; Kover and Clay 1998). When VT microbes reduce host fitness, they also reduce their transmission to future generations. Thus, VT pathogenic microbes, which harm their host, must enjoy a component of horizontal transmission sufficient to compensate for the reduction in host fitness. Without horizontal transmission, a pathogenic microbe would ensure its own extinction by reducing the fitness of the host lineages along which it was transmitted. Similarly, when two species of pathogen coexist in a single host, if one is strictly VT, it gains a transmission advantage by reducing the establishment of any HT pathogen that harms the host, even if there is not direct competition between the two parasites for host resources. Although theoretical models assume exclusive modes of transmission, many pathogens can be transmitted both vertically and horizontally. Thus, it is in the evolutionary interest of every VT microbe to exclude any hostdamaging pathogen from joining the community. Just as with deleterious mutations in asexual species, infection by a virulent pathogen condemns that host lineage and its VT community to extinction.

We have begun to extend the basic ideas of competition among pathogens to consider some of the complications that arise when microbial interactions within vectors are considered (Lively *et al.* 2005; Lively *et al.* in preparation., Box 4.2). The model is focused on microbial interactions within ticks but could be extended to other arthropod vectors. The model also assumes that nymphal and larval populations of ticks are limited by the number of mice (Van Buskirk and Ostfeld 1995) but the adult population is limited more by over-winter survival. Results of interaction between VT and HT microbes depended on the number of nymphs per mouse (Lively *et al.* in preparation). In general, successful invasion by the HT microbe into initially uninfected populations requires a threshold number of nymphs per mouse. This invasion by the HT microbe was followed by invasion by the VT microbe under most conditions, and coexistence of the two forms in the same tick population. In general, higher transmission probabilities favored coexistence of the two microbes within the same tick population. However, high numbers of nymphs per mouse and high probabilities of vertical transmission for the VT microbe led to the virtual elimination of the HT microbe and relatively stable temporal dynamics, with the frequency of HT infection greatly reduced (Box 4.2). These results show that interactions among microbes with different transmission routes can have dramatic effects on the frequency of ticks and mice infected

with human pathogens. The results correspond to our empirical findings of a high frequency of VT symbionts in tick populations but a low frequency of HT pathogens. Moreover, they strongly correspond to the pattern described by Burgdorfer *et al.* (1981) in the Bitterroot Valley of Montana. In a broader sense, this model may provide an alternative mechanism by which VT microbes are maintained in populations, in spite of their inherent metabolic cost to the host.

4.7 Conclusions

We suggest that microbial interactions affect pathogen prevalence and human disease, and that consideration of these interactions will lead to advances in epidemiology. Multispecies microbial communities are common in arthropod vectors and vertebrate hosts but have been largely ignored in past research. Data from the United States indicate that ticks are the most important vectors of human disease, including an ever-growing list of emerging diseases and novel pathogens. More than other arthropod vectors, ticks are long-lived, tolerant of environmental stress, and widespread. The extended periods between blood meals allow for the development of microbial communities potentially structured by interspecific interactions within ticks. Further research on how microbial interactions enhance or mitigate tick-borne disease risk will encourage new techniques for quantifying pathogen populations and microbial communities, and will inform applied control efforts.

References

Anderson, B. E., K. G. Sims, J. G. Olson, J. E., Childs, J. F. Piesman, C. M. Happ *et al.* (1993). *Amblyomma americanum*: a potential vector of human ehrlichiosis. *American Journal of Tropical Medicine and Hygiene* **49**:239–244.

Armstrong, P. M., S. M. Rich, R. D. Smith, D. L. Hartl, A. Spielman, and S. R. Telford. (1996). A new *Borrelia* infecting Lone Star ticks. *Lancet* **347**:67–68.

Atlas, R. M. (2002). Bioterrorism: from threat to reality. *Annual Review of Microbiology* **56**:167–185.

Barbour, A. G., G. O. Maupin, G. J. Teltow, C. J. Carter, and J. Piesman. (1996). Identification of an uncultivable *Borrelia* species in the hard tick *Amblyomma americanum*:

possible agent of a Lyme disease- like illness. *Journal of Infectious Diseases* **173**:403–409.

Brune, A. and M. Friedrich. (2000). Microecology of the termite gut: structure and function on a microscale. *Current Opinions in Microbiology* **3**:263–269.

Brunk, C. F., J. Li, and E. Avaniss-Aghajani. (2002). Analysis of specific bacteria from environmental samples using a quantitative polymerase chain reaction. *Current Issues in Molecular Biology* **4**:13–18.

Burgdorfer, W. (1975). A review of Rocky Mountain spotted fever (Tick-borne typhus), its agent, and its tick vectors in the United States. *Journal of Medical Entomology* **12**:269–278.

Burgdorfer, W., S. F. Hayes, and A. J. Mavros. (1981). Nonpathogenic rickettsiae in *Dermacentor andersoni*: a limiting factor for the distribution of *Rickettsia rickettsii*. In W. Burgdorfer and R. L. Anacker, eds. *Rickettsiae and Rickettsial Diseases*, pp. 585–594. Academic Press, New York.

Burkot, T. R., G. R. Mullen, R. Anderson, B. S. Schneider, C. M. Happ, and N. S. Zeidner. (2001). *Borrelia lonestari* DNA in adult *Amblyomma americanum* ticks, Alabama. *Emerging Infectious Diseases* **7**:471–473.

CDC. Centers for Disease Control and Prevention. (1998). Summary of notifiable diseases, United States, 1997. *Morbidity and Mortality Weekly Report* **46**(54):1–87.

Chang, C. C., B. B. Chomel, R. W. Kasten, V. Romano, and N. Tietze. (2001). Molecular evidence of *Bartonella* spp. in questing adult *Ixodes pacificus* ticks in California. *Journal of Clinical Microbiology* **39**:1221–1226.

Diamond, J. M. (1975). Assembly of species communities. In M. L. Cody and J. M. Diamond, eds. *Ecology and Evolution of Communities*, pp. 342–444. Harvard University Press, Cambridge, MA.

Dobson, A. P. (1985). The population dynamics of competition between parasites. *Parasitology* **91**:317–347.

Dobson, A. P. and M. Roberts. (1994). The population dynamics of parasitic helminth communities. *Parasitology* **109**:97–108.

Dumler, J. S. and D. H. Walker. (2001). Tick-borne ehrlichioses. *Lancet Supplement* **S**:21–28.

Esch, G., A. Bush, and J. Aho. (1990). *Parasite Communities: Patterns and Processes*. Chapman and Hall, New York.

Ewald, P. (1987). Transmission modes and evolution of the parasitism-mutualism continuum. *Annals of the New York Academy of Sciences* **503**:295–306.

Ewing, S. A., J. E. Dawson, R. J. Panciera, J. S. Mathew, K. W. Pratt, P. Katavolos *et al.* (1997). Dogs infected with a human granulocytotropic *Ehrlichia* spp. (Rickettsiales: Ehrlichieae). *Journal of Medical Entomology* **34**:710–718.

Feng, Z. L. and J. X. Velasco-Hernandez. (1997). Competitive exclusion in a vector-host model for the Dengue fever. *Journal of Mathematical Biology* **35**:523– 544.

Fingerle, V., U. G. Munderloh, G. Liegl, and B. Wilske. (1999). Coexistence of ehrlichiae of the phagocytophila group with *Borrelia burgdorferi* in *Ixodes ricinus* from South Germany. *Medical Microbiology and Immunology* **188**:145–149.

Fuqua, C., M. Parsek, and E. P. Greenberg. (2001). Regulation of gene expression by cell-to-cell communication: acyl-homoserine lactone quorum sensing. *Annual Review of Genetics* **35**:439–468.

Gage, K. L., R. S. Ostfeld, and J. G. Olson. (1995). Nonviral vector-borne zoonoses associated with mammals in the United States. *Journal of Mammalogy* **76**:695–715.

Gherna, R. L., J. H. Werren, W. Weisburg, R. Cote, C. R. Woese, L. Mandelco *et al.* (1991). *Arsenophonus nasoniae* gen. nov., sp. nov., the causative agent of the son-killer trait in the parasitic wasp *Nasonia vitripennis*. *International Journal of Systematic Bacteriology* **41**:563–565.

Gotelli, N. J. (2000). Null model analysis of species co-occurrence patterns. *Ecology* **81**:2606–2621.

Gotelli, N. J. and K. Rohde. (2002). Co-occurrence of ectoparasites of marine fishes: a null model analysis. *Ecology Letters* **5**:86–94.

Gotelli, N. J. and G. L. Entsminger. (2003). EcoSim: null models software for ecology. Version 7:available http://homepages.together.net/~gentsmin/ecosim.htm.

Grindle, N., J. J. Tyner, K. Clay, and C. Fuqua. (2003). Identification of *Arsenophonus*-type bacteria from the dog tick *Dermacentor variabilis*. *Journal of Invertebrate Pathology* **83**:264–266.

Herwaldt, B. L., D. H. Pershing, E. A. Precigout *et al.* (1996). A fatal case of babesiosis in Missouri: identification of another piroplasm that infects humans. *Annals of Internal Medicine* **124**:643–665.

Hofmeister, E. K., C. P. Kolbert, A. S. Abdulkarim, J. M. H. Magera, M. K. Hopkins, J. R. Uhl *et al.* (1998). Cosegregation of a novel *Bartonella* species with *Borrelia burgdorferi* and *Babesia microti* in *Peromyscus leucopus*. *Journal of Infectious Diseases* **177**:409–416.

Holmes, J. C. and P. W. Price. (1986). Communities of parasites. In D. J. Anderson and J. Kikkawa, eds. *Community Ecology: Patterns and Processes*, pp. 187–213. Blackwell Scientific, Oxford, England.

Hoogstraal, H. (1979). The epidemiology of tick-borne Crimean-Congo hemorrhagic fever in Asia, Europe and Africa. *Journal of Medical Entomology* **15**:307–417.

Hubbell, S. P. (2001). *The Unified Neutral Theory of Biodiversity and Biogeography*. Princeton University Press, Princeton, NJ.

Hugenholz, P., B. M. Goebel, and N. R. Pace. (1998). Impact of culture-independent studies on the emerging phylogenetic view of bacterial diversity. *Journal of Bacteriology* **180**:4765–4774.

Karabatsos, N. (1985). International catalogue of arboviruses including certain other viruses of vertebrates, 3rd edition. American Society of Tropical Medicine and Hygiene, San Antonio.

Kordick, S. K., E. B. Breitschwerdt, B. C. Hegarty, K. L. Southwick, C. M. Colitz, S. I. Hancock *et al.* (1999). Coinfection with multiple tick-borne pathogens in a Walker Hound kennel in North Carolina. *Journal of Clinical Microbiology* **37**:2631–2638.

Kover, P. X. and K. Clay. (1998). Trade-off between virulence and vertical transmission and the maintenance of a virulent plant pathogen. *American Naturalist* **152**:165–175.

Kuris, A. M. and K. D. Lafferty. (1994). Community structure: larval trematodes in snail hosts. *Annual Review of Ecology and Systematics* **25**:189–217.

Lafferty, K. D., D.T. Sammond, and A.M. Kuris. (1994). Analysis of larval trematode communities. *Ecology* **75**:2275–2285.

Lane, R. S. (1994). Competence of ticks as vectors of microbial agents with an emphasis on *Borrelia burgdorferi*. In D. E. Sonenshine and T. N. Mather, eds. *Ecological Dynamics of Tick-Borne Zoonoses*, pp. 45–67. Oxford University Press, New York.

Leutenegger, C. M., N. Pusterla, C. N. Mislin, R. Weber, and H. Lutz. (1999). Molecular evidence of coinfection of ticks with *Borrelia burgdorferi* sensu late and the human granulocytic ehrlichiosis agent in Switzerland. *Journal of Clinical Microbiology* **37**:3390–3391.

Levin, M. L. and D. Fish. (2000). Acquisition of coinfection and simultaneous transmission of *Borrelia burgdorferi* and *Ehrlichia phagocytophila* by *Ixodes scapularis* ticks. *Infection and Immunity* **68**:2183–2186.

Lipsitch, M., S. Siller, and M. A. Nowak. (1996). The evolution of virulence in pathogens with vertical and horizontal transmission. *Evolution* **50**:1729–1741.

Little, S. E., D. E. Stallknecht, J. M. Lockhart, J. E. Dawson, and W. R. Davidson. (1998). Natural coinfection of a white-tailed deer (*Odocoileus virginianus*) population with three *Ehrlichia* spp. *Journal of Parasitology* **84**:897–901.

Lively, C. M., K. Clay, M. J. Wade, and C. Fuqua. (2005). Competitive coexistence of vertically and horizontally transmitted parasites. *Evolutionary Ecology Research* (in press, available on-line).

Lockhart, J. M., W. R. Davidson, D. E. Stallknecht, J. E. Dawson, and E. W. Howerth. (1997). Isolation of *Ehrlichia chaffeensis* from wild white-tailed deer (*Odocoileus virginiainus*). *Journal of Clinical Microbiology* **35**:1681–1686.

Macaluso, K. R., D. E. Sonenshine, S. M. Ceraul, and A. F. Azad. (2002). Rickettsial infection in *Dermocentor variabilis* (Acari:Ixodidae) inhibits transovarial transmission of a second *Rickettsia*. *Journal of Medical Entomology* **39**:809–813.

Marchesi, J. R., Sato, T., Weightman, A. J., Fry, J. C., and Hiom, S. J. (1998). Design and evaluation of useful bacterial-specific PCR primers that amplify genes coding for bacterial 16s rRNA. *Applied and Environmental Microbiology* **64**:795–799.

Marsh, T. L. (1999). Terminal restriction fragment length polymorphism (T-RFLP): an emerging method for characterizing diversity among homologous populations of amplification products. *Current Opinions in Microbiology* **2**:323–327.

Mather, T. N. Riberiro, J. M. C., and Spielman, A. (1987). Lyme disease and babesiosis: acaricide focused on potentially infected ticks. *American Journal of Tropical Medicine and Hygiene* **36**:609–614.

McDade, J. E. (1990). Ehrlichiosis, a disease of animals and humans. *Journal of Infections Diseases* **161**:609–617.

McKenzie, F. E. and W. H. Bossert. (1997). Mixed-species *Plasmodium* infections of humans. *Journal of Parasitology* **83**:593–600.

McKenzie, F. E. and W. H. Bossert. (1999). Multispecies *Plasmodium* infections of humans. *Journal of Parasitology* **85**:12–18.

Mitchell, P. D., K. D. Reed, and J. M. Hofkes. (1996). Immunoserologic evidence of coinfection with *Borrelia burgdorferi*, *Babesia microti* and human granulocytic *Ehrlichia* species in residents of Wisconsin and Minnesota. *Journal of Clinical Microbiology* **34**:724–727.

Niebylski, M. L., M. G. Peacock, E. R. Fischer, S. F. Porcella, and T. G. Schwan. (1997a). Characterization of an endosymbiont infecting wood ticks, *Dermacentor andersoni*, as a member of the genus *Francisella*. *Applied and Environmental Microbiology* **63**:3393–3940.

Niebylski, M. L., M. E. Schrumpf, W. Burgdorfer, E. R. Fischer, K. L. Gage, and T. G. Schwan. (1997b). *Rickettsia peacockii* sp. nov., a new species infecting wood ticks, *Dermacentor andersoni*, in western Montana. *International Journal of Systematic Bacteriology* **47**:446–452.

Niebylski, M. L., M. G. Peacock, and T. G. Schwan. (1999). Lethal effect of *Rickettsia rickettsii* on its tick vector (*Dermacentor andersoni*). *Applied and Environmental Microbiology* **65**:773–778.

Noda, H., U. G. Munderloh, and T. J. Kurtti. (1997). Endosymbionts of ticks and their relationship to *Wolbachia* spp. and tick-borne pathogens of humans and animals. *Applied and Environmental Microbiology* **63**:3926–3932.

Ostfeld, R. S. (1997). The ecology of Lyme disease risk. *American Scientist* **85**:338–346.

Parola, P. and R. Didier. (2001). Ticks and tickborne bacterial diseases in humans: an emerging infectious threat. *Clinical Infectious Diseases* **32**:897–928.

Petney, T. N. and R. H. Andrews. (1998). Multiparasite communities in animals and humans: frequency, structure and pathogenic significance. *International Journal of Parasitology* **28**:377–393.

Philip, R. N., E. A. Casper, R. A. Ormsbee, M. G. Peacock, and W. Burgdorfer. (1976). Microimmuno-fluorescence test for the serological study of Rocky Mountain spotted fever and typhus. *Journal of Clinical Microbiology* **3**:51–61.

Piesman, J. and C. M. Happ. (2001). The efficacy of co-feeding as a means of maintaining *Borrelia burgdorferi*: a North American model system. *Journal of Vector Ecology* **26**:216–220.

Poulin, R. (1997). Species richness of parasite assemblages: evolution and patterns. *Annual Review of Ecology and Systematics* **28**:341–358.

Price, W. H. (1953). Interference phenomenon in animal infections with rickettsiae of Rocky Mountain spotted fever. *Proceedings of the Society for Experimental Biology and Medicine* **82**:180–184.

Richie, T. L. (1988). Interactions between malaria parasites infecting the same vertebrate host. *Parasitology* **96**:607–639.

Ricklefs R. E. and J. Travis. (1980). A morphological approach to the study of avian community organization. *The Auk* **97**:321–338.

Rikihisa, Y. (1991). The tribe Ehrlichieae and ehrlichial diseases. *Clinical Microbiology Reviews* **4**:286–308.

Rolain, J. M., F. Gouriet, P. Brouqui, D. Larrey, F. Janbon, S. Vene *et al.* (2005). Concomitant or consecutive infection with *Coxiella burnetii* and tickborne diseases. *Clinical Infectious Diseases* **40**:82–88.

Rondon, M. R., P. R. August, A. D. Bettermann, S. F. Brady, T. H. Grossman *et al.* (2000). Cloning the soil metagenome: a strategy for accessing the genetic and functional diversity of uncultured microorganisms. *Applied and Environmental Microbiology* **66**:2541–2547.

Sauer, J. R., J. L. McSwain, A. S. Bowman, and R. C. Essenberg. (1995). Tick salivary gland physiology. *Annual Review of Entomology* **40**:245–267.

Schabereiter-Gurtner, C., W. Lubitz, and S. Rolleke. (2003). Application of broad-range 16S rRNA PCR amplification and DGGE fingerprinting for detection of tick-infecting bacteria. *Journal of Microbiological Methods* **52**:251–260.

Schauber, E. M., S. J. Gertz, W. T. Maple, and R. S. Ostfeld. (1998). Coinfection with blacklegged ticks (*Acari:Ixodidae*) in Dutchess County, New York, with agents of Lyme disease and human granulocytic ehrlichiosis. *Journal of Medical Entomology* **35**:901–903.

Schouls, L. M., I. van De Pol, G. T. Rijpkema, and C. S. Schot. (1999). Detection and identification of *Ehrlichia*, *Borrelia burgdorferi* sensu lato, and *Bartonella* species in Dutch *Ixodes ricinus* ticks. *Journal of Clinical Microbiology* **37**:2215–2222.

Schoener, T.W. (1984). Size differences among sympatric, bird-eating hawks: a world-wide survey. In D. R. Strong, D. Simberloff, L. G. Abele, and A. B. Thistle, eds. *Ecological Communities: Conceptual Issues and the Evidence*, pp. 254–281. Princeton University Press, Princeton, NJ.

Smith, G., M-G Basanez, K. Dietz, M. A. Gemmel, B. T. Grefell, F. M. D Gulland *et al.* (1995). Macroparasite group report: problems in modeling the dynamics of macroparasite systems. In B. T. Grenfell and A. P. Dobson, eds. *Ecology of Infectious Diseases in Natural Populations.*, pp. 209–229. Cambridge University Press, Cambridge.

Sonenshine, D. E. (1991). *Biology of Ticks*, Vol. 1, 447 pp. New York: Oxford University Press.

Sonenshine, D. E. and T. N. Mather, eds. (1994). *Ecological Dynamics of Tick-Borne Zoonoses*. Oxford University Press, New York.

Sparagano, O. A. E., M. Allsopp, R. A. Mank, S. G. T. Rijpkema, J. V. Figueroa, and F. Jongejan. (1999). Molecular detection of pathogen DNA in ticks (Acari : Ixodidae): a review. *Experimental and Applied Acarology* **23**:929–960.

Stahl, D. A. (1995). Application of phylogenetically base hybridization probes to microbial ecology. *Molecular Ecology* **4**:535–542.

Steere, A. C., S. E. Malawista, D. R. Snydman, R. E. Shope, W. A. Andiman, M. R. Ross *et al.* (1977). Lyme Arthritis: an epidemic of oligoarticular arthritis in children and adults in three Connecticut communities. *Arthritis and Rheumatism* **20**:7–17.

Strong, D. R., L. A. Szyska, and D. Simberloff. (1979). Tests of community-wide character displacement against null hypotheses. *Evolution* **33**:897–913.

Sun, L. V., G. A. Scoles, D. Fish, and S. L. O'Neill. (2000). *Francisella*-like endosymbionts of ticks. *Journal of Invertebrate Pathology* **76**:301–303.

Tanaka, M. M. and M. W. Feldman. (1999). Theoretical considerations of cross-immunity, recombination and the evolution of new parasitic strains. *Journal of Theoretical Biology* **198**:145–163.

van Borm, S., A. Buschinger, J. J. Boomsma, and J. Billen. (2002). *Tetraponera* ants have gut symbionts related to nitrogen-fixing root-nodule bacteria. *Proceedings of the Royal Society of London B* **269**:2023–2027.

Van Buskirk, J. and R. S. Ostfeld. (1995). Controlling Lyme disease by modifying density and species composition of tick hosts. *Ecological Applications* **5**:1133–1140.

Varde, S., J. Beckley, and I. Schwartz. (1998). Prevalence of tick-borne pathogens in *Ixodes scapularis* in a rural New Jersey county. *Emerging Infectious Diseases* **4**:97–99.

Wormser, G. P., H. W. Horowitz, J. Nowakowski, D. McKenna, J. S. Dumler, S. Varde *et al.* (1997). Positive Lyme disease serology in patients with clinical and laboratory evidence of human granulocytic ehrlichiosis. *American Journal of Clinical Pathology* **107**:142–147.

Zeidner, N. S., T. R. Burkot, R. Massung, W. L. Nicholson, M. C. Dolan, J. S. Rutherford *et al.* (2000). Transmission of the agent of human granulocytic ehrlichiosis by *Ixodes spinipalpis* ticks: evidence of an enzootic cycle of dual infection with *Borrelia burgdorferi* in northern Colorado. *Journal of Infectious Diseases* **182**:616–619.

CHAPTER 5

Disease dynamics in plant communities

Charles E. Mitchell and Alison G. Power

5.1 Introduction

Mounting evidence indicates that plant pathogens can influence the population density, genetic structure, and spatial structure of their hosts (Gilbert 2002). At the same time, it is increasingly clear that the spread of plant pathogens is influenced not only by the density, genetic structure, and spatial structure of single-species host populations, but also by the structure of entire communities. Together, such reciprocal effects between plant and pathogen populations create the potential for dynamic feedbacks between the spread of plant pathogens and the structure of ecological communities. This chapter focuses on these feedbacks and the mechanisms that may drive them. To set the stage for summarizing such feedbacks, we first separately review recent evidence for effects of plant community structure on pathogen spread, and effects of pathogens on plant community structure. In each case, specialist and generalist pathogens (here defined as infecting one versus multiple species within a focal host community) are seen to produce contrasting dynamics. We also extend this community-level framework for plant–pathogen interactions to include other species in the biotic community, such as herbivores and microbial symbionts.

Why focus on plant pathogens? First, plants play a fundamental role in communities, as the primary producers on which most other organisms and ecological processes ultimately depend. This fundamental role of plants suggests that plant pathogens may have impacts that reverberate through entire communities. For example, the structure of plant communities, particularly their

species composition and diversity, can control aspects of ecosystem functioning (Loreau *et al.* 2001; Tilman *et al.* 2002; van Ruijven and Berendse 2003), so pathogens may influence ecosystem functioning through their impacts on plant community structure.

Second, plant–pathogen interactions provide excellent model systems for understanding general principles in disease ecology (Antonovics *et al.* 2002). They are ideal for directly testing theory about the effects of host community structure on pathogen spread, because host community structure can be readily manipulated on relevant spatial scales in the field (Mitchell *et al.* 2002; Mitchell *et al.* 2003; Power and Mitchell 2004). The presence or abundance of plant pathogens can also be manipulated in the field (Paul *et al.* 1989; Mitchell 2003; Power and Mitchell 2004), although typically this is more logistically challenging than manipulations of their plant hosts. A great strength of disease ecology to date is that theoretical and empirical progress have been tightly linked (Grenfell and Dobson 1995; Hudson *et al.* 2002; Dwyer *et al.* 2004). However, because of the relatively large spatial scale and mobility of many wildlife populations, independently manipulating multiple species in a community will often be impractical. Although other tools such as analysis of long-time series and parameterization of theoretical models can still provide direct tests of theory (Begon *et al.* 1999; Gilbert *et al.* 2001; Tompkins *et al.* 2003), experimentation is the most rigorous approach for understanding causality in complex feedbacks between hosts and pathogens. Thus, the potential to independently manipulate dozens of plant species on the spatial scale of several square meters provides an excellent opportunity to understand the dynamics of feedbacks between communities of hosts and pathogens.

What pathogens infect plants? There are over 10,000 named species of plant pathogens (Agrios 2004), but this is almost certainly an underestimate by at least an order of magnitude. For comparison, there are 250,000 species of vascular plants to serve as potential hosts (Whitton and Rajakaruna 2001). Plant pathogens are phylogenetically diverse as well, including fungi, viruses, bacteria, nematodes, and protists. Over three-quarters of known plant pathogens are fungi, but they have probably been more completely enumerated because they are typically more visually obvious.

Many, probably most, plant species are susceptible to infection by multiple pathogen species (Farr *et al.* 1989). The limited available theory, largely developed for animal hosts, suggests that specialist pathogen community structure and diversity will depend on host population density (Dobson 1990), and thus perhaps host community structure. However, there is a striking paucity of empirical studies that consider interactions among multiple pathogens infecting wild plant populations.

Plant pathogens have long been studied primarily because of their impact on agricultural production. Even with current efforts to control them, they reduce global crop production by approximately one-sixth, roughly equal to the respective impacts of herbivores and weeds (Oerke *et al.* 1994). Although crop diseases have been known since at least the time of the ancient Greeks (Agrios 2004), a substantial factor in their recent large impact is undoubtedly the common practice of growing crops as monocultures, often genetic monocultures. As a result, since the start of the green revolution over forty years ago, there has been rising interest in increasing diversity within cropping systems. This interest has led to the development of conceptual frameworks and an extensive body of empirical tests of the spread of plant pathogens in diverse host populations (Power 1987, 1991; Boudreau and Mundt 1997; Garrett and Mundt 1999; Zhu *et al.* 2000; Mundt 2002). While this interest in diversity was largely inspired by observations of natural plant communities, there have been few experimental tests of these processes in complex natural communities.

One major simplification in agricultural systems is that there is little potential for long-term feedbacks from pathogens to host population dynamics because the host population is directly controlled by humans. This has allowed models of disease in agricultural systems to assume that host abundance is not a dynamic variable (van der Plank 1963; Leonard 1969; Jeger *et al.* 1981; Garrett and Mundt 1999; Segarra *et al.* 2001). Because of such differences between agricultural and unmanaged systems, and because the spread of disease in agricultural mixtures has recently been reviewed (Mundt 2002), we focus here on disease in unmanaged plant communities. We note, however, that studies of unmanaged communities would be much more difficult were it not for the conceptual and methodological developments inspired by studies of crop pathogens. In particular, numerous studies show that the diversity and composition of crops both influence, and can be affected by, the spread of plant pathogens (Power 1987, 1990, 1991; Boudreau and Mundt 1997; Garrett and Mundt 1999; Zhu *et al.* 2000; Mundt 2002). These are the agricultural roots of plant community epidemiology.

5.2 Plant community effects on pathogens

Species richness (the number of species present) and species composition (the identity of species present) are two characteristics of plant communities that are likely to influence the spread of pathogens. The potential for species richness and composition to influence disease arises from the fact that species inherently vary in characteristics that influence disease dynamics. The greater the extent of such functional variation among species in a community, the greater is the potential for strong effects of species richness and composition (Tilman and Lehman 2002).

Many characteristics that vary among plant species—from defensive compounds to photosynthetic pathway to architecture to phenology—might influence pathogen spread either directly or indirectly. Surprisingly little work has examined variation among wild plant species in components of pathogen transmission such as susceptibility or infectiousness (Box 5.1). In a recent exception, a

Box 5.1 Transmission of fungi and viruses in diverse plant communities

Transmission of plant pathogens is necessarily a multistage process, which can be broadly divided into pre-dispersal events (production and liberation of propagules from an infected host), dispersal events (movement and survival of propagules), and post-dispersal events (survival and infection of a susceptible host). While all of these components are well studied in various crop-pathogen systems (McCartney 1997; Jones 1998; Garrett and Mundt 1999; Aylor 2003; Gray and Gildow 2003), they are likely to operate differently in species-rich, unmanaged plant communities (Boudreau and Mundt 1997; Garrett and Mundt 1999). Additionally, for a given plant pathogen, each stage is likely to depend on the species composition of the host community because host species will likely vary in traits influencing each component of transmission. The limited theory available on multi-host pathogen systems suggests that correlations among host species in their effects on these various components can strongly influence disease dynamics (Jeger *et al*. 1981; Garrett and Mundt 1999), and that transmission of specialist pathogens can be highly sensitive to the identity of non-host species in the community (Boudreau and Mundt 1997). Moreover, for most pathogens, each stage of the transmission process is highly dependent on abiotic conditions (McCartney 1997) and perhaps on interactions with other species, particularly vectors (Power and Gray 1995; Gray and Gildow 2003). This creates an enormous number of factors that could potentially control transmission processes, raising the question of which are essential for understanding particular systems. Notably, in the vast majority of agricultural studies, the details of transmission are not explicitly considered, and the simplifying assumption is made that observed patterns of disease prevalence or severity reflect the process of transmission.

More mechanistically, Garrett and Mundt (1999) have developed a conceptual framework for disease spread in genetically diverse crop populations, which we summarize here and seek to extend to unmanaged, multispecies communities. They conclude that five major traits of plant-pathogen systems should contribute to reduce spread of disease in more species-rich populations. Adapting their terminology for unmanaged multispecies communities, those traits are: (1) small contiguous area of each host species or small plant size; (2) shallow pathogen dispersal gradient; (3) small pathogen lesion size or large pathogen carrying capacity; (4) short pathogen generation time; and (5) strong host specialization by the pathogen. They also conclude that disease spread will depend on host species composition if plants vary in traits such as competitive ability and potential for compensatory growth. Finally, they argue that the importance of these various traits will vary among systems and among environments, for example, depending on whether climate is favorable to epidemic development, and whether epidemics in the focal populations are driven by inoculum from distant populations. Garrett and Mundt (1999) did not try to incorporate vector-transmitted pathogens into their framework. For vector-transmitted pathogens, vector behavior is likely to be a key control on pathogen transmission (Power 1991; Power and Gray 1995; Gray and Gildow 2003). For example, strong host specialization by a vector might substitute for pathogen specialization as a contributor to reduced disease spread in more diverse populations. For directly transmitted pathogens, the factors outlined by Garrett and Mundt (1999) provide the best starting point for a mechanistic understanding of the processes controlling pathogen transmission in species-diverse plant communities.

study of 18 wild clover species in California found that species with larger leaves retained more water on the surface, and species with greater water retention were more susceptible to infection by a generalist foliar fungal pathogen (Bradley *et al.* 2003). This study provides unusual mechanistic insight into sources of among-species variation in pathogen susceptibility. Having documented this variation at the species level, it would be interesting to see if this allows prediction of processes at the community level, e.g., how the richness and composition of communities of clover influence

spread of the shared pathogen, and how those processes vary along moisture gradients.

5.2.1 Specialist pathogens

For pathogens specialized on one or a few host species within a community, decreased species richness in that community is predicted to increase spread of directly transmitted pathogens (Leonard 1969; Burdon and Chilvers 1976; Chapin *et al.* 1997; Garrett and Mundt 1999). The primary hypothesized mechanism is that decreased species richness decreases competition for resources among the remaining species, allowing them to increase in abundance, on average (Burdon and Chilvers 1976; Boudreau and Mundt 1997; Chapin *et al.* 1997). In turn, increased abundance of those species increases disease transmission of their specialized pathogens by decreasing the average distance between host individuals (Burdon and Chilvers 1982; Gilbert 2002). Vector transmission may complicate this expectation by partially decoupling transmission rate from inter-host distance (e.g. Power 1990; Antonovics and Alexander 1992). While this long-standing hypothesis is supported by numerous tests with highly specialized pathogens of individual crop genotypes (Mundt 2002), whether the same process occurs in species-diverse unmanaged plant communities has only recently been tested experimentally.

In two field experiments with perennial grassland species in Minnesota, decreased plant richness increased pathogen load of foliar fungi (percentage of leaf area infected across the plant community) (Mitchell *et al.* 2002, 2003). In both experiments, pathogen load was nearly three times as high in monocultures than in communities of approximately natural species richness (i.e. 16–24 species). Species richness was manipulated directly by seeding plots with randomly chosen species numbers, then removing unplanted species by hand-weeding. Most individual diseases followed the same pattern as at the community level in that they were more severe in less species-rich plant communities. As predicted by theory, change in the relative abundance of individual host species was the chief mechanism for the effects of species richness on disease. Decreasing species richness increased transmission of individual diseases that persisted in the community by allowing their host species to increase in abundance.

When plant species richness changes through species loss or introduction, the species composition of the community necessarily changes as well. Thus, it is important to separate the effects of composition and richness. In the two experiments in Minnesota, species composition and richness both independently influenced pathogen load (Mitchell *et al.* 2002, 2003). Species composition more strongly influenced pathogen load than did

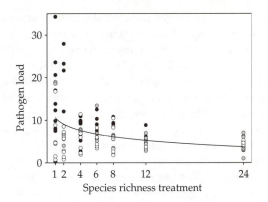

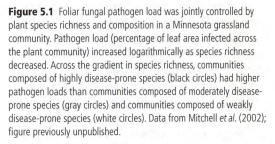

Figure 5.1 Foliar fungal pathogen load was jointly controlled by plant species richness and composition in a Minnesota grassland community. Pathogen load (percentage of leaf area infected across the plant community) increased logarithmically as species richness decreased. Across the gradient in species richness, communities composed of highly disease-prone species (black circles) had higher pathogen loads than communities composed of moderately disease-prone species (gray circles) and communities composed of weakly disease-prone species (white circles). Data from Mitchell *et al.* (2002); figure previously unpublished.

richness. In this case, species composition was quantified functionally in terms of the constituent species' disease proneness, or their percentage of leaf area infected in the most species-rich communities. Across the gradient in species richness, communities comprised of more disease-prone species had heavier pathogen loads and communities of less disease-prone species had lighter pathogen loads (Fig. 5.1), reflecting the joint control of pathogen load by species composition and richness. However, in contrast to the effects of plant species richness, the spread of individual diseases was not strongly influenced by community composition. Thus, the effect of species composition at the community level resulted not from an effect of species composition on transmission, but simply from the presence or absence of disease-prone host species and their associated pathogens.

5.2.2 Generalist pathogens

Several bodies of theory predict that the spread of generalist plant pathogens can be influenced by host community richness, but that this will depend critically on species composition. Theory developed for directly transmitted crop pathogens predicts that decreased richness can increase or decrease spread of generalist pathogens, depending on host species composition, particularly differences in resistance traits among hosts (Jeger *et al.* 1981; Garrett and Mundt 1999). Experimental tests with directly transmitted generalist crop pathogens have generally found weak, inconsistent reductions of disease at higher richness (Mundt 2002), perhaps because effects of richness are overridden by composition. Two more general theoretical investigations both recently concluded that decreased richness was more likely to decrease establishment of directly transmitted generalist pathogens and increase establishment of vector-transmitted generalist pathogens (Holt *et al.* 2003; Dobson 2004). Further, these two studies predict that the effects of richness depend on species composition, particularly host species' effects on the pathogen population (and the vector population in the vector-transmitted case).

Pathogen spillover among host species is thought to be one mechanism for effects of species composition on generalist pathogens. Pathogen spillover occurs when a pathogen population builds up in a highly susceptible host population, then is transmitted from individuals in that population to individuals in a more resistant host population (Daszak *et al.* 2000; Dobson 2004; Power and Mitchell 2004). Spillover results from asymmetries in transmission rates among species. It is thus predicted to be a common feature of generalist pathogens in communities including multiple host species because host species almost inevitably vary in key epidemiological traits that can generate such asymmetries (Woolhouse *et al.* 2001; Bradley *et al.* 2003; Holt *et al.* 2003; Dobson 2004; Power and Mitchell 2004). Spillover has been reported for numerous pathogens, but most examples center on domesticated populations, and the process has rarely been examined experimentally (Daszak *et al.* 2000; Power and Mitchell 2004).

In an experiment in 1999 with annual wild grasses in central New York State, community prevalence (percentage of individuals infected) of a generalist aphid-vectored virus was controlled by species composition, but not by species richness (Power and Mitchell 2004). Communities that contained one species previously identified as highly susceptible to the virus, *Avena fatua* (wild oats), were over 10 times more heavily infected than communities

lacking *Avena*. These results suggest that host species richness was a less important factor in pathogen spread than species composition, particularly the presence of a highly susceptible species. High community virus prevalence resulted in part from the high rate of infections in the population of *Avena* itself, but also—and more interestingly—because *Avena*'s presence increased prevalence in more resistant host populations through pathogen spillover. Spillover from *Avena* to some species was very strong—for example, presence of *Avena* in the community increased virus prevalence in *Setaria lutescens* (yellow foxtail) by about an order of magnitude (Power and Mitchell 2004).

To further investigate the dynamics and consequences of pathogen spillover, we conducted an additional experiment in 2001 in which *Avena* presence was factorially manipulated with virus presence and nitrogen addition. *Avena* presence increased virus prevalence across the rest of the community (three other species) by 60% (Fig. 5.2) (Power and Mitchell 2004). As a result of pathogen spillover, aboveground primary production was lower in communities that included *Avena* and that were inoculated with the virus (Mitchell and Power, *unpublished data*).

These experiments support the view that the spread of generalist pathogens is crucially dependent on host community species composition. The

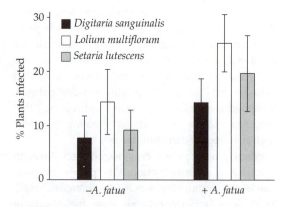

Figure 5.2 Virus prevalence across *D. sanguinalis* (black bars), *L. multiflorum* (white bars), and *S. lutescens* (gray bars) in experimental communities planted with *A. fatua* or lacking *A. fatua* in 2001. The presence of *A. fatua* increased virus prevalence across the other three species (*P* < 0.05), demonstrating pathogen spillover. Data shown are means ± SE. Redrawn from Power and Mitchell (2004).

epidemiology of generalist pathogens is inherently a community-level process—understanding disease dynamics in any host population, especially non-reservoir species, requires knowledge of disease dynamics in other host populations. Pathogen prevalence in a population is a function not just of factors intrinsic to a focal host population, such as genetically based resistance, physiological stress, and population abundance, but of the community context in which host and pathogen are embedded.

In complement to these few highly controlled experiments with annual grasses, many non-manipulative studies of generalist forest pathogens have revealed a strong dependence of disease dynamics on landscape-scale variation in plant community structure. For example, sudden oak death disease, caused by the protist *Phytophthora ramorum*, is of current public concern primarily because of its devastating effects on canopy trees, especially oaks (*Quercus* spp.) and tanoaks (*Lithocarpus densiflora*) in coastal forests of California and Oregon (Rizzo and Garbelotto 2003). Tanoaks appear capable of sustaining epidemics themselves, probably because the pathogen can infect almost any part of a tanoak, from leaves to trunk (Rizzo and Garbelotto 2003). However, the best biological predictor of disease-induced mortality of oaks across a California landscape was abundance of an understory shrub, bay laurel (*Umbellularia californica*) (Kelly and Meentemeyer 2002). Preliminary evidence suggests that bay laurel drives epidemics in oak populations (Rizzo and Garbelotto 2003; Meentemeyer *et al.* 2004; Davidson *et al.* 2005). The pathogen infects laurel leaves, where it can produce many spores, apparently without greatly increasing mortality. In contrast, oak infections are limited to the trunk and branches, which can girdle and kill trees, but produce no spores for further transmission (Davidson *et al.* 2005). Thus, variation in tolerance to the negative effects of disease, not just susceptibility to infection, can drive pathogen spillover. As a result, conservation of these endangered forests may hinge on understanding the community epidemiology of sudden oak death.

The sudden oak death pathogen appears to have been recently introduced to the United States, perhaps from Asia, although its native range remains undetermined (Ivors *et al.* 2004). Introduction of

species to new ranges is one of the most pervasive impacts of human activities on ecological communities. While some of the most devastating invaders are plant pathogens (Anderson *et al.* 2004), these introductions may be something of an exception to the rule. On average, when plant species are introduced to new habitats, surveys of host–pathogen associations indicate that they leave the vast majority of their pathogens behind (Wolfe 2002; Mitchell and Power 2003; Torchin and Mitchell 2004). Because most ecological communities are rapidly accumulating introduced plant species, the escape of introduced species from pathogens has important ramifications at the community level. It implies that species introductions are lowering the ratio of pathogen species to plant species within communities. This estimation needs further examination with data from the field, but if true, it may reduce the potential for the rich array of ecological effects of plant pathogens, to which we will now turn.

5.3 Impacts of pathogens on plant communities

In a recent review of plant pathogens in natural ecosystems, Gilbert (2002) concluded that pathogens can drive density-dependent plant population dynamics, cause rapid evolution in plant populations, mediate plant competition, accelerate plant community succession, and help maintain plant species diversity (e.g. Burdon 1991; Bever *et al.* 1997; Van der Putten and Peters 1997; Alexander and Mihail 2000; Packer and Clay 2000). We focus here on impacts of pathogens that were not emphasized in this and previous reviews (Augspurger 1987; Burdon 1987; Kranz 1990; Burdon 1991; Alexander 1992; Dickman 1992; Jarosz and Davelos 1995; Alexander and Holt 1998). In particular, most research on plant pathogens in natural communities, and thus most reviews of this topic, have focused on their evolutionary ecology (Gilbert 2002), rather than on processes operating at the community level.

5.3.1 Specialist pathogens

Specialist pathogens can influence community structure by decreasing the abundance of their host species, particularly if the host species is a dominant member of the community when relatively free of disease. Such effects of pathogens can be revealed by changes in other ecological processes. For example, global change may alter plant–pathogen interactions in ways that could fundamentally re-shape plant communities. Perhaps

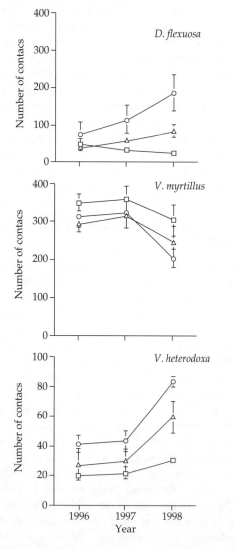

Figure 5.3 Vegetation responses to the three nitrogen treatments in a Swedish boreal forest (squares, control; triangles, 12.5 kg N ha^{-1} year^{-1}; circles, 50 kg N ha^{-1} year^{-1}) over the 3 years in terms of the abundance of *D. flexuosa*, *V. myrtillus* and disease prevalence of *V. heterodoxa* on *V. myrtillus* leaves. Vertical bars denote ± 1 SE (n = 6), where large enough to be visible. Reprinted from Strengbom *et al.* (2002).

the best example of this potential to date is a series of studies examining the effects of nitrogen deposition on the understory vegetation of Swedish forests. Increased rates of fertilizer production and fossil fuel burning result in the volatilization of reactive nitrogen compounds in the atmosphere, where they can be transported for thousands of kilometers (Vitousek *et al.* 1997; Galloway and Cowling 2002; Matson *et al.* 2002). In Sweden, the experimental addition of nitrogen nearly quadrupled prevalence of infection of leaves of the shrub *Vaccinium myrtillus* by the fungal pathogen *Valdensia heterodoxa* (Fig. 5.3(c); Strengbom *et al.* 2002). Within 3 years of starting the treatment, *Vaccinium* abundance declined by one-third, and the grass *Deschampsia flexuosa* also nearly quadrupled in abundance in disease foci (Fig. 5.3(b) and (a), respectively; Strengbom *et al.* 2002). A subsequent experiment indicated that this shift in community structure occurred because the disease reduced competition for light from the shrub (Strengbom *et al.* 2004). Furthermore, a national survey of the abundances of the plant species and the pathogen found the same patterns along geographic gradients of nitrogen deposition rate (Strengbom *et al.* 2003). These multiple lines of evidence suggest that increased disease due to nitrogen deposition is causing the conversion of forest understory from shrub-dominated to grass-dominated, a fundamental shift in species composition that could have dramatic impacts on processes from nutrient cycling to animal habitat use.

5.3.2 Generalist pathogens

Several studies of beach dune vegetation have shown that soil organisms, particularly pathogenic nematodes, can accelerate plant community succession by negatively affecting dominant early successional species (de Rooij-van der Goes 1995; Van der Putten and Peters 1997). However, these studies have primarily focused on the population dynamics of a single such species, *Ammophila arenaria* (marram grass). A recent study of grasslands has extended understanding of pathogen effects on plant succession to the community level (De Deyn *et al.* 2003). Inoculating experimental plant communities with soil biota from successional grasslands revealed that the soil microfauna, especially parasitic nematodes, inhibited growth of early- and mid-successional species and facilitated growth of late-successional species, increasing the rate of succession. Also, as a result of suppressing the otherwise dominant early-successional species, inoculation with soil microfauna increased the evenness of the plant community. This study suggests that pathogens may control the tempo of succession, maintain plant diversity, and aid in community restoration.

Aquatic community dynamics can also be driven by pathogens. While almost unstudied until the late 1980s, evidence has since been rapidly accumulating that viruses can control the dynamics of phytoplankton communities in both marine and freshwater systems. Initially, viruses were recognized and manipulated primarily as a filtered size-class, limiting the potential to understand species-level dynamics, but recent methodological advances are beginning to bring them out of the black box (Culley et al. 2003). Viruses can regulate individual phytoplankton populations, and mediate competition among species (Brussaard 2004). In the broader community context, viruses often increase in abundance during phytoplankton blooms, thus accelerating succession of phytoplankton, zooplankton, and bacteria populations (Park et al. 2004). As a result of these activities, aquatic viruses are major regulators of food web structure and nutrient dynamics (Fuhrman 1999; Wilhelm and Suttle 1999).

5.4 Feedbacks between plant and pathogen communities

Given the substantial evidence that plant community structure and pathogen spread can impact one another, we now turn to dynamic feedbacks that can result when such effects occur reciprocally. Several related conceptual models exist for such interactions (Janzen 1970; Connell 1971; Holt and Lawton 1994; Bever 2003). However, empirical work is still limited, perhaps due to the logistical challenges of simultaneously manipulating pathogens and plant community structure. The most venerable conceptual model is the Janzen–Connell hypothesis for the maintenance of

species diversity. The model predicts that specialist natural enemies, including pathogens, act as density-dependent regulators of plant populations, decreasing species dominance and maintaining diversity. Evidence that pathogens can drive Janzen–Connell dynamics in both high diversity tropical forests (the original focus) and other plant communities is substantial (Gilbert 2002).

More recently, Bever (Bever 1994, 2003 Bever et al. 1997) has developed a conceptual and mathematical model for feedbacks between plant species and soil biota, including pathogens. This model assumes that plant species differentially influence the functional composition of the soil biota (e.g. abundances of pathogens versus mutualists), and that plant species respond differentially to changes in the composition of the soil biota (e.g. the relative effects of pathogens and mutualists differ among plant hosts). Thus, local growth of a plant species fosters changes in the soil biota that result in either greater performance (positive feedback) or decreased performance (negative feedback) of that species relative to competitors. Negative feedback is predicted to maintain local species diversity. Available evidence indicates that feedback on plant species' growth is commonly negative, and can be caused by pathogens, but the consequences for community diversity and composition remain largely untested (Bever 2003).

Pathogen spillover (described above) also creates the potential for feedback to host community structure. When pathogen spillover decreases the performance of the focal host population, this is the process of apparent competition (Holt 1977; Holt and Lawton 1994; Alexander and Holt 1998) (Box 5.2). Apparent competition is so called because it is phenomenologically the same as direct competition (one population decreases performance of another), but is mediated by the two populations' interactions with the shared natural enemy (Fig. 5.4), not the mechanisms of direct competition, such as resource reduction. Apparent competition is a positive feedback in that a population can promote its own growth by inhibiting competing populations via their shared enemy, so it has the potential to decrease community diversity. It thus contrasts with the Janzen–Connell hypothesis and Bever's model of plant–soil feedback, both of which

Box 5.2 Detecting apparent competition among plant species

Apparent competition (Holt 1977) is an indirect effect involving at least two host species and one shared enemy (Fig. 5.4). Its magnitude can be estimated through a variety of approaches, all of which have advantages and disadvantages that make them suitable for different study systems and circumstances. First, theoretical models may be used to elucidate apparent competition. Greenman and Hudson (Hudson and Greenman 1998; Greenman and Hudson 2000) have developed an intriguing analytic approach called gateway analysis, which is used to understand the equilibrium dynamics of systems such as multiple-host parasite models that are too algebraically complex for standard mathematical analyses. While promising in its generality, as yet it has been little applied. A more common method is to develop a dynamic model of the interacting species and parameterize it with data from the field, literature, inoculation experiments, or a combination thereof (Gilbert *et al*. 2001; Tompkins *et al*. 2003). A major advantage of this approach is its ability to predict the equilibrium outcome of the interaction, but it is limited by the assumption that dynamics of the system are driven solely by the species in the model (typically just two hosts and one parasite). In systems with long-term observational time series data, temporal correlations among host abundances and prevalences can be used to infer the importance of apparent competition and other forms of interaction (Begon *et al*. 1999). This approach is strong in that it integrates all interactions operating within the community, but difficult to implement because few studies have been run for sufficiently long periods to generate the required data.

Finally, there are numerous experimental approaches to test for apparent competition, which generally involve independent manipulations of apparent competition and direct competition. First, when one host species is suspected to be the main reservoir for the shared pathogen, its direct and indirect effects on the rest of the host community can be dissected by factorially constructing communities with/without the suspected reservoir species (through selectively removing that species, adding it, or planting communities *de novo*) and with/without the pathogen (Grosholz 1992; Power and Mitchell 2004). The difference in the effect of the reservoir on the other host species with and without the pathogen is the effect of apparent competition. Smaller-scale field experiments can be used to detect the effects of apparent competition on individual plants of a focal species by planting them with/without neighbors of the hypothesized reservoir species. This approach was recently implemented for salt marsh forbs sharing a beetle herbivore (Rand 2003), and could be applied to pathogens expected to be transmitted chiefly between nearest neighbors, such as many soil pathogens. Both of these approaches only allow assessment of the effects of the hypothesized reservoir species on the others. To elucidate all of the pairwise direct and indirect effects in a community, an appropriate experiment would include monocultures of each species and all possible bicultures, each with/without the shared pathogen. This design would allow collection of data to directly parameterize simple models of apparent competition, and thereby predict the equilibrium outcome. This design could be expanded to a multispecies context using the "combined-monocultures" approach, which can also be further elaborated to partition the effects of direct competition into root and shoot competition (Rajaniemi *et al*. 2003). The combined-monocultures approach would also allow more direct assessment of apparent competition by constructing plots which allowed apparent competition, but not direct competition. In contrast, the previous approaches quantify the magnitude of apparent competition by subtraction. Finally, a simple approach recently employed to detect parasitoid-mediated apparent competition among insects (Morris *et al*. 2004), might also be extended to plants. In this experiment, the only manipulation was experimental removal of the putative reservoir species, the effect of which was interpreted as the effect of apparent competition because the reservoir and focal host were known not to compete directly. In circumstances where two plant species are known not to compete directly (e.g. because of habitat specificity or phenology), this approach could be employed.

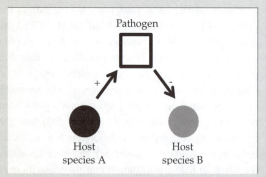

Figure 5.4 Apparent competition in a simple community module consisting of two host species (circles) and a shared pathogen species (square). Here, host species A can indirectly suppress host species B by acting as a reservoir for the shared pathogen.

emphasize negative feedbacks that limit the abundance of individual species, promoting diversity at the community level. However, these theoretical predictions are all for well-mixed or spatially homogenous communities. In spatially heterogeneous habitats, positive feedbacks that operate on a restricted spatial scale can promote diversity at larger spatial scales (Bever *et al.* 1997).

Although apparent competition is predicted to be a common phenomenon (Holt 1977; Holt and Lawton 1994; Alexander and Holt 1998), it has rarely been demonstrated in field experiments (Grosholz 1992; Rand 2003; Morris *et al.* 2004), especially with plant pathogens (Alexander and Holt 1998; Gilbert 2002; Power and Mitchell 2004). A recent field experiment in the Netherlands raised the possibility that parasite-mediated apparent competition can play a key role in community resistance to invasion by introduced species (van Ruijven *et al.* 2003). In an experiment that manipulated the species diversity and composition of a grassland community, one of the best predictors of resistance to invasion was presence of the species *Leucanthemum vulgare* (Asteraceae). This was noteworthy because *Leucanthemum* had very low biomass in monoculture. In contrast, other species that increased community resistance to invasion had large biomass in monoculture, suggesting they decreased invasibility through direct competition. Moreover, the abundance of root nematodes was several times higher in communities including *Leucanthemum*, suggesting that nematode-mediated apparent competition contributed to community invasion resistance. If this was the case, then pathogen spillover and apparent competition provided a positive feedback at the community level, maintaining abundance of resident species and decreasing abundance of invaders. However, nematodes were not experimentally manipulated, so other factors could have been responsible for the effect (van Ruijven *et al.* 2003).

Another recent field experiment independently manipulated plant community species composition and pathogen prevalence, thereby confirming the occurrence of apparent competition. As discussed above, this experiment factorially manipulated presence of barley yellow dwarf virus, presence of a highly susceptible plant species (*A. fatua*, wild oats),

and soil nitrogen availability, and found strong virus spillover from *Avena* to the three other planted species (Power and Mitchell 2004). Moreover, pathogen spillover from *Avena* resulted in negative effects of apparent competition on aboveground biomass of two of the three other species, *Digitaria sanguinalis* (hairy crabgrass) and *Lolium multiflorum* (Italian ryegrass), although not *S. lutescens* (yellow foxtail). By providing a positive feedback on its abundance, apparent competition served to maintain *Avena* as a dominant species in the community despite being the most heavily infected. Thus, this experiment suggests that apparent competition can be a key determinant of biotic community structure.

5.5 Interactions with other components of biotic communities

Interactions between pathogens and other microbes or animal herbivores can have important impacts at scales from the leaf to the ecosystem (Blomqvist *et al.* 2000; Olff *et al.* 2000; Arnold *et al.* 2003; Silliman and Newell 2003). Starting at the leaf scale, Arnold *et al.* (2003) recently documented that infection of leaves of the tropical tree *Theobroma cacao* ("cacao," the source of chocolate) by naturally occurring assemblages of fungal endophytes reduced leaf mortality caused by a fungal pathogen by two-thirds. Fungal endophytes of woody angiosperms spread within plant leaves without obvious external symptoms. They are evolutionarily distinct from endophytes of grasses (Clay and Schardl 2002). Many are closely related to pathogens, and were not previously thought to have a defensive function against pathogens, although they can reduce insect damage (Faeth and Hammon 1997a,b). A survey of natural infections of cacao by endophytes revealed that they were present in close to 100% of mature leaves, and endophyte species diversity was astoundingly high—344 unique morphotaxa were isolated from 125 leaves. While previous studies have emphasized interactions among pathogenic and nonpathogenic microbes on leaf surfaces (Lindow *et al.* 2002), these results show that community-level interactions within plant leaves can also be important determinants of pathogen impact.

At the scale of a grassland community, recent field experiments suggest that complex interactions between herbivores and pathogens can drive plant community dynamics. In the Netherlands, digging by rabbits and ants decreased abundances of root-infecting parasitic nematodes, and allowed *Carex arenaria* to dominate (Blomqvist *et al.* 2000; Olff *et al.* 2000). In undisturbed areas, these nematodes strongly inhibited growth of *Carex* favoring growth of the other dominant species, *Festuca rubra*. Unidentified soil pathogens were also implicated in patchy declines of *Festuca*. Over 17 years, this complex web of interactions (Fig. 5.5) resulted in a spatio-temporal mosaic of dominance by these two species. Local sites within the grassland cycled between dominance by *Carex* and *Festuca*. Cycles in each site were out-of-phase with other sites, creating a perpetually shifting pattern. Such dynamics have been predicted by spatial simulations of Bever's plant–soil feedback model (Molofsky *et al.* 2002). Further, the key role of rabbits and ants illustrates how plant–pathogen interactions are embedded within a broader web of interactions within a community.

As well as inhibiting pathogens, herbivores can facilitate their growth or transmission, even directly cultivating them in a mutualistic attack on the plant. Preliminary grazing by snails in a salt marsh increased leaf infection by pathogenic fungi ("probably primarily ascomycetes in the genera *Phaeosphaeria* and *Mycosphaerella*") (Silliman and Newell 2003). Snail fecal pellets increased fungal growth via a fertilizer effect. The snails then fed preferentially on infected tissue, indicating that they were essentially farming the fungal pathogens. Factorially removing snails and fungi revealed that when snails and fungi acted in concert, they reduced plant biomass to only one-third of what it would be in their absence. Interestingly, the pathogens were responsible for half of the biomass reduction in the presence of snails, but did not reduce biomass in the absence of snails (Fig. 5.6). Effects of the pathogens were strictly contingent on the presence of their snail "farmers." Thus, snails and pathogens jointly regulated net primary

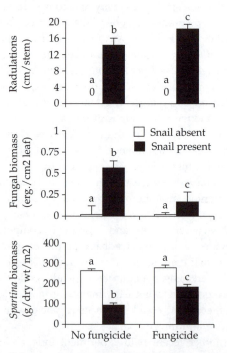

Figure 5.6 Interactive and separate effects of snail presence and fungicide on the total length of grazer-induced wounds per stem (*A*), fungal biomass (micrograms of ergosterol (erg.) per square centimeter of leaf blade) on green leaves (*B*), and *Spartina* aboveground biomass (*C*). Different letters denote significant pairwise differences in mean values at *P* = 0.05 as determined from Tukey's post hoc test. Error bars represent ± SE. Reprinted from Silliman and Newell (2003).

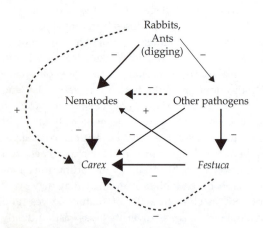

Figure 5.5 Proposed interaction web depicting the possible relationships between the two investigated plant species (*F. rubra* and *C. arenaria*), soil-borne pathogens, and organisms causing soil disturbances (rabbits, ants). *Thicker arrows* depict larger effects. *Solid arrows* indicate direct effects, *dashed arrows* indicate indirect effects. The direct negative effect of *Festuca* on *Carex* (competitive dominance in the absence of pathogens) was not investigated, but is postulated on the outcome of pilot experiments. Reprinted from Olff *et al.* (2000).

productivity, showing that community level interactions between pathogens and other organisms can have major consequences at the scale of entire ecosystems.

5.6 Conclusions

Interactions between a focal plant species and a focal pathogen species are embedded in a broader community of species, many of which can influence the plant–pathogen interaction. Although there are some cases in which plant–pathogen dynamics can be sufficiently understood without reference to this broader community, in many cases—particularly with generalist pathogens—consideration of community-level processes will be essential for understanding dynamics within any single plant–pathogen system. Specifically, we have seen that plant–pathogen interactions can be modified by competing plant species, reservoir plant species, microbial symbionts of plants, and animal herbivores. Thus, parasitism, competition, mutualism, and herbivory will all potentially interact in ecological communities, arguing for approaches that integrate these interactions.

Expanding the focal system from a single host and pathogen to a multispecies complex or the community as a whole opens up a wealth of interactions with potentially profound ecological consequences, both for pathogen dynamics and for community structure. This potential for linked disease and community dynamics is perhaps best illustrated by generalist pathogen spillover from reservoir species to more resistant species, and resulting apparent competition. The range of possible community-level dynamics involving specialist pathogens is somewhat more limited than with generalist pathogens, but pathogen suppression of otherwise dominant host species can have large repercussions. Also, the available evidence suggests that specialists and generalists are sensitive to different aspects of host community structure. Specialist pathogens appear more sensitive to host community species richness, and generalist pathogens more sensitive to the species composition of the host community. However, changes in richness and composition are linked, and so both specialist and generalist pathogens are likely to be impacted by changes in plant community structure. Finally, several studies have shown that plant community disease dynamics can be driven by global change, either in terms of abiotic variables such as nitrogen availability, or biotic variables such as species diversity and composition. The increasing pace of human-induced environmental alterations (Vitousek *et al.* 1997) suggests that the influence of global change on community disease dynamics will only increase.

Acknowledgments

This work was funded by an NSF Postdoctoral Research Fellowship in Microbial Biology (CEM), and Cornell University, the USDA and NSF (AGP).

References

Agrios, G. N. (2004). *Plant Pathology*, 5th edition. Academic Press, San Diego, CA.

Alexander, H. M. (1992). Fungal pathogens and the structure of plant populations and communities. In G. C. Carroll and D. T. Wicklow, ed. *The Fungal Community: Its Organization and Role in the Ecosystem*, pp. 481–497. Dekker, New York.

Alexander, H. M. and R. D. Holt. (1998). The interaction between plant competition and disease. *Plant Ecology, Evolution, and Systematics* **1**:206–220.

Alexander, H. M. and J. D. Mihail. (2000). Seedling disease in an annual legume: consequences for seedling mortality, plant size, and population seed production. *Oecologia* **122**:346–353.

Anderson, P. K., A. A. Cunningham, N. G. Patel, F. J. Morales, P. R. Epstein, and P. Daszak. (2004). Emerging infectious diseases of plants: pathogen pollution, climate change and agrotechnology drivers. *Trends in Ecology & Evolution* **19**:535–544.

Antonovics, J. and H. M. Alexander. (1992). Epidemiology of anther-smut infection of *Silene alba* (= *S. latifolia*) caused by *Ustilago violacea*: patterns of spore deposition in experimental populations. *Proceedings of the Royal Society of London B* **250**:157–163.

Antonovics, J., M. Hood, and J. Partain. (2002). The ecology and genetics of a host shift: *Microbotryum* as a model system. *American Naturalist* **160**:S40–S53.

Arnold, A. E., L. C. Mejia, D. Kyllo, E. I. Rojas, Z. Maynard, N. Robbins, and E. A. Herre. (2003). Fungal endophytes limit pathogen damage in a tropical tree. *Proceedings of the National Academy of Sciences, USA* **100**:15649–15654.

Augspurger, C. K. (1987). Impact of pathogens on natural plant populations. In A. J. Davy, M. J. Hutchings, and A. R. Watkinson, eds. *Plant Population Ecology*, pp. 413–433. Blackwell Scientific Publications, Oxford.

Aylor, D. E. (2003). Spread of plant disease on a continental scale: role of aerial dispersal of pathogens. *Ecology* 84:1989–1997.

Begon, M., S. M. Hazel, D. Baxby, K. Bown, R. Cavanagh, J. Chantrey, T. Jones, and M. Bennett. (1999). Transmission dynamics of a zoonotic pathogen within and between wildlife host species. *Proceedings of the Royal Society of London, B* 266:1939–1945.

Bever, J. D. (1994). Feedback between plants and their soil communities in an old field community. *Ecology* 75:1965–1977.

Bever, J. D. (2003). Soil community feedback and the coexistence of competitors: conceptual frameworks and empirical tests. *New Phytologist* 157:465–473.

Bever, J. D., K. M. Westover, and J. Antonovics. (1997). Incorporating the soil community into plant population dynamics: the utility of the feedback approach. *Journal of Ecology* 85:561–573.

Blomqvist, M. M., H. Olff, M. B. Blaauw, T. Bongers, and W. H. van der Putten. (2000). Interactions between above- and belowground biota: importance for small-scale vegetation mosaics in a grassland system. *Oikos* 90:582–598.

Boudreau, M. A. and C. C. Mundt. (1997). Ecological approaches to disease control. In N. A. Rechcigl and J. E. Rechcigl, eds. *Environmentally Safe Approaches to Crop Disease Control*, pp. 33–62. CRC Press, Boca Raton, FL.

Bradley, D. J., G. S. Gilbert, and I. M. Parker. (2003). Susceptibility of clover species to fungal infection: the interaction of leaf surface traits and environment. *American Journal of Botany* 90:857–864.

Brussaard, C. P. D. (2004). Viral control of phytoplankton populations—a review. *Journal of Eukaryotic Microbiology* 51:125–138.

Burdon, J. J. (1987). *Diseases and Plant Population Biology*. Cambridge University Press, Cambridge.

Burdon, J. J. (1991). Fungal pathogens as selective forces in plant populations and communities. *Australian Journal of Ecology* 16:423–432.

Burdon, J. J. and G. A. Chilvers. (1976). Epidemiology of Pythium-induced damping-off in mixed species seedling stands. *Annals of Applied Biology* 82:233–240.

Burdon, J. J. and G. A. Chilvers. (1982). Host density as a factor in plant disease ecology. *Annual Review of Phytopathology* 20:143–166.

Chapin, F. S., III, B. H. Walker, R. J. Hobbs, D. U. Hooper, J. H. Lawton, O. E. Sala, and D. Tilman. (1997). Biotic control over the functioning of ecosystems. *Science* 277:500–504.

Clay, K. and C. Schardl. (2002). Evolutionary origins and ecological consequences of endophyte symbiosis with grasses. *American Naturalist* 160:S99–S127.

Connell, J. H. (1971). On the role of natural enemies in preventing competitive exclusion in some marine animals and in rain forest trees. In P. J. den Boer and G. R. Gradwell, eds. *Dynamics of Populations*, pp. 298–313. Centre for Agricultural Publishing and Documentation, Wageningen, The Netherlands.

Culley, A. I., A. S. Lang, and C. A. Suttle. (2003). High diversity of unknown picorna-like viruses in the sea. *Nature* 424:1054–1057.

Daszak, P., A. A. Cunningham, and A. D. Hyatt. (2000). Emerging infectious diseases of wildlife—threats to biodiversity and human health. *Science* 287:443–449.

Davidson, J. M., A. C. Wickland, H. A. Patterson, K. R. Falk, and D. M. Rizzo. (2005). Transmission of *Phytophthora ramorum* in mixed-evergreen forest in California. *Phytopathology* 95:587–596.

De Deyn, G. B., C. E. Raaijmakers, H. R. Zoomer, M. P. Berg, P. C. de Ruiter, H. A. Verhoef, T. M. Bezemer, and W. H. van der Putten. (2003). Soil invertebrate fauna enhances grassland succession and diversity. *Nature* 422:711–713.

de Rooij-van der Goes, P. C. E. M. (1995). The role of plant-parasitic nematodes and soil-borne fungi in the decline of *Ammophila arenaria* (L.) Link. *New Phytologist* 129:661–669.

Dickman, A. (1992). Plant pathogens and long-term ecosystem changes. In G. C. Carroll and D. T. Wicklow, eds. *The Fungal Community: Its Organization and Role in the Ecosystem*. Marcel Dekker, New York.

Dobson, A. P. (1990). Models for multi-species parasite-host communities. In G. W. Esch, A. O. Bush, and J. M. Aho, eds. *Parasite Communities: Patterns and Processes*, pp. 261–288. Chapman and Hall, New York.

Dobson, A. P. (2004). Population dynamics of pathogens with multiple host species. *American Naturalist* 164:S64–S78.

Dwyer, G., J. Dushoff, and S. H. Yee. (2004). The combined effects of pathogens and predators on insect outbreaks. *Nature* 430:341–345.

Faeth, S. H. and K. E. Hammon. (1997a). Fungal endophytes in oak trees: experimental analyses of interactions with leafminers. *Ecology* 78:720–727.

Faeth, S. H. and K. E. Hammon. (1997b). Fungal endophytes in oak trees: long-term patterns of abundance and association with leafminers. *Ecology* 78:810–819.

Farr, D. F., G. F. Bills, G. P. Chamuris, and A. Y. Rossman. (1989). *Fungi on plants and plant products in the United States*. APS Press, St Paul MN.

Fuhrman, J. A. (1999). Marine viruses and their biogeochemical and ecological effects. *Nature* 399:541–548.

Galloway, J. N. and E. B. Cowling. (2002). Reactive nitrogen and the world: 200 years of change. *Ambio* **31**:64–71.

Garrett, K. A. and C. C. Mundt. (1999). Epidemiology in mixed host populations. *Phytopathology* **89**:984–990.

Gilbert, G. S. (2002). Evolutionary ecology of plant diseases in natural ecosystems. *Annual Review of Phytopathology* **40**:13–43.

Gilbert, L., R. Norman, K. M. Laurenson, H. W. Reid, and P. J. Hudson. (2001). Disease persistence and apparent competition in a three-host community: an empirical and analytical study of large-scale, wild populations. *Journal of Animal Ecology* **70**:1053–1061.

Gray, S. and F. E. Gildow. (2003). Luteovirus-aphid interactions. *Annual Review of Phytopathology* **41**:539–566.

Greenman, J. V. and P. J. Hudson. (2000). Parasite-mediated and direct competition in a two-host shared macroparasite system. *Theoretical Population Biology* **57**:13–34.

Grenfell, B. T. and A. P. Dobson, eds. (1995). *Ecology of infectious diseases in natural populations*. Cambridge University Press, Cambridge.

Grosholz, E. D. (1992). Interactions of intraspecific, interspecific, and apparent competition with host–pathogen population dynamics. *Ecology* **73**:507–514.

Holt, R. D. (1977). Predation, apparent competition, and the structure of prey communities. *Theoretical Population Biology* **12**:197–229.

Holt, R. D. and J. H. Lawton. (1994). The ecological consequences of shared natural enemies. *Annual Review of Ecology and Systematics* **25**:495–520.

Holt, R. D. A. P. Dobson, M. Begon, R. G. Bowers, and E. M. Schauber. (2003). Parasite establishment in host communities. *Ecology Letters* **6**:837–842.

Hudson, P. and J. Greenman. (1998). Competition mediated by parasites: biological and theoretical progress. *Trends in Ecology and Evolution* **13**:387–390.

Hudson, P. J., A. Rizzoli, B. T. Grenfell, H. Heesterbeek, and A. P. Dobson, eds. (2002). *The Ecology of Wildlife Diseases*. Oxford University Press, Oxford.

Ivors, K. L., K. J. Hayden, P. J. M. Bonants, D. M. Rizzo, and M. Garbelotto. (2004). AFLP and phylogenetic analyses of North American and European populations of *Phytophthora ramorum*. *Mycological Research* **108**:378–392.

Janzen, D. H. (1970). Herbivores and the number of tree species in tropical forests. *American Naturalist* **104**:501–527.

Jarosz, A. M. and A. L. Davelos. (1995). Effects of disease in wild plant populations and the evolution of pathogen aggressiveness. *New Phytologist* **129**:371–387.

Jeger, M. J., E. Griffiths, and D. G. Jones. (1981). Disease progress of non-specialised fungal pathogens in intraspecific mixed stands of cereal cultivars. I. Models. *Annals of Applied Biology* **89**:187–198.

Jones, D. G., ed. (1998). *The Epidemiology of Plant Diseases*. Kluwer, Dordrecht.

Kelly, M. and R. K. Meentemeyer. (2002). Landscape dynamics of the spread of sudden oak death. *Photogrammetric Engineering and Remote Sensing* **68**:1001–1009.

Kranz, J. (1990). Fungal diseases in multispecies plant communities. *New Phytologist* **116**:383–405.

Leonard, K. J. (1969). Factors affecting rates of stem rust increase in mixed plantings of susceptible and resistant oat varieties. *Phytopathology* **59**:1845–1850.

Lindow, S. E., E. I. Hecht-Poinar, and V. J. Elliott, eds. (2002). *Phyllosphere Microbiology*. APS Press, St Paul, MN.

Loreau, M., S. Naeem, P. Inchausti, J. Bengtsson, J. P. Grime, A. Hector, D. U. Hooper, M. A. Huston, D. Raffaelli, B. Schmid, D. Tilman, and D. A. Wardle. (2001). Biodiversity and ecosystem functioning: current knowledge and future challenges. *Science* **294**:804–808.

Matson, P., K. A. Lohse, and S. J. Hall. (2002). The globalization of nitrogen deposition: consequences for terrestrial ecosystems. *Ambio* **31**:113–119.

McCartney, H. A. (1997). The influence of environment on the development and control of disease. In N. A. Rechcigl and J. E. Rechcigl, eds. *Environmentally Safe Approaches to Crop Disease Control*, pp. 3–31. CRC Press, Boca Raton, FL.

Meentemeyer, R., D. Rizzo, W. Mark, and E. Lotz. (2004). Mapping the risk of establishment and spread of sudden oak death in California. *Forest Ecology and Management* **200**:195–214.

Mitchell, C. E. (2003). Trophic control of grassland production and biomass by pathogens. *Ecology Letters* **6**:147–155.

Mitchell, C. E. and A. G. Power. (2003). Release of invasive plants from fungal and viral pathogens. *Nature* **421**:625–627.

Mitchell, C. E., D. Tilman, and J. V. Groth. (2002). Effects of grassland species diversity, abundance, and composition on foliar fungal disease. *Ecology* **83**:1713–1726.

Mitchell, C. E., P. B. Reich, D. Tilman, and J. V. Groth. (2003). Effects of elevated CO_2, nitrogen deposition, and decreased species diversity on foliar fungal plant disease. *Global Change Biology* **9**:438–451.

Molofsky, J., J. D. Bever, J. Antonovics, and T. J. Newman. (2002). Negative frequency dependence and the importance of spatial scale. *Ecology* **83**:21–27.

Morris, R. J., O. T. Lewis, and H. C. J. Godfray. (2004). Experimental evidence for apparent competition in a tropical forest food web. *Nature* **428**:310–313.

Mundt, C. C. (2002). Use of multiline cultivars and cultivar mixtures for disease management. *Annual Review of Phytopathology* **40**:381–410.

Oerke, E. -C., H. -W. Dehne, F. Schonbeck, and A. Weber. (1994). *Crop Production and Crop Protection: Estimated Losses in Major Food and Cash Crops*. Elsevier, Amsterdam.

Olff, H., B. Hoorens, R. G. M. de Goede, W. H. van der Putten, and J. M. Gleichman. (2000). Small-scale shifting mosaics of two dominant grassland species: the possible role of soil-borne pathogens. *Oecologia* **125**:45–54.

Packer, A. and K. Clay. (2000). Soil pathogens and spatial patterns of seedling mortality in a temperate tree. *Nature* **404**:278–281.

Park, M. G., W. Yih, and D. W. Coats. (2004). Parasites and phytoplankton, with special emphasis on dinoflagellate infections. *Journal of Eukaryotic Microbiology* **51**:145–155.

Paul, N. D., P. G. Ayres, and L. E. Wyness. (1989). On the use of fungicides for experimentation in natural vegetation. *Functional Ecology* **3**:759–769.

Power, A. G. (1987). Plant community diversity, herbivore movement, and an insect-transmitted disease of maize. *Ecology* **68**:1658–1669.

Power, A. G. (1990). Cropping systems, insect movement, and the spread of insect-transmitted diseases in crops. In S. R. Gliessman, ed. *Agroecology: Researching the Ecological Basis for Sustainable Agriculture*, pp. 47–69. Springer-Verlag, New York.

Power, A. G. (1991). Virus spread and vector dynamics in genetically diverse plant populations. *Ecology* **72**:232–241.

Power, A. G. and S. M. Gray. (1995). Aphid transmission of barley yellow dwarf viruses: Interactions between viruses, vectors, and host plants. In C. D'Arcy and P. A. Burnett, eds. *Barley Yellow Dwarf: 40 Years of Progress*, pp. 259–289. APS Press, St. Paul, MN.

Power, A. G. and C. E. Mitchell. (2004). Pathogen spillover in disease epidemics. *American Naturalist* **164**:S79–S89.

Rajaniemi, T. K., V. J. Allison, and D. E. Goldberg. (2003). Root competition can cause a decline in diversity with increased productivity. *Journal of Ecology* **91**:407–416.

Rand, T. A. (2003). Herbivore-mediated apparent competition between two salt marsh forbs. *Ecology* **84**:1517–1526.

Rizzo, D. M. and M. Garbelotto. (2003). Sudden oak death: endangering California and Oregon forest ecosystems. *Frontiers in Ecology and the Environment* **1**:197–204.

Segarra, J., M. J. Jeger, and F. van den Bosch. (2001). Epidemic dynamics and patterns of plant diseases. *Phytopathology* **91**:1001–1010.

Silliman, B. R. and S. Y. Newell. (2003). Fungal farming in a snail. *Proceedings of the National Academy of Sciences, USA* **100**:15643–15648.

Strengbom, J., A. Nordin, T. Nasholm, and L. Ericson. (2002). Parasitic fungus mediates change in nitrogen-exposed boreal forest vegetation. *Journal of Ecology* **90**:61–67.

Strengbom, J., M. Walheim, T. Nasholm, and L. Ericson. (2003). Regional differences in the occurrence of understorey species reflect nitrogen deposition in Swedish forests. *Ambio* **32**:91–97.

Strengbom, J., T. Nasholm, and L. Ericson. (2004). Light, not nitrogen, limits growth of the grass *Deschampsia flexuosa* in boreal forests. *Canadian Journal of Botany-Revue Canadienne De Botanique* **82**:430–435.

Tilman, D. and C. L. Lehman. (2002). Biodiversity, composition, and ecosystem processes: theory and concepts. In A. Kinzig, D. Tilman, and S. Pacala, eds. *Functional Consequences of Biodiversity: Empirical Progress and Theoretical Extensions*, pp. 9–41. Princeton University Press, Princeton, NJ.

Tilman, D., J. M. H. Knops, D. Wedin, and P. Reich. (2002). Experimental and observational studies of diversity, productivity, and stability. In A. Kinzig, D. Tilman, and S. Pacala, eds. *Functional Consequences of Biodiversity: Empirical Progress and Theoretical Extensions*, pp. 42–70. Princeton University Press, Princeton, NJ.

Tompkins, D. M., A. R. White, and M. Boots. (2003). Ecological replacement of native red squirrels by invasive greys driven by disease. *Ecology Letters* **6**:189–196.

Torchin, M. E. and C. E. Mitchell. (2004). Parasites, pathogens, and invasions by plants and animals. *Frontiers in Ecology and the Environment* **2**:183–190.

van der Plank, J. E. (1963). *Plant Diseases: Epidemics and Control*. Academic Press, New York.

Van der Putten, W. H. and B. A. M. Peters (1997). How soil-borne pathogens may affect plant competition. *Ecology* **78**:1785–1795.

van Ruijven, J. and F. Berendse. (2003). Positive effects of plant species diversity on productivity in the absence of legumes. *Ecology Letters* **6**:170–175.

van Ruijven, J., G. B. De Deyn, and F. Berendse. (2003). Diversity reduces invasibility in experimental plant communities: the role of plant species. *Ecology Letters* **6**:910–918.

Vitousek, P. M., H. A. Mooney, J. Lubchenco, and J. M. Melillo. (1997). Human domination of Earth's ecosystems. *Science* **277**:494–499.

Whitton, J. and N. Rajakaruna. (2001). Plant biodiversity, overview. In S. A. Levin, ed. *Encyclopedia of Biodiversity*, pp. 621–630. Academic Press, San Diego.

Wilhelm, S. W. and C. A. Suttle. (1999). Viruses and nutrient cycles in the sea. *BioScience* **49**:781–788.

Wolfe, L. M. (2002). Why alien invaders succeed: support for the escape-from-enemy hypothesis. *American Naturalist* **160**:705–711.

Woolhouse, M. E. J., L. H. Taylor, and D. T. Haydon. (2001). Population biology of multihost pathogens. *Science* **292**:1109–1111.

Zhu, Y., H. Chen, J. Fan, Y. Wang, Y. Li, J. Chen, J. Fan, S. Yang, L. Hu, H. Leung, T. W. Mew, P. S. Teng, Z. Wang, and C. C. Mundt. (2000). Genetic diversity and disease control in rice. *Nature* **406**:718–722.

CHAPTER 6

Host selection and its role in transmission of arboviral encephalitides

Robert S. Unnasch, Eddie W. Cupp, and Thomas R. Unnasch

6.1 Background

Arthropod-borne viruses (or arboviruses) are transmitted primarily between vertebrate hosts by blood-feeding arthropods (e.g. insects, ticks, and mites), which serve as vectors for these infections. Because arboviruses infect two very different types of hosts (vertebrates and invertebrates) the dynamics of these infections are often quite complex. The successful transmission of these viruses involves many factors, including the ability of the virus to multiply in the different host species, the interactions of the different host species, and important environmental factors such as temperature and rainfall. The interaction between the vertebrate host species and the insect vectors is one of the most important variables in determining whether an arboviral infection can be sustained in a given environment (Monath 1988). Thus, understanding the dynamics of arboviral transmission ultimately requires an understanding of the community ecology in the areas endemic for these viruses.

In North America the most important arboviral infections from the public health perspective are those that cause encephalitis, or the arboviral encephalitides. These are viral infections that cause inflammation of the membranes of the central nervous system, which often result in permanent neurological damage or death. There are five major arboviral encephalitides in North America (Table 6.1): eastern equine encephalomyelitis (EEE), St Louis encephalomyelitis (SLE), La Crosse encephalomyelitis (LAC), western equine encephalomyelitis (WEE) and West Nile encephalomyelitis (WNV) (Tsai 1991). These five viruses are classified in several different taxonomic groups, but all share many important features of their life cycles. For example, with the exception of LAC, all of these viruses are common infections of the endemic avifauna, and birds are thought to be the primary or sole enzootic vertebrate hosts for these viruses. Transmission from bird to bird in the enzootic cycle of transmission is generally thought to occur primarily through the action of "ornithophilic" mosquito species that feed primarily or exclusively upon birds (Tsai 1991). With the exception of WNV, these infections are usually nonfatal and self-limiting in the bird population. Occasionally, the virus is capable of escaping the strict ornithological pattern of transmission and goes on to infect mammals, including humans. This expansion from the bird-to-bird cycle is effected by so-called bridge vectors, such as "catholic-feeding" mosquito species that prey on a variety of vertebrate taxa, including both birds and mammals. Unlike birds, mammals generally do not develop circulating viral titers high enough to infect mosquitoes (Morris 1988; Bunning et al. 2002). Thus, mammals are generally considered to be dead-end hosts for these viruses.

6.2 Stability and maintenance of arboviruses

An interesting feature of many of the endemic arboviral infections is that they appear to be maintained in relatively stable foci from year to year. The mechanism through which these viruses

Table 6.1 Major arboviral viruses infecting humans in the United States

Virus	Acronym	Genus	North American distribution	Major vector
Eastern equine encephalomyelitis	EEE	*Alphavirus*	Northeast, Gulf Coast and Northern Mid-west (United States)	*Culiseta melanura*
Western equine encephalomyelitis	WEE	*Alphavirus*	West of Mississippi River	*Culex tarsalis*
Saint Louis encephalomyelitis	SLE	*Flavivirus*	Continental United States except Northern New England and Alaska	*Culex* spp.
West Nile encephalomyelitis	WNV	*Flavivirus*	Continental United States (except Alaska), Canada and Northern Mexico	*Culex pipiens* complex
La Crosse encephalomyelitis	LAC	*Bunyavirus*	United States east of Texas	*Ochlerotatus triseriatus*

are maintained through the winter months remains unclear. Several means have been proposed. First, it is possible that the virus is maintained in the vector population. This might occur through infected, hibernating mosquitoes. Such mosquitoes might harbor the virus through the winter and transmit it to a susceptible host upon taking a blood meal in the spring. Alternatively, the virus might be vertically transmitted from an infected over-wintering mosquito directly to her offspring, if the virus is capable of directly infecting the eggs in the ovaries of the infected mosquito. A third mechanism might be that the virus in question is maintained in a vertebrate host. This could occur through long-term infection of vertebrate hosts that are capable of maintaining circulating virus levels in their blood and they either remain resident at the site throughout the winter or migrate back to the site each year.

Over-wintering of EEE virus remains particularly enigmatic throughout its range in the United States. Attempts to find infected, hibernating adult mosquitoes in established foci have failed. Similarly, attempts to demonstrate trans-ovarial transmission of EEE virus in both ornithophilic (*Culiseta melanura*) and bridge (*Coquillettidia perturbans*) vectors have to date been unsuccessful (Clark *et al.* 1985; Morris 1988). Thus, it seems unlikely that the virus over-winters in the mosquito vector population. The hypothesis that EEE is re-introduced every year by migrating birds is equally unsatisfying for several reasons. First, the foci of EEE appear to remain stable from year to year, both in those northern states endemic for the virus (Grady *et al.* 1978; Ross and Kaneene 1996) and in Florida (Bigler *et al.* 1976), and this would demand

a high rate of site fidelity for both adult and first-year birds. Second, molecular genetic studies have suggested that dispersal of EEE throughout North America is not complete, suggesting that there is little genetic flow between foci (Weaver 1993). Again, such genetic isolation would demand high site fidelity for returning migrants. Finally, field studies aimed at invoking re-introduction of the virus into foci by migrating passerine birds have failed to support this hypothesis. Longitudinal serological studies of migrating birds suggest that they do not appear to be exposed to EEE to a significant extent in their winter resident areas (Emord and Morris 1984). Together, these studies suggest that the virus is capable of over-wintering in its endemic foci, and is not reintroduced annually.

The mechanism involved in the maintenance of SLE in the avian population is somewhat clearer. Some studies suggest that SLE might be capable of over-wintering in the vector. For example, there is some evidence for ongoing transmission of SLE during the winter months in California. This suggests that the relative stability of SLE foci in this state may be due to maintenance of the virus through year-round transmission (Gruwell *et al.* 2000). In addition, several laboratory studies have demonstrated that SLE can be vertically transmitted in various vector mosquitoes (Nayar *et al.* 1986; Rosen 1988), and the virus has been isolated from over-wintering *Culex pipiens* (Bailey *et al.* 1978). These results, when taken together, suggest that SLE might be stably maintained at endemic foci, either through ongoing low-level transmission in the winter months, or through vertical transmission in over-wintering mosquitoes.

West Nile encephalomyelitis has rapidly expanded its range in the United States since its introduction in 1999, and therefore is seemingly capable of over-wintering as well. However, as is the case with EEE, the mechanism for over-wintering remains somewhat obscure. WNV, like SLE and yellow fever, is a member of the flavivirus group and one might expect that the over-wintering mechanism of WNV would be similar to that seen in SLE. In support of this, laboratory studies have demonstrated that WNV is capable of being vertically transmitted in mosquitoes (Baqar *et al.* 1993; Turell *et al.* 2001; Dohm *et al.* 2002b; Goddard *et al.* 2003), and WNV has been detected in hibernating mosquitoes (Centers for Disease Control and Prevention 2000). Together these data suggest that WNV, like SLE, may over-winter in the vector mosquito population.

6.3 Vectorial capacity

The transmission of arboviruses involves a vertebrate host and an arthropod vector. Thus, the parameters that influence the transmission of these viruses can be broadly divided into three categories. The first of these is the ability of an infected vertebrate host to infect a mosquito vector. This is defined as "reservoir competence". A complementary factor, "vector competence", is the ability of a given mosquito species, once it has fed upon an infected vertebrate, to infect a naive vertebrate host. Finally, transmission depends critically upon the interaction of the vertebrate reservoir and vector mosquito communities.

The latter two factors (vector competence and the interaction of the reservoir and vector communities) are combined in a concept known as vectorial capacity (Garret-Jones 1964). Vectorial capacity can be expressed mathematically by the following equation:

$$V = \frac{ma^2 p^n b}{-\ln p} \qquad (6.1)$$

where V = vectorial capacity, m = the density of the vector species, a = the probability of successful feeding on the vertebrate viral reservoir species, p = the daily survival probability of the vector, n = the extrinsic incubation time (the time in days

from when a mosquito takes a virus-laden blood meal to when the virus reaches a concentration in the mosquito that renders it infectious to another vertebrate host), and b = the vector competence. Of the five terms in this equation, three refer to an inherent property of the vector (daily survival probability, vector competence and extrinsic incubation period) while the other two refer to the interaction of the vector and vertebrate communities (vector density and the probability of feeding success). See Chapter 7, this volume, for additional discussion of vectorial capacity in the context of malaria transmission.

Equation (6.1) suggests that the two factors which will most affect the vectorial capacity of a given mosquito species will be the daily survival probability and the probability that the mosquito will successfully feed upon the vertebrate reservoir host species. The probability of feeding upon the vertebrate reservoir species can in turn be expressed as a product of the intrinsic host preference of the mosquito and the probability of success of feeding upon a given host.

Vector competence is essentially a measurement of the ability of a given mosquito species to serve as a vector for a given virus. Vector competence is affected by several variables, including the probability that a given mosquito will become infected with the virus upon feeding on an infected vertebrate host, the probability that once infected, the virus will be capable of disseminating throughout the mosquito, and finally, the probability that a mosquito with a disseminated infection will be capable of transmitting the infection to another susceptible host. Vector competence is most easily measured in the laboratory, and laboratory studies have shown that vector competence can vary dramatically between different mosquito species and even within populations of the same species. For example, vector competence values for potential North American vectors of WNV were found to vary by as much as 25-fold (Sardelis *et al.* 2001).

In addition to the inherent susceptibility of a vector species to infection with a given virus, other factors can also affect vector competence. For example, ambient temperature has been shown to affect the competence of *Cx. pipiens* for WNV (Dohm *et al.* 2002a). When *Cx. pipiens* infected with

WNV were held at 30°C, >90% of the infected mosquitoes developed a disseminated infection after as little as 4 days. In contrast, when held at 18°C, fewer than 30% of the infected mosquitoes developed a disseminated infection, even at 28 days post-infection.

Apart from the factors mentioned above, vector competence is also affected by the concentration of viral particles in the blood of the infected vertebrate host, a measure of the reservoir competence of the vertebrate host. Infection of mosquitoes by viremic hosts exhibits both threshold and saturation effects. Thus, at viremias below the threshold, none of the mosquitoes feeding upon the infected host will become infected. Above this threshold, the proportion of mosquitoes of a competent vector species that are infected increases as the viral titer in the blood increases (Komar *et al.* 1999). This relationship eventually reaches a plateau, after which essentially every mosquito feeding upon the infected host becomes infected, and further increases in the viral titer in the blood of the infected host have no effect on transmission. For example, Komar and co-workers (1999) found that the minimum infectious dose of EEE for a single female *Cs. melanura* was three plaque forming units (PFU) of virus, while 100% of the *Cs. melanura* became infected when exposed to 5000 PFU. Thus, the most efficient vertebrate reservoirs are those species which produce a viremia sufficient to efficiently infect the mosquito vector and maintain an infectious viremia for a prolonged period of time. With this in mind, Komar and coworkers have proposed that reservoir competence can be best estimated by multiplying the proportion of mosquitoes that are infected when feeding on a given vertebrate host by the number of days that the host maintains an infectious viremia (Komar *et al.* 1999).

Chamberlin (1958) has suggested that differences in transmission efficiency of the mosquito vectors may affect the virulence of the virus infection in the vertebrate host. For example, viruses that are transmitted by vectors having a low threshold of infection will be under little selective pressure to develop high viremias in the vertebrate host. Conversely, viruses transmitted by vectors with a high infection threshold will be under selective pressure to produce high viremias in their verte-brate hosts. These more actively replicating viruses might be predicted to exhibit an enhanced pathogenicity, both in their normal vertebrate reservoir and in accidental vertebrate hosts, such as humans.

The factors affecting vector competence described above all play an important role in determining the probability that a vector mosquito that has fed upon an infected vertebrate host will actually become infected with the virus. However, once a vector becomes *infected*, it must then convert to an *infectious* state, that is it must be able to infect another naive vertebrate host. The extrinsic incubation period (n) represents the amount of time (measured in days) from when a mosquito takes an infected blood meal until the infection becomes disseminated and the mosquito is able to infect a susceptible vertebrate host. It appears as an exponent to the daily survival probability in the vectorial capacity formula. The entire term (p^n) is an estimate of the proportion of infected mosquitoes that survive long enough to become infectious to a susceptible host. The extrinsic incubation period can vary depending upon environmental conditions, such as the local ambient temperature (Dohm *et al.* 2002a), as in the above example.

The second exponential variable in the vectorial capacity formula is the probability that a mosquito will successfully feed upon the vertebrate reservoir host. This variable (a) is squared because an individual vector mosquito must successfully feed twice upon the vertebrate reservoir species to complete the transmission cycle; once on an infected vertebrate host to obtain the virus and once on a susceptible host to transmit the infection. The probability of feeding on the vertebrate reservoir is in turn a function of two variables, the density of the vertebrate host and the host-feeding preference of the mosquito vector.

The host-feeding preferences of vector mosquitoes are most accurately measured by directly identifying the source of blood meals in wild-caught mosquitoes. Blood-meal identification methods have historically exploited antigen–antibody reaction based assays, using polyclonal antibodies raised against blood components from potential hosts (Tempelis 1975; Staak *et al.* 1981; Washino and Tempelis 1983; Hunter and Bayly 1991; Chow *et al.* 1993). Preparation of antibodies against each potential host is often laborious and difficult, and pre-adsorption steps are often necessary to prevent cross reactions (Hunter and Bayly 1991). Furthermore, despite extensive pre-absorption steps, antibody-based assays are often limited in their taxonomic resolution, identifying only the Order of any host species represented in a blood meal. Thus, these assays could not be used to study the feeding profiles of ornithophilic mosquitoes at the species level. Recently, we have developed alternative methods for blood-meal identification which rely upon the specific polymerase chain reaction (PCR) amplification of vertebrate cytochrome B sequences that are present in the DNA of the blood meal, as described in Box 6.1. (Boakye *et al.* 1999; Lee *et al.* 2002). Because the cytochrome B sequences are unique to a given species, this approach permits the identification of the source of blood meals to the species level (Lee *et al.* 2002).

As discussed above, mosquito host-choice should depend on the relative availability of various host species and the innate feeding preference of the mosquito when faced with a choice of potential hosts. The null hypothesis is that mosquitoes would not exhibit any innate host preference, and host choice would therefore be based solely upon the relative abundance of the various host species. It is possible to estimate the relative host preference for different species using a feeding index (Kay *et al.* 1979), as follows:

$$FI = \left[\frac{(B_a/B_b)}{(A_a/A_b)} \right]$$

Here, B_a = number of blood meals taken from host species a, B_b = number of meals taken from host species b A_a = abundance of host a and A_b = abundance of host b. If the feeding index is 1, mosquitoes show no preference for a given species, and the proportion of blood meals from each species is the same as the relative abundance of the two species. If the feeding index is >1, mosquitoes feed on host 'a' to a greater extent than would be predicted based upon the relative abundance of *a*. In cases where the abundance of all potential host species is known, it is possible to use

---

Box 6.1 Identification of blood meals using molecular methods

The source of blood meals can be identified to the species level using the polymerase chain reaction (PCR). In the first step in this process, DNA prepared from mosquitoes that have taken a blood meal is used as a template in a PCR amplification reaction targeting the cytochrome B gene. The cytochrome B gene is targeted because it tends to exhibit a good deal of DNA sequence variation among species, but tends to be conserved within species. The PCR amplification reaction is carried out using primers and amplification conditions that support the amplification of cytochrome B sequences from vertebrate but not from invertebrate organisms. Thus, only the cytochrome B sequences that are derived from the blood meal DNA and not the vector mosquito DNA are amplified.

In the second step in the process, the PCR amplification products derived from the blood meals (e.g. blood meal A and blood meal B in Fig. 6.1) are mixed with a driver PCR product. The driver is produced by amplification of the cytochrome B sequence from a species that is related to those to be identified. The mixture of PCR products is

heated to denature the DNA and cooled to allow the complementary strands of the PCR product to re-anneal. This results in the formation of four DNA duplexes. Two of these, known as homoduplexes, are formed when the two strands of the driver re-anneal to themselves and the two strands of the blood-meal derived PCR product anneal to themselves. These products are identical to those in the original mixture. In addition, two new molecules are formed, one consisting of the upper strand of the driver annealed to the lower strand of the blood meal product, and the second consisting of the lower strand of the driver annealed to the upper strand of the blood meal product. These chimeric molecules are known as heteroduplexes. Each heteroduplex will contain mismatches between strands. The number, type, and position of these mismatches will vary depending upon the species from which the blood meal was derived.

In the third step, the products are subjected to electrophoresis on a partially denaturing polyacrylamide gel. The denaturing conditions in such a gel are insufficient

continues

Box 6.1 *continued*

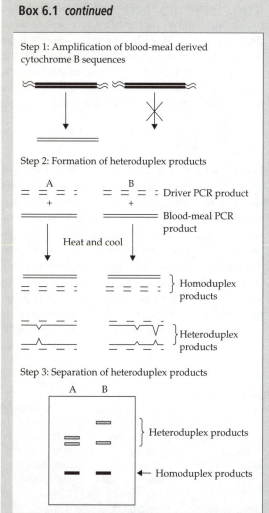

Step 1: Amplification of blood-meal derived cytochrome B sequences

Step 2: Formation of heteroduplex products

A   B
= = = =   = = = = :   Driver PCR product
  +   +
_____   _____   Blood-meal PCR
                       product

Heat and cool

} Homoduplex products

} Heteroduplex products

Step 3: Separation of heteroduplex products

A   B

} Heteroduplex products

← Homoduplex products

Figure 6.1 Diagram of PCR amplification and molecular analysis of mosquito blood meals to identify avian hosts.

to denature regions of DNA duplex that are perfectly matched, but do support localized denaturation (i.e. "bubble" formation) in regions surrounding a mismatch. All homoduplex molecules exhibit the same mobility in the partially denaturing gel. However, the mobility of the heteroduplexes is retarded relative to the homoduplexes. The degree of retardation is a function of the number, type, and position of the mismatches in each heteroduplex molecule. Thus, each species will exhibit a distinct pattern of three bands, consisting of the homoduplex band (both homoduplexes, since they are perfectly matched run with identical mobilities) and two additional bands representing the two heteroduplex molecules. The two heteroduplex molecules exhibit different mobilities because the mismatches present in each heteroduplex molecule are distinct from one another.

In practice, each sample is generally tested with two different drivers. This serves two purposes. First, experience has shown that samples that produce similar heteroduplex patterns (mobilities) with one driver do not produce similar patterns with another. Second, samples that are identical to the driver will only produce a homoduplex. The use of two drivers permits unambiguous identification of such samples.

Finally, the assignment of each sample to a particular species can be accomplished in two ways. First, assignments can be made by comparison of the heteroduplex patterns from each sample to a standard gel containing patterns derived from all known species at the site. Alternatively, the heteroduplex assay may be used to arrange the samples into groups, where all samples within a given group exhibit identical heteroduplex patterns with the two drivers used. The DNA sequence of a representative of each group may then be determined for comparison with available sequence databases in order to identify the group taxon.

Equation (6.2) and to calculate a global feeding index for each potential host. On the other hand, if the abundance of all hosts is not known, the feeding index can be used to compare the relative preference for two or more focal host species of known abundance (Kay *et al*. 1979). The feeding index calculation in its most basic version uses the relative abundance of the host species to calculate relative feeding. However, the index can easily be weighted by other factors, such as the relative size or mass of the host species in question.

6.4 Integrating ornithology, entomology and molecular biology to study transmission of EEE in south-central Alabama

Outside of Florida (Bigler *et al*. 1976; Day and Stark 1996; Mitchell *et al*. 1996) the ecology of EEE in the southeastern United States is much less understood than in other endemic locations in the eastern United States. This is problematic because habitat fragmentation is occurring rapidly throughout the region due to increased population movement and expansive peri-urban development in the south Atlantic and southeastern states (Deming 1996). Consequently, susceptible human populations are migrating into or near sylvatic areas, wetlands and permanent standing water habitats where the virus may be endemic.

In 2001, we began a study to document EEE transmission at one site in south-central Alabama. The goals of this study were to produce a comprehensive picture of EEE transmission at the site, to identify the mosquito species responsible for transmitting EEE at the site, and to relate the timing of EEE transmission to changes in the feeding patterns of the resident vector mosquito species.

The study site was located in Tuskegee National Forest (TNF) in Macon County, Alabama. This general area is within the narrow Fall Line transition zone from the Piedmont to the Black Belt, a physiographic region that is characterized by heavy calcareous soils of Cretaceous origin. Within the site, there has been extensive regeneration of forest over depleted farmland that was abandoned in the early 1900s. Hazel alder (*Alnus serrulata*) is prevalent in thickets along the wet margins of the ponds and the edges of temporary pools in the forest islands. This shrub and its codominant, red maple (*Acer rubrum*), have open, above-ground root mats that serve as excellent resting places for adult mosquitoes.

Mosquito collections were undertaken twice a week from March through October in 2001 and in 2002. Mosquitoes were collected using a number of different methods, including CO_2-baited light traps, vegetation sweeps with a backpack aspirator, resting boxes, and aspiration from natural resting sites, in order to ensure that the collections were as unbiased by the sampling methods used as possible. The mosquitoes were sorted according to species, collection site, and collection date and aggregated into pools with a maximum of 50 individuals per pool. Blooded mosquitoes were identified and preserved individually. Pooled mosquitoes were assayed for the presence of EEE virus by reverse transcriptase polymerase chain reaction (RT-PCR),

and blood meals were identified to the species level using the vertebrate-specific PCR assay as described in Box 6.1 (Lee *et al.* 2002).

A total of 34 different mosquito species were collected at the site, and EEE virus was found in 6 species (Fig. 6.2) (Cupp *et al.* 2003). The most commonly infected mosquito was *Culex erraticus* (Fig. 6.2(b)). When normalized for the number of mosquitoes collected, *Cs. melanura* was found to have the highest rate of infection, with an infection rate of 20/1000 mosquitoes collected in 2001 and 40/1000 in 2002 (Fig. 6.2(c)). *Cs. melanura* is the major enzootic vector for EEE virus in the northeastern United States (Crans 1962). However, this mosquito species was quite rare at the TNF site, representing <1% of the vector mosquitoes collected (Fig. 6.2(a)). Thus, although *Cs. melanura* exhibited a high infection rate, its rarity probably means that it played a relatively minor role in EEE transmission at the site, as its low density would have greatly reduced its vectorial capacity.

Culex erraticus was the most common mosquito collected at the site, and it was also the species producing the largest number of positive pools (Fig. 6.2(a, b)). Because of its density, it is likely that *Cx. erraticus* plays a major role in perpetuating EEE transmission at this site. *Cx. erraticus* is a member of the subgenus *Melanoconion*, a largely tropical group of mosquitoes (Pecor *et al.* 1992). This species is the most common member of that subgenus in the United States and is distributed throughout the eastern United States, the upper mid-west, and westward to California (Lothrop *et al.* 1995). It is a competent vector of EEE virus (Chamberlin *et al.* 1954), and the habitat in which it occurs in the TNF is generally similar to that described for *Cx.* (*Mel.*) *taeniopus* and *Cx.* (*Mel.*) *ferreri*, known enzootic vectors of EEE virus in the humid forests of Brazil, Trinidad, Panama (Downs *et al.* 1959; Shope *et al.* 1966; Srihingse and Galindo 1967), and Venezuela (Walder *et al.* 1984). If *Cx. erraticus*, a neotropical species, plays a major role in the transmission of EEE virus at TNF, then the ecology of EEE virus in Alabama might resemble that seen in EEE foci in South America more closely than the pattern found in the northeastern United States.

Apart from *Cs. melanura* and *Cx. erraticus*, EEE infections were detected in four other species

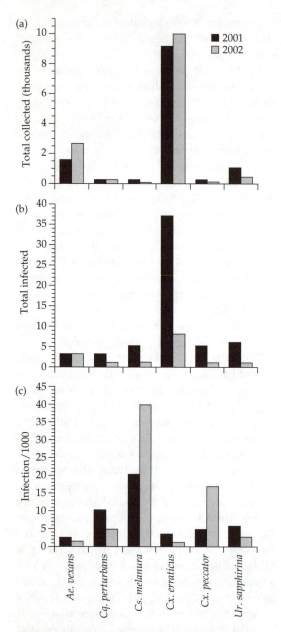

Figure 6.2 Mosquitoes carrying eastern equine encephalomyelitis (EEE) virus collected at TNF in 2001 and 2002. (a) total number of individual mosquitoes from each species found to be infected with EEE virus, (b) total number of EEE-positive pools (see text) detected in each species, and (c) minimum infection rates (infected mosquitoes per 1000 collected) for each species.

(Fig. 6.2). These included *Aedes vexans* and *Cq. perturbans*, both of which have been implicated as potential bridge vectors for EEE in previous studies (Crans and Schulze 1986). Interestingly, EEE virus was also detected in *Culex peccator* and *Uranotaenia sapphirina*. Reports of EEE infections in *U. sapphirina* are rare (Morris 1988), and EEE virus has not been previously reported in *Cx. peccator*. The finding that EEE was present in these species is of interest, as these species were previously reported to feed primarily upon heterothermic animals, such as reptiles and amphibians (Morris 1988).

We determined the identity of the avian-derived blood meals in the four species thought to feed frequently upon birds (*Cs. melanura*, *Cx. erraticus*, *A. vexans*, and *Cq. perturbans*) (Hassan *et al.* 2003). The numbers of blooded *A. vexans* and *Cq. perturbans* collected were low, and a large majority of the meals collected from these species were non-avian in origin. Thus, the analysis of the avian-derived meals was restricted to *Cx. erraticus* and *Cs. melanura*, in which significant numbers of avian-derived blood meals were detected.

Overall, blood from 21 different avian species were detected in the blooded mosquitoes in 2001 and 2002. Interestingly, however, we found a striking pattern of host preference. In both years, blood from just three avian species made up nearly 50% or more of all of the avian blood meals detected (Fig. 6.3(a)). This result suggested that the mosquitoes were preferentially targeting certain host species. It was possible that the apparent host preference exhibited by the mosquitoes feeding upon birds reflected the abundance of the different bird species at the site. To determine if this was the case, the local bird community was surveyed and population sizes estimated for all species encountered at the site (Ralph *et al.* 1995). A total of 71 bird species were found at the site. These abundance data were used directly to calculate feeding indices for all those avian species fed upon. However, mosquito attraction to hosts involves a variety of factors, including CO_2 output, heat, and moisture, that enable the mosquito to distinguish the potential host from the background (Khan 1977). These factors are all related to the overall size of the potential host. Similarly, once a mosquito has identified a host, successful feeding is affected by the exposed surface area of the host available to the mosquito. For these reasons, abundance data were normalized for the mass and surface area of each bird

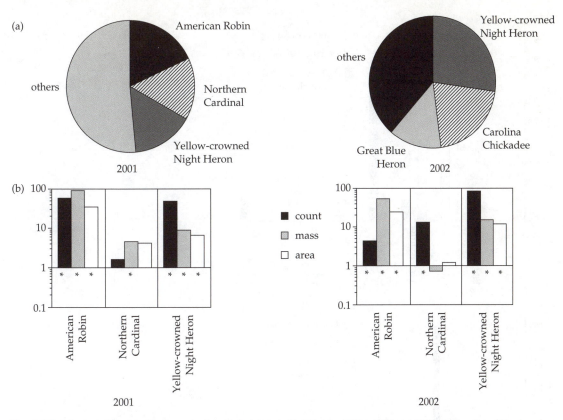

Figure 6.3 Avian host choice in mosquito species found to be infected with EEE virus at TNF in 2001 and 2002: (a) Proportion of blood meals taken from the three most commonly targeted bird species and all other avian species combined, (b) Feeding indices (calculated according to Equation (6.2)) of the three most commonly targeted species. Asterisks indicate feeding indices that are significantly > 1 ($p < 0.05$).

species, and the adjusted abundance data were compared with the blood-meal prevalence data.

The feeding indices calculated for the three species most commonly fed upon in 2001 and 2002 are shown in Fig. 6.3(b). Interestingly, one of the most commonly targeted avian hosts in 2001 was the American robin (*Turdus migratorus*), which was not observed at the study site, although this bird was commonly found in the open fields nearby. This finding suggested that at least some of the mosquitoes might leave the wetland to forage for blood meals and return to the wetland to digest their blood meals and oviposit. Of the other avian hosts, the most frequently targeted species were wading birds, including the great blue heron (*Ardea herodias*), the green heron (*Butorides virescens*), and the Yellow-crowned Night Heron (*Nyctnassa violacea*). The latter species was consistently over-represented in blood meals in both 2001 and 2002, whether the

abundance data were analyzed directly or normalized for either biomass or surface area (Fig. 6.3(b)).

These feeding index calculations suggest that the vectors of EEE virus preferentially targeted ciconiiform birds (wading birds of the order *Ciconiiforma*), and in particular the Yellow-crowned Night-Heron. Given the apparent high degree of contact between Yellow-crowned Night Herons and local vector populations, these data suggest that this species may play an important role in the ecology of EEE virus in central Alabama and probably elsewhere in the southeastern United States where the Yellow-crowned Night Heron and EEE are co-endemic. Previous studies have shown that the Yellow-crowned Night Heron is susceptible to EEE virus (Stamm 1963).

Earlier studies have suggested that some ciconiiform birds are particularly susceptible to mosquito attack, as they do not exhibit defensive

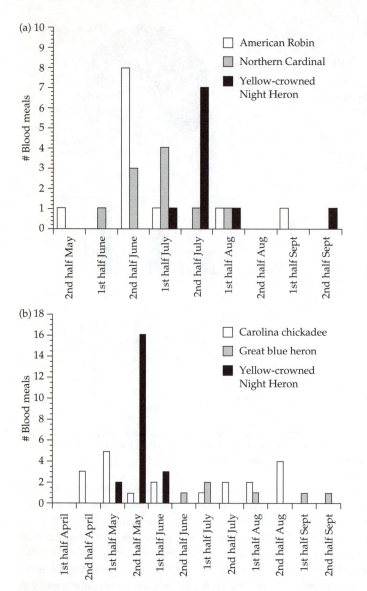

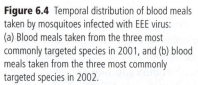

Figure 6.4 Temporal distribution of blood meals taken by mosquitoes infected with EEE virus: (a) Blood meals taken from the three most commonly targeted species in 2001, and (b) blood meals taken from the three most commonly targeted species in 2002.

behaviors (Edman 1974). One reason for this lack of defensive behavior is the fact that herons are ambush predators, which stand motionless for long periods of time and would thus be particularly vulnerable to mosquitoes. If this were the case, one would predict that the meals taken from the Yellow-crowned Night Heron would have been distributed fairly evenly throughout the year. However, an analysis of the temporal distribution of the blood meals taken from the Yellow-crowned Night Heron suggests that the hunting behavior of this species is not what is making it vulnerable to mosquito attack. The meals

taken from this species were temporally clustered in both 2001 and 2002 (Fig. 6.4), suggesting that this species was particularly vulnerable to attack only for a short period of time. In this regard, it is interesting to note that observations of mosquito feeding on avian hosts has suggested that nestlings are more readily fed upon than are adult birds, but then this preferential feeding success on nestlings declines dramatically as the nestlings fledge and begin to exhibit the defensive behaviors typical of adult birds (Kale *et al.* 1972). It is thus possible that the tight temporal clustering of the Yellow-crowned

Night Heron meals reflects an intensive feeding upon recently hatched nestlings, and that this feeding pattern disappears as the nestlings grow older.

In support of this hypothesis, the temporal distributions of the blood meals taken from the most frequently fed-upon species were generally found to be consistent with the breeding life history of most of the commonly targeted avian species. For example, Yellow-crowned Night Herons raise one brood of young per year in late spring through mid-summer, consistent with the short period during which mosquitoes were seen to feed upon this species. In contrast, cardinals and chickadees raise two or even three broods per season. Thus, nestlings of these species are potentially present during an extended period from mid-spring to late summer, again consistent with the wide temporal distribution of blood meals taken from these species. Robins were an exception to this pattern. They can produce multiple broods, but all robin blood meals were collected during a narrow period of time. However, as mentioned above, robins were not observed at the TNF study site in 2001, and a single unobserved nest on the edge of the site may have been the source of all the blood meals, causing robin blood meals to appear only when this nest was active.

Two species thought to feed primarily upon reptiles and amphibians, *Ur. sapphirina* and *Cx. peccator* were also found to be infected with EEE virus. The source of the blood meals in these species were examined using a variation on the vertebrate-specific PCR assay described in Box 6.1 (Cupp *et al.* 2004). Amplification of the DNA contained in the blood meals of *Ur. sapphirina* was generally unsuccessful, with just 2/35 mosquito samples tested producing a detectable PCR product. In contrast, 62% of the 210 blooded *Cx. peccator* examined produced a detectable amplification product. The vast majority of these blood meals (97%) were taken from heterothermic taxa, while the remaining 3% were from avian hosts (Fig. 6.5). Among reptiles, *Agkistrodon piscivorous* (the cottonmouth snake) was selected 81% of the time. Only species belonging to the genus *Rana* were selected among amphibians. More than half of those (58%) were taken from *Rana catesbiana* (bullfrog). The avian blood meals were derived

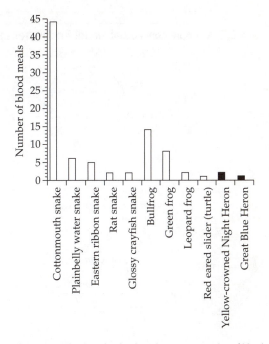

Figure 6.5 Blood meals taken by *Culex peccator*. Number of blood meals taken from each species. Blood meals from heterothermic species are indicated by white bars and those from avian species by black bars.

from the Yellow-crowned Night Heron and the great blue heron, in keeping with the preference for ciconiiform birds found in the ornithophilic mosquito species described above.

These findings, when taken together, suggest that reptiles and amphibians may serve as reservoir hosts for EEE virus in the southeastern United States. These heterothermic species may play an important supplemental role in the transmission of EEE virus at TNF, and may be instrumental in the winter maintenance of the virus at this site. A model incorporating exothermic taxa into the EEE viral transmission cycle is presented in Box 6.2. In this regard, it is interesting to note that studies in EEE endemic foci in Panama demonstrated that 13% of the lizard species in the genera *Ameiva* and *Cnemidophorus* and 30% of lizards of the genus *Basiliscus* had antibodies to EEE virus (Craighead *et al.* 1962). Berezin (1977) also isolated EEE virus from the blood of an iguana in Cuba. These observations suggest that *Cx. peccator* may become infected with EEE as a consequence of feeding upon a reptile or an amphibian reservoir

Box 6.2 A simple conceptual model for the transmission of eastern equine encephalomyelitis virus

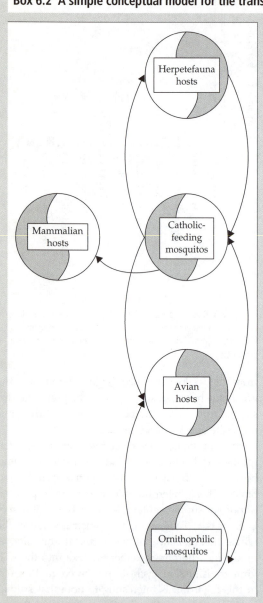

In Fig. 6.6, the circles represent populations of viral hosts, with the shaded portions reflecting the infectious portion. Viral infections are transmitted from the infectious portion of one population to the uninfected portion of another. Viral transmission is mediated through the feeding of the mosquito vector, and thus is controlled by the proportion of each host population that is infectious, the relative feeding success of the mosquitoes, and the vectorial capacity of each mosquito species. Transmission only occurs when an infectious mosquito feeds upon an uninfected host, or when an uninfected mosquito feeds upon an infectious host. In early spring the majority of hosts are uninfected, and thus the growth of the virus is dependent on its rapid cycling between different host populations.

Classically, arboviral infections have been thought to be mediated primarily through an enzootic cycle involving only an avian vertebrate reservoir and ornithophilic mosquitoes (species that feed primarily or exclusively upon birds). Escape of the virus from this cycle to infect mammals was thought to be mediated by catholic-feeding mosquitoes (species that feed upon a variety of hosts, including both birds and mammals). However, recent data described in the text has suggested a potential addition to this cycle, involving heterotherms. Here, the cycle is maintained by mosquitoes that feed primarily on reptiles and amphibians (e.g. *Culex peccator*). Virus may escape from the heterothermic cycle when *Cx. peccator* feeds upon an avian host, as it occasionally does.

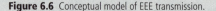

Figure 6.6 Conceptual model of EEE transmission.

of the virus. Furthermore, it is interesting to note that when *Cx. peccator* fed upon birds, they targeted ciconiiforms, the same species targeted by the ornithophilic vector species. Thus, it is possible that *Cx. peccator* plays an important role as a bridge vector between the heterothermic and

avian host populations for EEE virus at the TNF site.

The data collected from the studies described above demonstrate that the vectors of EEE virus at the TNF site do not feed opportunistically, but appear to target certain species the majority of the time. Furthermore, host choice was not strictly dependent upon the density of available hosts, as some host species were fed upon to a much greater extent than was predicted based upon abundance alone (cf. Fig. 6.3). Because the probability that a mosquito will feed on a reservoir host is one of the most influential variables in the calculation of vectorial capacity, mosquito host preferences may play a significant role in driving the development of avian enzootics of EEE.

6.5 Host-feeding preferences in *Culex pipiens*

The studies described above were restricted to a single site in southeastern Alabama and involved only mosquito species that were implicated in the transmission of EEE virus at that particular site. However, a recent study of the host-feeding patterns of potential vectors for WNV in the eastern United States (Apperson *et al.* 2004) suggests that the phenomenon of selective feeding of mosquitoes on certain avian species is a generalized one. In this study, over 1700 blooded mosquitoes were examined individually. Of the 21 mosquito species represented in the study, 19 were previously shown to have been infected with WNV. These mosquitoes were collected at three geographically separate areas, in the Hudson River Valley of New York state, in southern New Jersey, and in the city of Memphis and sites in nearby Shelby County in Tennessee. The vertebrate host of each meal taken by the mosquitoes was determined to the class level using an ELISA-based method, and the avian meals were then further identified to the species level by PCR.

Only four of the mosquito species examined contained significant numbers of meals derived from avian sources. These included *Cs. melanura*, the *Culex pipiens* complex, *Cx. restuans* and *Cx. salinarius*. Mosquitoes in the *Cx. pipiens* complex are thought to be the most important vectors of WNV in the eastern United States (Centers for Disease Control and Prevention 2002). The proportion of avian-derived blood meals detected in *Cx. pipiens* varied by location, ranging from 35% in New Jersey to 85% in New York.

Blood from 24 avian species was detected in the blooded mosquitoes. Three different collections (i.e.

single mosquito species collected at particular locations) contained 20 or more identifiable avian-derived blood meals. These included *Cs. melanura* from New Jersey and *Cx. pipiens* from New Jersey and Tennessee. Within each of these collections, the three most common avian hosts together represented over 60% of the blood meals identified (data not shown). The northern cardinal was among the three most common hosts in all the three collections. The American robin was one of the most common hosts in both collections from New Jersey, while the northern mockingbird was the most common host in mosquitoes from Tennessee.

Because avian censuses were not undertaken in this study, it was not possible to accurately estimate feeding indices for the blood meal data. However, the data suggest that the frequency with which particular species were targeted exceeded levels that might be predicted based upon the abundance of the species alone. For example, the northern cardinal was host for $22.5 \pm 8.4\%$ of the avian blood meals identified in New Jersey, while representing just $1.5 \pm 0.26\%$ of the birds identified in nearby observation routes by the north American Breeding Bird Survey (Sauer *et al.* 2003). Similar differences were noted for the tufted titmouse in New Jersey ($16.2 \pm 8.0\%$ of the avian derived blood meals versus $1.4 \pm 0.25\%$ abundance) and the northern mockingbird in Tennessee ($29 \pm 14.4\%$ of the avian derived blood meals versus $4.0 \pm 0.64\%$ abundance). Because the bird abundance data presented above are derived from the Breeding Bird Survey, and not from data collected at each collection point, it is possible that some of these differences might have reflected variations in the local abundance of the bird species in question. However, local variation in host abundance is not likely to explain all of the differences seen. For example, the blood meal data from New Jersey were derived from collections from seven geographically separated sites, while the bird abundance data were collected from ten separate survey routes. Among these 10 routes, the proportion of northern cardinals ranged from 0.9% to just 2.8%. Taken together, these data suggest certain of the more common bird species are fed upon more or less frequently than would be predicted based solely upon their local abundance.

These results are similar to those of our study in the Tuskagee National Forest described above.

Since WNV was first detected in the United States, examining dead American crows for WNV has become a common surveillance strategy (CDC 2003; Eidson *et al.* 2001). However, crow-derived blood meals were relatively rare in this study, despite the fact that the crow was the most abundant bird noted in the north American Breeding Bird Survey in Westchester County, New York, and was among the five most abundant species in New Jersey. In this regard, it is interesting to note that Komar and coworkers have documented contact transmission of WNV between crows (Komar *et al.* 2003). This observation brings into question whether the high level of crow mortality observed during WNV epizootics results from virus transmitted via mosquito bites or by bird-to-bird contact. Thus, while representing good sentinels for WNV, crows may not be important vertebrate reservoirs for the virus, given the low level of contact between crows and the established mosquito vectors for WNV.

6.6 Summary and conclusions

The successful transmission of an arbovirus requires the interaction of two communities: the vertebrate reservoir and the vector mosquito. These communities interact through the host-seeking and blood-feeding activities of the mosquito vector population. As described above, recent developments in the identification of blood meals to the species level have been quite useful in shedding light on this interaction. The data clearly demonstrate that vector mosquitoes target certain vertebrate species, and that this choice is not just a factor of relative host abundance. These studies have provided some important clues about the factors that may be important in the dynamics of arboviral transmission. For example, the finding that *Cx peccator*, a species regularly found to be carrying EEE virus, fed almost exclusively upon heterotherms suggests that reptiles and amphibians may represent an additional vertebrate reservoir for EEE virus, and that these hosts may play a role in the over-winter maintenance of the virus (cf. Box 6.2). Furthermore, the data suggest that vector mosquitoes for both EEE virus and WNV preferentially feed upon certain bird species, and the temporal pattern of feeding upon the most frequently targeted species is consistent with preferential feeding upon nestlings and young of the year.

Although the data already collected offer some clues to the importance of vector–reservoir interactions for the dynamics of EEE virus transmission, they open up many additional questions. For example, further work is necessary before we will be able to determine why particular host species are targeted by mosquitoes. It is likely that many different factors play a role in the host selection process. Mosquito species differ in the times of day that they are most active in seeking blood meals and the heights at which they forage (Bosak *et al.* 2001; Horsfall and Fowler 1973; Irby and Apperson 1988; Morris *et al.* 1991; Nasci and Edman 1981). Similarly, bird species differ in the height at which they forage, nest, and roost. They also differ in whether they nest in cavities, in vegetation, or on the ground. Finally, different species and different age classes vary in how actively they attack and kill mosquitoes that approach them. Any or all of these factors may play a role in determining which species are most frequently fed upon by mosquitoes.

Another question that remains to be answered is how a feeding pattern resulting in the preferential feeding upon young of the year may affect the dynamics of viral transmission. Laboratory studies have suggested that nestlings and young of the year of some species also develop infectious circulating viremias more rapidly than adult birds, and that peak viral titers present in nestlings are as high as or higher than those seen in adult birds (McLean *et al.* 1995). These observations, combined with our own, suggest that vector mosquitoes might be feeding intensively on young of the year of the chosen host species and that this concentration might increase the intensity of EEE virus transmission. Further work will be needed to test this hypothesis.

References

Apperson, C. S., H. K. Hassan, B. A. Harrison, S. E. Aspen, H. M. Savage, A. Farajollahi, W. Crans, T. J. Daniels,

R. C. Falco, M. Benedict, M. Anderson, L. McMillen, and T. R. Unnasch. (2004). Host feeding patterns of probable vector mosquitoes of West Nile Virus in the Eastern United States. *Vector-Borne and Zoonotic Diseases* **4**:71–82.

Bailey, C. L., B. F. Eldridge, D. E. Hayes, D. M. Watts, R. F. Tammariello, and J. M. Dalrymple. (1978). Isolation of St. Louis encephalitis virus from overwintering *Culex pipiens* mosquitoes. *Science* **199**:1346–1349.

Baqar, S., C. G. Hayes, J. R. Murphy, and D. M. Watts. (1993). Vertical transmission of West Nile virus by Culex and Aedes species mosquitoes. *American Journal of Tropical Medicine and Hygiene* **48**:757–762.

Berezin, V. V. (1977). Characteristics of the ecology of the eastern equine encephalomyelitis virus in the Republic of Cuba. *Voprosy Virusologii* **1**:62–70.

Bigler, W. J., E. B. Lassing, E. E. Buff, E. C. Prather, E. C. Beck, and G. L. Hoff. (1976). Endemic eastern equine encephalomyelitis in Florida: a twenty-year analysis, 1955–1974. *American Journal of Tropical Medicine and Hygiene* **25**:884–890.

Boakye, D., J. M. Tang, P. Truc, A. Merriweather, and T. R. Unnasch. (1999). Identification of blood meals in hematophagous Diptera by polymerase chain reaction amplification and heteroduplex analysis. *Medical and Veterinary Entomology* **13**:282–287.

Bosak, P. J., L. M. Reed, and W. J. Crans. (2001). Habitat preference of host-seeking *Coquillettidia perturbans* (Walker) in relation to birds and eastern equine encephalomyelitis virus in New Jersey. *Journal of Vector Ecology* **26**:103–109.

Bunning, M. L., R. A. Bowen, C. B. Cropp, K. G. Sullivan, B. S. Davis, N. Komar, M. S. Godsey, D. Baker, D. L. Hettler, D. A. Holmes, B. J. Biggerstaff, and C. J. Mitchell. (2002). Experimental infection of horses with West Nile virus. *Emerging Infectious Diseases* **8**:380–386.

Centers for Disease Control and Prevention. (2000). Update: Surveillance for West Nile virus in overwintering mosquitoes—New York, 2000. *Morbidity and Mortality Weekly Report* **49**:178–179.

Centers for Disease Control and Prevention. (2002). Provisional surveillance summary of the West Nile virus epidemic—United States, January–November 2002. *Morbidity and Mortality Weekly Report* **51**:1129–1133.

Centers for Disease Control and Prevention. (2003). Report. *Epidemic/Epizootic West Nile virus in the United States: Guidelines for Surveillance, Prevention and Control.* 3rd revision. Centers for Disease Control and Prevention, Fort Collins, CO.

Chamberlin, R. W. (1958). Vector relationships of the arthropod borne encephalitides in North America. *Annals of the New York Academy of Sciences* **70**:312–319.

Chamberlin, R. W., R. K. Sikes, D. B. Nelson, and W. D. Sudia. (1954). Studies on the North American arthropod-borne encephalitides: VI. Quantitative determinations of virus-vector relationships. *American Journal of Hygiene* **60**:278–285.

Chow, E., R. A. Wirtz, and T. W. Scott. (1993). Identification of blood meals in *Aedes aegypti* by antibody sandwich enzyme-linked immunosorbent assay. *Journal of the American Mosquito Control Association* **9**:196–205.

Clark, G. G., W. J. Crans, and C. L. Crabbs. (1985). Absence of eastern equine encephalitis (EEE) virus in immature *Coquillettidia perturbans* associated with equine cases of EEE. *Journal of the American Mosquito Control Association* **1**:540–542.

Craighead, J. E., A. Shelokov, and P. H. Peralta. (1962). The lizard: A possible host for eastern equine encephalitis virus in Panama. *American Journal of Hygiene* **76**:82–87.

Crans, W. J. (1962). Bloodmeal preference studies with New Jersey mosquitoes. *Proceedings of the New Jersey Mosquito Exterminators Association* **49**:120–126.

Crans, W. J. and T. L. Schulze. (1986). Evidence incriminating *Coquillettidia perturbans* (Diptera: Culicidae) as an epizootic vector of eastern equine encephailitis. I. Isolation of EEE virus from *C. perturbans* during an epizootic among horses in New Jersey. *Bulletin of the Society of Vector Ecology* **11**:178–184.

Cupp, E. W., K. Klinger, H. K. Hassan, L. M. Viguers, and T. R. Unnasch. (2003). Eastern Equine Encephalomyelitis virus transmission in central Alabama. *American Journal of Tropical Medicine and Hygiene* **68**:495–500.

Cupp, E. W., D. Zhang, X. Yue, M. S. Cupp, C. Guyer, T. Korves, and T. R. Unnasch. (2004). Identification of reptilian and amphibian bloodmeals from mosquitoes in an eastern equine encephalomyelitis virus focus in Central Alabama. *American Journal of Tropical Medicine and Hygiene* **71**:272–276.

Day, J. F. and L. M. Stark. (1996). Transmission patterns of St. Louis encephalitis and eastern equine encephalitis viruses in Florida: 1978–1993. *Journal of Medical Entomology* **33**:132–139.

Deming, W. G. (1996). A decade of economic change and population shifts in U.S. regions. *Monthly Labor Review* **119**:3–12.

Dohm, D. J., M. L. O'Guinn, and M. J. Turell. (2002a). Effect of environmental temperature on the ability of *Culex pipiens* (Diptera: Culicidae) to transmit West Nile virus. *Journal of Medical Entomology* **39**:221–225.

Dohm, D. J., M. R. Sardelis, and M. J. Turell. (2002b). Experimental vertical transmission of West Nile virus by *Culex pipiens* (Diptera: Culicidae). *Journal of Medical Entomology* **39**:640–644.

Downs, W. G., T. H. G. Aitken, and L. Spence. (1959). Eastern equine encephalitis virus isolated from *Culex nigripalpus* in Trinidad. *Science* **130**:1471.

Edman, J. D. (1974). Host-feeding patterns of Florida mosquitoes III. *Culex (Culex)* and *Culex (Neoculex)*. *Journal of Medical Entomology* **11**:95–104.

Eidson, M., N. Komar, F. Sorhage, R. Nelson, T. Talbot, F. Mostashari, and R. McLean. (2001). Crow deaths as a sentinel surveillance system for West Nile virus in the Northeastern United States, 1999. *Emerging Infectious Diseases* **7**:615–620.

Emord, D. E. and C. D. Morris. (1984). Epizootiology of eastern equine encephalomyelitis virus in upstate New York, USA. VI. Antibody prevalence in wild birds during an interepizootic period. *Journal of Medical Entomology* **21**:395–404.

Garret-Jones, C. (1964). Prognosis for the interruption of malaria transmission through assessment of a mosquito's vectorial capacity. *Nature* **204**:1173–1175.

Goddard, L. B., A. E. Roth, W. K. Reisen, and T. W. Scott. (2003). Vertical transmission of West Nile Virus by three California Culex (Diptera: Culicidae) species. *Journal of Medical Entomology* **40**:743–746.

Grady, G. F., H. K. Maxfield, S. W. Hildreth, R. J. Timperi, Jr., R. F. Gilfillan, B. J. Rosenau, D. B. Francy, C. H. Calisher, L. C. Marcus, and M. A. Madoff. (1978). Eastern equine encephalitis in Massachusetts, 1957–1976. A prospective study centered upon analyses of mosquitoes. *American Journal of Epidemiology* **107**: 170–178.

Gruwell, J. A., C. L. Fogarty, S. G. Bennett, G. L. Challet, K. S. Vanderpool, M. Jozan, and J. P. Webb. (2000). Role of peridomestic birds in the transmission of St. Louis encephalitis virus in southern California. *Journal of Wildlife Diseases* **36**:13–34.

Hassan, H. K., E. W. Cupp, G. E. Hill, C. R. Katholi, K. Klingler, and T. R. Unnasch. (2003). Avian host preference by vectors of eastern equine encephalomyelitis virus. *American Journal of Tropical Medicine and Hygiene* **69**:641–647.

Horsfall, W. R. and H. W. Fowler. (1973). Bionomics. In W. R. Horsfall, H. W. Fowler, L. J. Moretti, and J. R. Larsen, eds. *Bionomics and Embryology of the Inland Floodwater Mosquito Aedes vexans*, pp. 3–134. University of Illinois Press, Urbana, IL.

Hunter, F. F. and R. Bayly. (1991). ELISA for identification of blood meal source in black flies (Diptera: Simuliidae). *Journal of Medical Entomology* **28**:527–532.

Irby, W. S. and C. S. Apperson. (1988). Hosts of mosquitoes in the Coastal Plain of North Carolina. *Journal of Medical Entomology* **25**:85–93.

Kale, H. W., J. D. Edman, and L. A. Webber. (1972). Effect of behavior and age of individual ciconiiform birds on mosquito feeding success. *Mosquito News* **32**:343–350.

Kay, B. H., P. F. L. Boreham, and J. D. Edman. (1979). Application of the "feeding index" concept to studies of mosquito host-feeding patterns. *Mosquito News* **39**:68–72.

Khan, A. A. (1977). Mosquito attractants and repellants. In H. H. Shorey and M. J.J., eds. *Chemical control of insect behavior: theory and application*, pp. 305–325. John Wiley & Sons, New York.

Komar, N., D. J. Dohm, M. J. Turell, and A. Spielman. (1999). Eastern equine encephalitis virus in birds: relative competence of European starlings (*Sturnus vulgaris*). *American Journal of Tropical Medicine and Hygiene* **60**:387–391.

Komar, N., S. Langevin, S. Hinten, N. Nemeth, E. Edwards, D. Hettler, B. Davis, R. Bowen, and M. Bunning. (2003). Experimental infection of North American birds with the New York 1999 strain of West Nile virus. *Emerging Infectious Diseases* **9**: 311–322.

Lee, J. H., H. Hassan, G. Hill, E. W. Cupp, T. B. Higazi, C. J. Mitchell, M. S. Godsey, and T. R. Unnasch. (2002). Identification of mosquito avian-derived blood meals by polymerase chain reaction-heteroduplex analysis. *American Journal of Tropical Medicine and Hygiene* **66**:599–604.

Lothrop, B. B., R. P. Meyer, W. K. Reisen, and L. H. (1995). Occurence of *Culex (Melanoconion) erraticus* (Diptera: Culicidae) in California. *Journal of the American Mosquito Control Association* **11**:367–368.

McLean, R. G., W. J. Crans, D. F. Caccamise, J. McNelly, L. J. Kirk, C. J. Mitchell, and C. H. Calisher. (1995). Experimental infection of wading birds with eastern equine encephalitis virus. *Journal of Wildlife Diseases* **31**:502–508.

Mitchell, C. J., C. D. Morris, G. C. Smith, N. Karabatsos, D. Vanlandingham, and E. Cody. (1996). Arboviruses associated with mosquitoes from nine Florida counties during 1993. *Journal of the American Mosquito Control Association* **12**:255–262.

Monath, T. P., ed. (1988). *The arboviruses: epidemiology and ecology*. CRC Press, Boca Raton, FL.

Morris, C. D. (1988). Eastern equine encephalomyelitis. In T. P. Monath, ed. *The Arboviruses: Epidemiology and Ecology*, pp. 1–20. CRC Press, Boca Raton, FL.

Morris, C. D., V. L. Larson, and L. P. Lounibos. (1991). Measuring mosquito dispersal for control programs. *Journal of the American Mosquito Control Association* **7**:608–615.

Nasci, R. S. and J. D. Edman. (1981). Vertical and temporal flight activity of the mosquito *Culiseta melanura* (Diptera: Culicidae) in southeastern Massachusetts. *Journal of Medical Entomology* **18**:501–504.

Nayar, J. K., L. Rosen, and J. W. Knight. (1986). Experimental vertical transmission of Saint Louis encephalitis virus by Florida mosquitoes. *American Journal of Tropical Medicine and Hygiene* **35**: 1296–1301.

Pecor, J. E., V. L. Mallampalli, R. E. Harbach, and E. L. Peyton. (1992). Catalog and illustrated review of the subgenus *Melanoconion* of *Culex* (Diptera: Culicidae). *Contributions of the American Entomological Institute* **27**:1–228.

Ralph, C. J., S. Droege, and J. R. Sauer. (1995). Managing and monitoring birds using point counts: standards and applications. In C. J. Ralph, J. R. Sauer, and S. Droege, eds. *Monitoring bird populations by point counts*, pp. 161–168. US Department of Agriculture, Forest Service, Washington, D.C.

Rosen, L. (1988). Further observations on the mechanism of vertical transmission of flaviviruses by *Aedes* mosquitoes. *American Journal of Tropical Medicine and Hygiene* **39**:123–126.

Ross, W. A. and J. B. Kaneene. (1996). Evaluation of outbreaks of disease attributable to eastern equine encephalitis virus in horses. *Journal of the American Veterinary Medical Association* **208**:1988–1997.

Sardelis, M. R., M. J. Turell, D. J. Dohm, and M. L. O'Guinn. (2001). Vector competence of selected North American *Culex* and *Coquillettidia* mosquitoes for West Nile virus. *Emerging Infectious Diseases* **7**:1018–1022.

Sauer, J. R., J. E. Hines, and J. Fallon. (2003). *The North American Breeding Bird Survey, Results and Analysis 1966–2002*. USGS Patuxent Wildlife Research Center, Laurel, MD.

Shope, R. E., A. H. P. de Andrade, G. Bensabath, O. R. Causey, and P. S. Humphrey. (1966). The epidemiology of EEE, WEE, SLE and Turlock viruses, with special reference to birds, in a tropical rain forest near Belem, Brazil. *American Journal of Epidemiology* **84**:467–477.

Srihingse, S. and P. Galindo. (1967). The isolation of eastern equine encephalitis virus from *Culex* (*Melanoconion*) *taeniopus* Dyar and Knab in Panama. *Mosquito News* **27**:74–76.

Staak, C., B. Allmang, U. Kampe, and D. Mehlitz. (1981). The complement fixation test for the species identification of blood meals from tsetse files. *Tropical Medicine and Parasitology* **32**:97–98.

Stamm, D. D. (1963). Susceptibility of bird populations to eastern, western, and Saint Louis encephalitis viruses. *Proceedings of the XIII International Ornithology Conference*, pp. 591–603.

Tempelis, C. H. (1975). Host-feeding patterns of mosquitoes, with a review of advances in analysis of blood meals by serology. *Journal of Medical Entomology* **11**:635–653.

Tsai, T. F. (1991). Arboviral infections in the United States. *Infectious Disease Clinics of North America* **5**:73–102.

Turell, M. J., M. L. O'Guinn, D. J. Dohm, and J. W. Jones. (2001). Vector competence of North American mosquitoes (Diptera: Culicidae) for West Nile virus. *Journal of Medical Entomology* **38**:130–134.

Walder, R., O. M. Suarez, and C. H. Calisher. (1984). Arbovirus studies in southwestern Venezuela during 1973–1981. II Isolations and further studies of Venezuelan and Eastern Equine encephalitis, Una, Itaqui and Moju viruses. *American Journal of Tropical Medicine and Hygiene* **33**:483–491.

Washino, R. K. and C. H. Tempelis. (1983). Mosquito host bloodmeal identification: Methodology and data analysis. *Annual Review of Entomology* **28**: 179–201.

Weaver, S. C., L. A. Bellew, L. Gousset, P. M. Repik, T. W. Scott and J. J. Holland. (1993). Diversity within natural populations of eastern equine encephalomyelitis virus. *Virology* **195**:700–709.

CHAPTER 7

Freshwater community interactions and malaria

Eliška Rejmánková, John Grieco, Nicole Achee, Penny Masuoka,
Kevin Pope, Donald Roberts, and Richard M. Higashi

7.1 Background

Human activities can positively or negatively affect disease occurrence. In the case of preventive measures, human activities can exert powerful control over incidence of disease. In the absence of preventive measures, human modifications of the environment may actually improve conditions for disease vectors and exacerbate the problem of disease burden. Malaria is one of the vector-borne diseases potentially impacted by ecological community changes. Many countries are experiencing long-term increases in the number of cases and in the geographical distribution of malaria (Roberts *et al.* 1997; Mouchet *et al.* 1998; Courtis and Lines 2000) and other arthropod-borne diseases. These increases reflect on one hand a progressive de-emphasis of preventive measures (e.g. the virtual elimination of vector-control approaches to disease control) and on the other hand a change in ecology. As preventive measures are abandoned, the arthropod-borne diseases are intensifying in endemic areas and extending into new areas. Indeed, these diseases now seem to be seeking new limits of expansion, as defined by climate, ecology, and interrelationships between environmental conditions and human activities.

Malaria in humans is caused by four species of protozoan parasite of the genus *Plasmodium*, and is transmitted by mosquito species from the genus *Anopheles*. Both the parasite and the vector have quite complex life cycles (Oaks *et al.* 1991). The parasite requires both human and mosquito to complete its developmental cycle. The mosquito goes through four stages: egg, larva, pupa, and adult. The adult female lays eggs in the aquatic environment. After hatching, anopheline larvae live and feed along the water–air interface, pass through four instars, pupate, and emerge as adults. In order to lay eggs a female mosquito must first obtain a blood meal from its host. Thus, when studying the ecology of malaria transmission we have to consider the ecology of a parasite as well as the ecology of the vector and human host.

The distribution of malaria cases and intensities of malaria transmission have long been influenced by anthropogenic changes. As described by Hackett (1949), malaria increased in Malaya as jungle was cleared for rubber plantations. Where forest was removed, the sun penetrated and populations of *Anopheles maculates* mosquitoes proliferated, greatly increasing the incidence of human malaria. Likewise, Hackett attributes to human activities the proliferation of an efficient malaria vector in New Delhi, which ultimately led to increased malaria in the urban environments. Human-induced changes continue to influence the distributions of vectors and disease today. Wetland rice cultivation provides optimal habitats for important vectors. For example, in a forest zone of Côte d'Ivoire, the population density of *Anopheles gambiae* is strongly correlated with wetland rice cultivation (Briët *et al.* 2003). However, rice cultivation does not always correlate with increased malaria transmission: malaria incidence in the irrigated Sahel of Mali has been measured as only half that of nonirrigated savannah areas (Sissoko *et al.* 2004). Anthropogenic ecosystem changes resulting in changes in community structure, malaria vectors, and disease occurrence are the subjects of our contribution to this book.

The presence and abundance of mosquito larvae in aquatic habitats and, consequently, the number of adult mosquitoes capable of malaria transmission are regulated by a variety of ecosystem processes operating and interacting at several organizational levels and spatial/temporal scales. Presence of water, food, and protection are the key variables. Aquatic plants (both micro- and macrophytes) provide protection from predators and, together with nearby trees and shrubs, contribute detritus that supports the bacterial community, which, in turn, serves as food for mosquito larvae. A change in any component in this complex structure may have a substantial impact on the mosquito population and can even lead to a replacement of one species with another. Because not all mosquito species are equally efficient in transmission of malaria, replacement of a less efficient vector with a more efficient one would have serious negative consequences.

Our study site, the country of Belize, is one of the least environmentally impacted countries in Central America, yet it is experiencing increasing deforestation, coupled with intensified production of existing crops, specifically sugarcane. These environmental changes have a strong potential to affect malaria vector populations and malaria incidence. Malaria is a persistent health problem in Belize, although control efforts in the north have prevented severe outbreaks in recent years (Hakre 2003). Nevertheless, changing land use and demographics in the north may increase malaria risks.

In this chapter, we provide data in support of the hypothesis that freshwater community changes can lead to changes in malaria transmission. Two community processes leading to changes in abundance of malaria vectors are documented here: (1) nutrient-mediated change in freshwater plant communities and (2) habitat selection by female mosquitoes. In addition, we show evidence of differences in the vectorial capacity of mosquitoes that transmit malaria.

7.2 Study system

7.2.1 Location and land use

Belize is a malaria-endemic, Central American country populated with approximately 230,000 people in a geographic area of 22,963 km^2. Slightly less than half of the country is low-lying coastal plain; the rest is hilly and mountainous. The lowlands consist of a variety of relatively undisturbed wetland ecosystems including several types of swamp forest, both freshwater and mangrove, and extensive herbaceous marshes (King *et al.* 1992).

Until the mid-nineteenth century, agriculture in Belize was rather insignificant. Sugarcane cultivation was established in the 1850s but most of its development, preceded by extensive deforestation, has occurred during the last 30 years. Sugarcane has become the most important cash crop in northern Belize with some 30,000 ha cultivated in 1987. Areas under sugarcane cultivation are spreading into more and more marginal soils, requiring increased fertilization. Inefficient application of fertilizers results in substantial losses through runoff after heavy rains. Deforestation of central and southern Belize has accelerated in recent years because of increases in citrus farming and logging concessions to international logging companies (Wright 1996).

7.2.2 Plant communities

Herbaceous wetlands of northern Belize are part of a group of phytogeographically related limestone-based marshes that cover extensive areas on the Yucatan Peninsula, Caribbean Islands and parts of the US state of Florida (Estrada-Loera 1991; Borhidi 1991, Chiappy-Jhones *et al.* 2001). Of the plant communities present, two types sketched in Fig. 7.1 are particularly relevant to disease ecology in this region: (1) sparse, short macrophytes, represented mainly by several species of rush from the genus *Eleocharis* interspersed with floating mats of cyanobacteria (Rejmankova *et al.* 1996b). *Eleocharis* spp. are occasionally accompanied by floating and submersed macrophytes such as *Nymphaea* and *Utricularia*, low mangrove shrubs, and sparsely growing sawgrass (*Cladium jamaicense*).

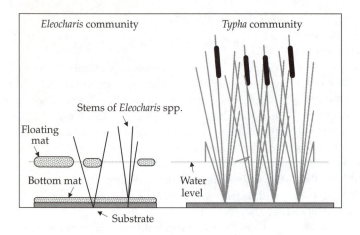

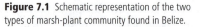

Figure 7.1 Schematic representation of the two types of marsh-plant community found in Belize.

The cyanobacterial mats consist of fine filaments of cyanobacteria from the genus *Leptolyngbya* that form most of the biomass and are intermingled with many other species of cyanobacteria, diatoms, and bacteria (Rejmánková and Komárková 2000). Typically, these communities occur in phosphorus-poor soils with medium to high interstitial water conductivity (2–10 mS cm⁻1). Above-ground biomass production is low (minimum, mean, and maximum dry mass: 2, 120, and 500 gm^{-2}), which, together with fast decomposition ($t_{1/2}$ = 200–250 days), results in a low accumulation of organic material. These communities are probably the first successional stages of macrophytic vegetation in shallow lakes in Belize. Here, we refer to this community as "*Eleocharis*". (2) Tall, dense macrophytes, represented mostly by cattails, *Typha domingensis* with occasional additions of *C. jamaicense, Phragmites australis*, and *Rhynchospora* spp. These macrophytes are usually 2–3 m tall and quite dense (cover > 50%, usually close to 80%). They typically grow on clay soils with relatively high concentrations of phosphorus and fresh to mid-conductivity waters. *Typha* marshes are characterized by rapid growth and decomposition (minimum, mean, and maximum dry weight of above-ground live biomass: 5, 261, and 844 gm^{-2}, respectively; $t_{1/2}$ = 170–200 days). Cyanobacterial mats are rarely present in dense *Typha* marshes due to shading. Here, we refer to this community as "*Typha*".

7.2.3 Phosphorus limitation

Phosphorus limitation is the most conspicuous characteristic of *Eleocharis* communities and is responsible for low primary production and sparse growth. The severe P limitation results in high P resorption and high P use efficiency (Rejmánková 2001). When P input increases, *Eleocharis* spp. respond quite rapidly with increased growth, resulting in higher plant density and subsequent elimination of cyanobacterial mats. In the long run, the tall, dense macrophytes of *Typha* communities usually outcompete *Eleocharis* communities.

7.2.4 Mosquito habitats

Natural wetlands in northern Belize provide breeding sites for a variety of *Anopheles* mosquito species (Rejmánková *et al*. 1993, 1995, 1998). Historically, *Anopheles albimanus* has been considered the major malaria vector in Belize (Kumm and Ram 1941). However, other species of importance include *A. vestitipennis* and *A. darlingi* (Roberts *et al*. 1996). Research aimed at delineating the ecological determinants for temporal and spatial distributions of larvae of the primary vectors of malaria in Belize showed a distinct habitat diversification among individual anopheline species. Investigations revealed that the important variables determining the presence or absence of larvae of specific anopheline species are hydrology and habitat composition in terms of live aquatic micro- and macrophytes and detritus. Other characteristics, especially physical and chemical, of larval habitats do not seem as important and, unless these particular characteristics exceed critical limits, the ranges of values for different species often overlap (Rejmánková *et al.* 1993, 1998).

Anopheles albimanus is a common anopheline species inhabiting a wide range of larval habitats (Marten *et al.* 1996). In northern Belize, it is mainly associated with shallow marshes of *Eleocharis* type (see above and Fig. 7.1). In an earlier paper (Rejmánková *et al.* 1996a), we reported results of a field oviposition experiment conducted in a marsh in northern Belize that showed a strong preference of *A. albimanus* for ovipositing in water with floating mats of cyanobacteria.

Anopheles vestitipennis is less common than *A. albimanus*. Larvae of *A. vestitipennis* generally occur in two types of communities, *Typha* marsh and swamp forest (Rejmánková *et al.* 1998). These two habitats share common characteristics such as shade and decomposing organic material in water; however, *Typha* marshes provide more permanent habitats than seasonally flooded forests, so most of our research concentrates on *Typha* communities.

Anopheles darlingi is found in riverine habitats associated with detritus assemblages. This contribution is focused mainly on *A. albimanus* and *A. vestitipennis*, although research on *A. darlingi* is in progress (Achee 2004).

Recent studies focusing on the vector competence of *A. albimanus* and *A. vestitipennis* have found differences in their transmission potential. It has been demonstrated that *A. vestitipennis* exhibits both strong endophagic (feeding indoors) and anthropophagic (feeding on human) behaviors (Grieco *et al.* 2002), while *A. albimanus* exhibits weak endophagic and anthropophagic feeding behaviors. In vector surveys conducted throughout Belize, Achee *et al.* (2000) have shown higher minimum field infection rates for *A. vestitipennis* than for *A. albimanus*, suggesting that *A. vestitipennis* is a more efficient malaria vector.

Given this background information, an increase in sugarcane cultivation resulting in nutrient enrichment of natural wetland ecosystems poses a significant environmental impact relevant to malaria transmission in Belize. Changes in wetland ecosystems are potentially responsible for an increase in availability of larval habitats for *A. vestitipennis*.

7.2.5 Conceptual framework

A conceptual scheme illustrating the connection between anthropogenic environmental change (increased P input to marshes) and mosquito larval habitats is shown in Fig 7.2 (Box 7.1). A change in any component of this complex structure may have a substantial impact on mosquito populations and can lead to a replacement of one species with another.

The potential scenario is as follows: anthropogenically mediated P enrichment of wetland plant communities (i.e. introduction of fertilizers) causes a switch from sparse macrophytes to tall, dense macrophytes. Tall, dense macrophytes provide favorable habitat for *A. vestitipennis*, which demonstrates characteristics of a more efficient vector of malaria (see below); thus, human-caused nutrient enrichment of marshes can lead to increased risk of malaria transmission in human settlements near the impacted marshes. Based on this scenario we formulated the following hypotheses:

H1: Phosphorus-enriched runoff from agricultural lands (pasture, sugarcane, and other crops) and human settlements causes an expansion of *Typha* communities in wetlands of northern Belize.

H2: *Typha* marshes provide more productive habitat for *A. vestitipennis* than for *A. albimanus*.

7.3 Methods

To document the plant and subsequent mosquito community change we employed both correlative and experimental approaches. Using detailed maps of the study area based on satellite imagery and incorporated into a geographic information system (GIS) database, we determined the spatial relationships between *Typha* marshes and land use (Box 7.2). We then executed a transect-based

Box 7.1 Conceptual scheme of mosquito population change and potential malaria transmission as a consequence of plant community change

Abundance and behavior of malaria vectors are regulated by a variety of processes operating and interacting at several organizational levels and spatial/temporal scales. Mosquito larvae are found in a wide range of habitats defined by hydrology and habitat composition in terms of live aquatic micro- and macrophytes and detritus (Clements 1999). Mosquito species distribution among various types of habitats is not random, on the contrary, there is a tight relationship between individual species and particular habitats (Rejmánková *et al.* 1992) given by a well-developed sense of ovipositing females for habitat selection.

Our research has provided data in support of the hypothesis that freshwater community changes can lead to changes in malaria transmission. Two broad community processes are critical for the changes in abundance of malaria vectors: (1) nutrient mediated change in the aquatic vegetation communities and (2) habitat selection by female mosquitoes.

Wetlands generally tend to be dominated by clonal macrophyte species, often forming monocultures. Oligotrophic, limestone-based marshes of the Caribbean region are limited by phosphorus and characterized by dominance of sparse stands of rush (*Eleocharis* spp.) combined with floating mats of cyanobacteria (CBM). Addition of P triggers a relatively rapid change towards replacement of sparse *Eleocharis* by a stronger competitor, cattail, *Typha domingensis*, resulting in formation of tall dense macrophytes communities (Fig. 7.2). *Eleocharis* and CBM dominated marshes are typical habitats for *Anopheles albimanus* mosquitoes while tall dense macrophytes provide favorable habitat for *Anopheles vestitipennis*. The "bottom-up" mediated transition in plant communities leads to the replacement of *A. albimanus* with *A. vestitipennis*, which is a more efficient vector of malaria, thus human-caused nutrient enrichment of marshes can lead to increased risk of malaria transmission.

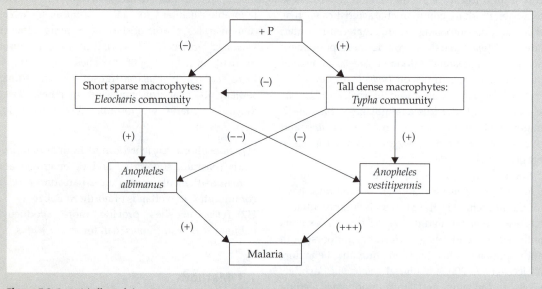

Figure 7.2 Potential effects of plant community structure on malaria transmission to humans.

sampling program, analyzing sediment and plant tissue to determine spatial patterns of P loading in and around marshes. A detailed description of the transect study is provided in Grieco *et al.* (*in preparation*). At each established transect location we sampled for the presence of anopheline larvae and recorded the preference of each mosquito species for a particular type of habitat. Four rounds of larval sampling were conducted to correspond with the "early wet" (August–September), "late wet" (October–November), "early dry" (February–March) and "late dry" (May–June) seasons. To explain mosquito habitat selection, we also have conducted field experiments on larval growth and survival

Box 7.2 Remote sensing and GIS for mapping marsh communities

Traditional field mapping can only be used to survey limited areas on the ground. In addition, some remote field sites may be difficult to access. Use of remote sensing and GIS allows large areas to be mapped. A combination of a multispectral system (French satellite "Probatoire de l'Observation de la Terre" or "SPOT") and radar imagery (Radarsat C) produce good classification maps (Fig. 7.3(a)) of marsh (pink, purple, red, black), forest (green), and agricultural areas (orange, yellow, brown). The classification maps are imported to a GIS system where buffer zones are created around the marshes (Fig. 7.3(b)). GIS programs are run to determine the amount of different types of vegetation within each marsh and the amount and type of land cover surrounding each marsh in the buffer zone. The resulting data are examined with a statistical program to determine correlations between surrounding land cover and marsh vegetation. In Fig. 7.3(c), *Typha* marsh is shown to be positively correlated to agriculture and negatively correlated to forest. These correlations demonstrate that the conversion of forest to cropland may be causing and increase in *Typha* marshes, which are an important *Anopheles* mosquito breeding habitat.

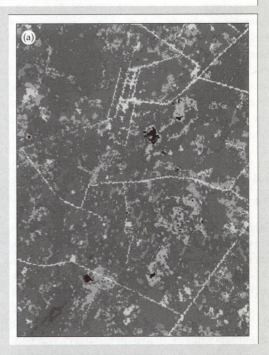

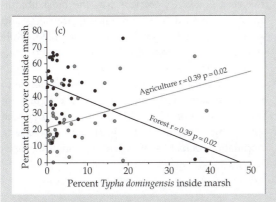

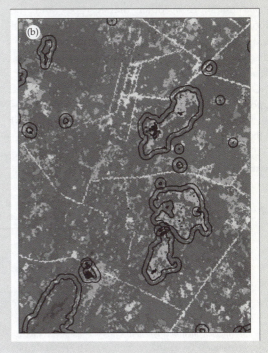

Figure 7.3 Remote sensing and GIS tools for monitoring plant community change and malaria vector abundance. (a) Classification maps of marsh (pink, purple, red, black), forest (green), and agricultural areas (orange, yellow, brown). (b) Marsh buffer zones, outlined in black. (c) Correlation between *Typha* cover inside the marsh with agricultural or forest cover within the buffer zone adjacent to the marsh. Orange circles and orange line indicate agricultural cover, green circles and green line indicate forest cover. (See also color Plate 1.)

and laboratory experiments on oviposition. Effects of the spatial distribution of larval habitats on movement of adult malaria vectors to human habitations have been assessed in a series of mark recapture experiments (Achee 2004). A long-term, manipulative field experiment is in progress, following changes in ecosystem processes and community structure upon nutrient additions along a salinity gradient. This experiment has already proven a strong response of vegetation to P enrichment (Rejmánková, unpublished results).

7.4 Results

7.4.1 Land use and mosquito habitats

Satellite images of Belize have been used to examine the relationship between land use and larval habitats of *A. albimanus* and *A. vestitipennis* (details of this study are presented in Pope *et al.*, 2005). A landcover classification based on multispectral SPOT imagery of northern Belize identified major cover classes, including agricultural, forest, and several marsh types (Box 7.2). Radarsat imagery was used to further refine the classification by separating the *Typha* marsh from other marsh types and the flooded forest from other forest types. *Typha* marsh and flooded forest are *A. vestitipennis* larval habitats, while *Eleocharis* marsh is the larval habitat for *A. albimanus*.

GIS-based analyses were used to estimate the amount and type of land cover within buffer zones surrounding individual marshes, transects, and villages. In all three buffer types, the amount of *T. domingensis* in a marsh was positively correlated with the amount of agricultural land in the adjacent

upland area, and negatively correlated with the amount of adjacent forest (Table 7.1). In general, the strongest correlations were found in the marsh-buffer analysis when only marshes with *T. domingensis* were included, and for the association of *Typha* marsh and sugarcane. These results are consistent with the hypothesis that nutrient (P) runoff from agricultural lands is causing an expansion of *T. domingensis* in northern Belize. Thus, the agriculture-induced expansion of *A. vestitipennis* larval habitat may be increasing malaria risk in Belize and in other countries where this species is a malaria vector.

7.4.2 Vegetation and mosquito species in impacted and unimpacted marshes

Larvae of the three dominant *Anopheles* species, *A. albimanus*, *A. vesititpennis*, and *A. crucians* (this latter species is not a malaria vector), were collected along transects during both wet and dry seasons. All three species were present in highest densities during the wet season (August–December), when there was an abundance of larval habitat. *Anopheles crucians* and *A. albimanus* maintained moderate population densities throughout the remainder of the year. *Anopheles crucians* was the most ubiquitous with regard to its presence in transects and was collected in 90% of all transects sampled, while *A. albimanus* was present in 83% and *A. vestitipennis* was present in only 73% of transects.

Analysis of the ecological variables in relation to the larval data showed that there was a significant linear correlation ($R^2 = 0.188$, $P < 0.001$) between increasing densities of *Typha* and increasing population densities of *A. vestitipennis*. *Anopheles*

Table 7.1 Pearson correlation coefficients (*R*) and significance (*P*) for the amount of *Typha domingensis* in a marsh versus the amount of various land-cover types in the adjacent upland

	Typha versus forest		*Typha* versus pasture/crop		*Typha* versus sugarcane		*Typha* versus agriculture	
	R	P	R	P	R	P	R	P
Transect (*n* = 40)	−0.22	0.18	—	—	0.41	<0.01	—	—
Marsh buffer, all (*n* = 112)	−0.14	0.13	0.17	0.07	0.23	0.01	0.25	<0.01
Marsh buffer, with *Typha* (*n* = 37)	−0.48	<0.01	0.33	0.05	0.35	0.03	0.39	0.02
Village buffer (*n* = 52)	−0.21	0.14	0.05	0.71	0.23	0.10	0.23	0.11

albimanus was positively correlated with cyanobacterial mats ($R^2 = 0.334$, $P < 0.0001$), and negatively correlated with cover of any species of emergent macrophytes. *Anopheles crucians* occurred most often in heavily shaded areas of the marsh. The larvae of this species were positively correlated with *Eleocharis* density ($R^2 = 0.324$, $P < 0.0001$) and showed a negative association with cyanobacterial mats. More than 82% of the larvae of *A. vestitipennis* occurred where *Typha* cover was 40% or greater (Fig. 7.4). When *A. vestitipennis* larvae occurred among lower densities of *Typha*, they were always associated with dense biomass above the water surface. *Anopheles vestitipennis* was the least abundant mosquito species and showed the highest preference for one habitat. This species was very rarely found in habitat other than very dense *Typha* and, when it was, it was usually in association with dense vegetation that provided high above-water biomass. The strong habitat preference exhibited by this species makes it a relatively easy target for potential larval control. Control measures aimed at *Typha* management could significantly influence the larval population, thereby reducing adult mosquito densities.

7.4.3 Vegetation and mosquito population changes following nutrient addition

Figure 7.5 summarizes the impacts of nutrient increase on marsh vegetation and, consequently, mosquito habitat availability. Previous results and ongoing experiments confirm that when the oligotrophic, P-limited *Eleocharis* marshes receive higher doses of P, the growth of *Eleocharis* rapidly increases, and cyanobacterial mats are eliminated through shading. If the macrophyte *T. domingensis* gets established in P-enriched plots, it soon outcompetes *Eleocharis*. This transition in the plant community is then followed by changes in mosquito populations. In Fig. 7.5 (a–c), we present results of the above-described transect study, and in Fig. 7.6, we show changes in *Eleocharis* density resulting from nutrient enrichment (note that nitrogen additions do not cause any change in this P-limited system). There is also a close correlation between *Eleocharis* cover and larval densities of *A. albimanus* and *A. crucians* (Fig. 7.6(b)). This nutrient-enrichment experiment has not achieved the stage of *Typha* dominance, so the expected changes in larval distribution have not yet been confirmed.

7.4.4 Habitat selection

Habitats occupied by the immature stages of a mosquito species are evidence of the oviposition sites used by females of these species (Clements 1999). Studies of specific larval habitats are therefore good starting points for gaining understanding of the oviposition choices of gravid females. We have previously characterized the habitats of primary vectors of malaria in Belize,

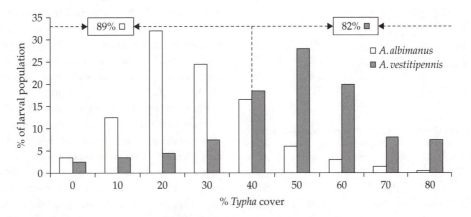

Figure 7.4 Relationship between density of mosquito larvae and density of *Typha domingensis*. The majority of *Anopheles vestitipennis* larvae (82%) were collected in habitats containing at least 40% cover of *Typha*, while the majority of *A. albimanus* larvae (89%) were collected from habitats containing less than 40% cover of *Typha*.

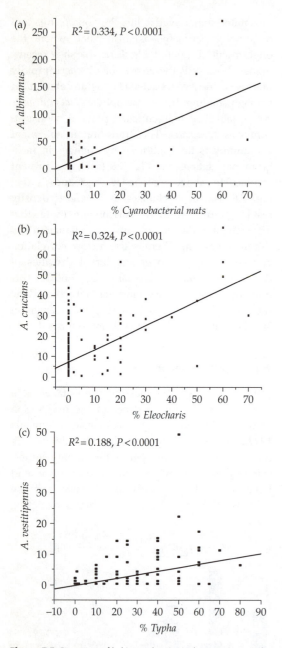

Figure 7.5 Responses of habitat and mosquito larvae to increased phosphorus loading. Results from transect sampling indicating the correlation between successive plant communities and larval densities of (a) *A. albimanus*, (b) *A. crucians* and (c) *A. vestitipennis*. Phosphorus loading increases from (a) to (b) to (c).

through correlative studies that suggested possible cues used by the different species for selecting oviposition sites (Manguin *et al.* 1996; Rejmánková *et al.* 1993, 1996b, 1998).

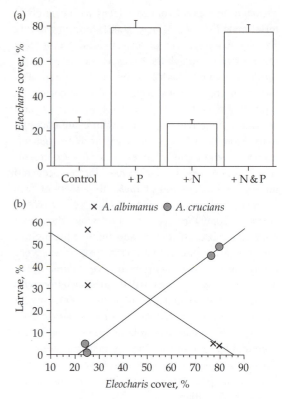

Figure 7.6 Results from a nutrient addition experiment indicating changes in (a) *Eleocharis* cover and (b) the correlation between *Eleocharis* cover and larval densities of *A. albimanus* and *A. crucians*.

Our studies suggest that volatile substances, for example, from protein degradents or bacterial cultures, released from these larval habitats could serve as oviposition stimulants (Rejmánková *et al.* 2000a). We collected materials from larval habitats of both *A. albimanus* and *An. vestitipennis*, that is cyanobacterial mats and *T. domingensis* litter, respectively. Volatile compounds were extracted by freeze-drying the material and trapping the volatilized material on a –55°C titanium condenser. For oviposition trials conducted with wild-caught females, these volatile materials were pipetted onto filters floating on the surface of deionized water in Teflon beakers that were placed within oviposition cages. For both species, volatile materials in low concentrations increased oviposition (assessed as egg density), but reduced oviposition at higher concentrations. To test whether the activity of volatile materials from different habitats was species-specific, we conducted reciprocal treatment

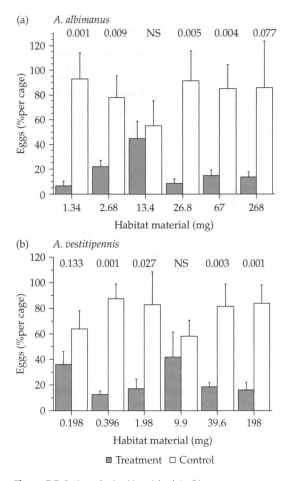

Figure 7.7 Reciprocal oviposition trials. a) *A. albimanus* response to volatile material from a primary habitat of *A. vestitipennis*. Treatment (*x*-axis): a range of concentrations of the volatile material from *A. vestitipennis* habitats, expressed as equivalent mass of habitat material in milligrams. Control: volatile material from *A. albimanus* habitats, concentrated at 0.99 mg equivalent mass of habitat material. b) *A. vestitipennis* response to volatile material from a primary habitat of *A. albimanus*. Treatment (*x*-axis): a range of concentrations of the volatile materials from *A. albimanus* habitats, expressed as equivalent mass of habitat material in milligrams. Control: volatile material from *A. vestitipennis* habitats, concentrated at 1.34 mg equivalent mass of habitat material. Oviposition expressed as percentage of eggs per cage, plus standard error. Dark bars = treatment, white bars = control. Significance of differences between each treatment and control indicated by *P*-values in the upper part of the graph; NS = non significant.

experiments. Females of each species were given a choice of volatile materials from their own habitat (positive control) and from the other species' habitat (treatment). Volatile materials proved to be clearly species-specific, that is, each species responded positively only to volatile materials from its own habitat (Fig. 7.7). In two separate trials, out of six doses of *Typha* volatiles tested against control volatiles from cyanobacterial mats, *A. albimanus* females laid significantly more eggs in the control beakers. Similarly, *A. vestitipennis* females preferentially oviposited into control beakers containing filters treated with *Typha* volatiles as compared to six different cyanobacterial treatment doses. For more details see Rejmánková *et al.* (2005).

After oviposition, one of the main factors determining larval survival is food availability. Merritt and coauthors (1992) pointed out that an understanding of the spatial and temporal distribution of the dietary resources available to larval mosquitoes in their natural habitats is needed to clarify the relationships among food availability, vector competence, and mosquito fitness. In the water column of aquatic ecosystems, bacteria are the major decomposers of organic matter (Merritt *et al.* 1992; Cottingham and Butzler, Chapter 8 this volume). The presence of particulate heterotrophic bacterial biomass represents an important link between detritus, dissolved organic matter, and higher trophic levels. This bacterial production is controlled or directly related to the supply of decomposable organic material. Our previous surveys (Rejmánková *et al.* 2000b) indicated a close correlation between particulate organic matter, dissolved organic carbon (DOC), and bacterial numbers—all potential nutritional components for larvae.

To assess the response of larvae to various habitat conditions, we conducted mosquito transplant experiments (Grieco *et al.*, in preparation). First-instar larvae of *A. albimanus*, *A. vestitipennis*, and *A. darlingi* were placed in floating containers in the respective habitats of each species. Habitat suitability was evaluated by time of development, survival rate, growth rate, sex, adult size, and protein and lipid content. Numbers of bacteria, POC (particulate organic carbon), DOC, total nitrogen and fatty acids were measured as environmental variables (data not shown). Several fourth-instar larvae of each species/habitat were examined for protein and lipid content. Response of mosquito species to environmental conditions in its own and

References

Achee, N. (2004). A study on the bionomics of *Anopheles darlingi* Root (Diptera: Culicidae) in Belize, Central America. Doctoral Dissertation, Uniformed Services University of the Health Sciences. 300 pp.

Achee, N. L., C. T. Korves, M. J. Bangs, E. Rejmánková, M. Lege, D. Curtin, H. Lenares, Y. Alonzo, R. G. Andre, and D. R. Roberts. (2000). *Plasmodium vivax* polymorphs and *Plasmodium falciparum* circumsporozoite proteins in Anopheles (Diptera: Culicidae) from Belize, Central America. *Journal of Vector Ecology* 25:203–211.

Aerts, R. and F. S. Chapin. (2000). The mineral nutrition of wild plants revisited: A re-evaluation of processes and patterns. *Advances in Ecological Research* 30:1–67.

Angelon, K. A, and J. W. Petranka. (2002). Chemicals of predatory mosquitofish (*Gambusia affinis*) influence selection of oviposition site by *Culex* mosquitoes. *Journal of Chemical Ecology* 28:797–806.

Borhidi, A. (1991). *Phytogeography and vegetation ecology of Cuba*. Akademiai Kiado, Budapest.

Briët, O. J., J. Dossou-Yovo, E. Akoda, N. V. de Giesen, and T. M. Teuscher. (2003). The relationship between *Anopheles gambiae* density and rice cultivation in the savannah zone and forest zone of Cote d'Ivoire. *Tropical Medicine and International Health* 8:439–448.

Chiappy-Jhones, C., V. Rico-Gray, L. Gama, and L. Giddings. (2001). Floristic affinities between the Yucatan Peninsula and some karstic areas of Cuba. *Journal of Biogeography* 28: 535–542.

Clements, A. N. (1999). *The biology of mosquitoes*. CABI Publ., New York.

Curtis, C. F. and J. D. Lines. (2000). Should DDT be banned by international treaty? *Parasitology Today* 16:119–121.

Edgerly, J. S., M. McFarland, P. Morgan, and T. Livdahl. (1998). A seasonal shift in egg-laying behaviour in response to cues of future competition in a treehole mosquito. *Journal of Animal Ecology* 67:805–818.

Estrada-Loera, E. (1991). Phytogeographic relationships of the Yucatan Peninsula. *Journal of Biogeography* 18:687–697.

Goddard, M. R. and M. A. Bradford. (2003). The adaptive response of a natural microbial population to carbon- and nitrogen-limitation. *Ecology Letters* 6:594–598.

Grieco, J. P., N. L. Achee, R. G. Andre, and D. R. Roberts. (2000). A comparison study of house entering and exiting behavior of *Anopheles vestitipennis* (Diptera: Culicidae) using experimental huts sprayed with DDT or deltamethrin in the southern district of Toledo, Belize, CA. *Journal of Vector Ecology* 25:62–73.

Grieco, J. P., N. L. Achee, R. G. Andre, and D. R. Roberts. (2002). Host feeding preferences of Anopheles species collected by manual aspiration, mechanical aspiration, and from a vehicle-mounted trap in the Toledo District, Belize, Central America. *Journal of the American Mosquito Control Association* 18:307–315.

Griew, J. P., N. L. Achee, I. Briceno, R. King, R. Andre, D. Roberts and E. Rejmánková. (2003). Comparison of life table attributes from newly established colonies of *Anopheles albimanus* and *Anopheles vestitipennis* in northern Belize. *Journal of Vector Ecology* 28:200–207.

Hackett, L. W. (1949). Distribution of malaria. In M. F. Boyd, ed. *Malariology*, pp. 722–735. Saunders, Philadelphia, PA.

Hakre, S. (2003). Household risk factors for malaria in selected villages in Belize, Central America. Doctoral Dissertation, Uniformed Services University of the Health Sciences, Bethesda, MD.

Harrington, R. A., J. H. Fownes, and P. M. Vitousek. (2001). Production and resource use efficiencies in N- and P-limited tropical forests: A comparison of responses to long-term fertilization. *Ecosystems* 4:646–657.

Johnson, P. T. J. and J. M. Chase. (2004). Parasites in the food web: linking amphibian malformations and aquatic eutrophication. *Ecology Letters* 7:521–526.

Kiflawi, M., L. Blaustein, and M. Mangel. (2003). Oviposition habitat selection by the mosquito *Culiseta longiareolata* in response to risk of predation and conspecific larval density. *Ecological Entomology* 28:168–173.

King, R. B., I. C. Baillie, T. M. B. Abell, J. R. Dunsmore, D. A. Gray, J. H. Pratt, H. R. Versey, A. C. S. Wright, and S. A. Zisman. (1992). Land resources assessment of northern Belize. Natural Resources Institute, Belize City, Belize, Bulletin 43.

Kumm, H. and L. Ram. (1941). Observations on the *Anopheles* of British Honduras. *American Journal of Tropical Medicine* 21:559–566.

Manguin, S., D. R. Roberts, R. G. Andre, E. Rejmánková, and S. Hakre. (1996). Characterization of *Anopheles darlingi* (Diptera: Culicidae) larval habitats in Belize, Central America. *Journal of Medical Entomology* 33: 205–211.

Marten, G. G., M. F. Suarez, and R. Astaeza. (1996). An ecological survey of *Anopheles albimanus* larval habitats in Colombia. *Journal of Vector Ecology* 21:122–131.

Merritt, R. W., R. H. Dadd, and E. D. Walker. (1992). Feeding-behavior, natural food, and nutritional relationships of larval mosquitoes. *Annual Review of Entomology* 37:349–376.

Mokany, A. and R. Shine. (2003). Oviposition site selection by mosquitoes is affected by cues from conspecific larvae and anuran tadpoles. *Austral Ecology* **28**:33–37.

Mordue Luntz, A. J. (2003). Arthropod semiochemicals: mosquitoes, midges and sealice. *Biochemical Society Transactions* **31**:128–133.

Morris, D. W. (2003). Toward an ecological synthesis: a case for habitat selection. *Oecologia* **136**:1–13.

Mouchet, J., S. Manguin, J. Sircoulon, S. Laventure, O. Faye, A. W. Onapa, P. Carnevale, J. Julvez, and D. Fontenille. (1998). Evolution of malaria in Africa for the past 40 years: Impact of climatic and human factors. *Journal of the American Mosquito Control Association* **14**:121–130.

Navarro, D. M. A. F., P. E. S. de Oliveira, R. P. J. Potting, A. C. Brito, S. J. F. Fital, and A. E. G. Sant'Ana. (2003). The potential attractant or repellent effects of different water types on oviposition in *Aedes aegypti* L. (Dipt., Culicidae). *Journal of Applied Entomology-Zeitschrift Fur Angewandte Entomologie* **127**:46–50.

Oaks, S. C., V. S. Mitchell, G. W. Pearson, and C. C. J. Cerpenter, eds. (1991). *Malaria, Obstacles and Opportunities*. National Academy Press, Washington, DC.

Orr, B. K. and V. H. Resh. (1992). Influence of *Myriophyllum aquaticum* cover on *Anopheles* mosquito abundance, oviposition, and larval microhabitat. *Oecologia* **90**:474–482.

Polis, G. A. and D. R. Strong. (1996). Food web complexity and community dynamics. *American Naturalist* **147**: 813–846.

Poonam, S., K. P. Paily, and K. Balaraman. (2002). Oviposition attractancy of bacterial culture filtrates response of *Culex quinquefasciatus*. *Memorias Do Instituto Oswaldo Cruz* **97**:359–362.

Pope, K., P. Masuoka, E. Rejmánková, J. Grieco, S. Johnson, and D. Roberts. (2005). Mosquito habitats, land use, and malaria risk in Belize. *Ecological Applications.* **15**:1223–1232.

Portielje, R. and D. T. Van der Molen. (1999). Relationships between eutrophication variables: from nutrient loading to transparency. *Hydrobiologia* **409**:375–387.

Rejmánková, E. (2001). Effect of experimental phosphorus enrichment on oligotrophic tropical marshes in Belize, Central America. *Plant and Soil* **236**:33–53.

Rejmánková, E., and J. Komarkova. (2000). A function of cyanobacterial mats in phosphorus-limited tropical wetlands. *Hydrobiologia* **431**:135–153.

Rejmánková, E., H. M. Savage, M. H. Rodriguez, D. R. Roberts, and M. Rejmanek. (1992). Aquatic vegetation as a basis for classification of *Anopheles albimanus* Weideman (Diptera, Culicidae) larval habitats. *Environmental Entomology* **21**:598–603.

Rejmánková, E., D. R. Roberts, R. E. Harbach, J. Pecor, E. L. Peyton, S. Manguin, R. Krieg, J. Polanco, and

L. Legters. (1993). Environmental and regional determinants of *Anopheles* (Diptera, Culicidae) larval distribution in Belize, Central-America. *Environmental Entomology* **22**:978–992.

Rejmánková, E., D. R. Roberts, A. Pawley, S. Manguin, and J. Polanko. (1995). Predictions of adult *Anopheles albimanus* in villages based on distance from remotely sensed larval habitats. *American Journal of Tropical Medicine and Hygiene* **53**:482–488.

Rejmánková, E., K. O. Pope, R. Post, and E. Maltby. (1996a). Herbaceous wetlands of the Yucatan Peninsula: Communities at extreme ends of environmental gradients. *Internationale Revue Der Gesamten Hydrobiologie* **81**:223–252.

Rejmánková, E., D. R. Roberts, S. Manguin, K. O. Pope, J. Komarek, and R. A. Post. (1996b). *Anopheles albimanus* (Diptera: Culicidae) and cyanobacteria: An example of larval habitat selection. *Environmental Entomology* **25**:1058–1067.

Rejmánková, E., K. O. Pope, D. R. Roberts, M. G. Lege, R. Andre, J. Greico, and Y. Alonzo. (1998). Characterization and detection of *Anopheles vestitipennis* and *Anopheles punctimacula* (Diptera: Culicidae) larval habitats in Belize with field survey and SPOT satellite imagery. *Journal of Vector Ecology* **23**:74–88.

Rejmánková, E., R. Higashi, D. Roberts, M. Lege, and R. Andre. (2000a). Detection of a potential oviposition attractant for *Anopheles albimanus* Wiedemann using solid-phase microextraction fibers *in situ*. *Aquatic Ecology* **34**:413–420.

Rejmánková, E., A. Harbin-Ireland, and M. Lege. (2000b). Bacterial abundance in larval habitats of four species of *Anopheles* (Diptera: Culicidae) in Belize, Central America. *Journal of Vector Ecology* **25**:229–239.

Rejmánková, E., R. Higashi, J. Grieco, N. Achee, and D. Roberts. Volatile substances from larval habitats as species specific oviposition stimulants for *Anopheles* mosquitoes. *Journal of Medical Entomology* **42**:95–103.

Roberts, D. R., L. L. Laughlin, P. Hsheih, and L. J. Legters. (1997). DDT, global strategies, and a malaria control crisis in South America. *Emerging Infectious Diseases* **3**:295–302.

Roberts, D. R., J. F. Paris, S. Manguin, R. E. Harbach, R. Woodruff, E. Rejmánková, J. Polanco, B. Wullschleger, and L. J. Legters. (1996). Predictions of malaria vector distribution in Belize based on multispectral satellite data. *American Journal of Tropical Medicine and Hygiene* **54**:304–308.

Rubio-Palis, Y. and R. H. Zimmerman. (1997). Ecoregional classification of malaria vectors in the neotropics. *Journal of Medical Entomology* **34**:499–510.

Sissoko, M. S., A. Dicko, O. J. T. Briet, M. Sissoko, I. Sagara, H. D. Keita, M. Sogoba, C. Rogier, Y. T. Toure, and O. K. Doumbo. (2004). Malaria incidence in relation to rice cultivation in the irrigated Sahel of Mali. *Acta Tropica* **89**:161–170.

Takken, W. (1999). Chemical signals affecting mosquito behaviour. *Invertebrate Reproduction & Development* **36**:67–71.

Timmermann, E. E. and H. Briegel. (1996). Water depth and larval density affect development and accumulation of reserves in laboratory populations of mosquitoes. *Bulletin of the Society of Vector Ecology* **18**:174–187.

Wasserberg, G., Z. Abramsky, B. P. Kotler, R. S. Ostfeld, I. Yarom, and A. Warburg. (2003). Anthropogenic disturbances enhance occurrence of cutaneous leishmaniasis in Israel deserts: patterns and mechanisms. *Ecological Applications* **13**:868–881.

Wright, C. (1996). The Columbia River Forest Reserve. *Belize Review* **4**:5–9.

CHAPTER 8

The community ecology of *Vibrio cholerae*

Kathryn L. Cottingham and Julia M. Butzler

8.1 Background

The intestinal disease cholera is caused by certain strains of the heterotrophic bacterium *Vibrio cholerae*, an abundant, naturally occurring component of freshwater, estuarine, and marine ecosystems worldwide (reviewed by Islam *et al.* 1997). Interestingly, most strains of *V. cholerae* do not cause disease in humans: although some strains can cause intestinal upsets (e.g. Islam *et al.* 1992), strains from only two, relatively rare, serogroups are known to be capable of causing epidemic disease (Faruque *et al.* 1998). Humans come into contact with virulent (disease-causing) *V. cholerae* by ingesting contaminated water or food. Ingested *V. cholerae* make their way to the small intestine, where they attach to the host using a structure called pilus (Faruque *et al.* 1998). Attached *V. cholerae* begin cell division, and when sufficient numbers of cells have accumulated, they begin to produce an enterotoxin called cholera toxin which causes severe diarrhea and the shedding of many bacteria into the environment—up to 10^{13} bacteria per infected individual per day (Mintz *et al.* 1994). Fortunately, cholera is treatable as long as affected individuals have rapid access to rehydration therapy.

Unfortunately, cholera is a more persistent and global health problem now than it was a few decades ago (Colwell 1996). The disease remains endemic to South Asia, and is emerging or reemerging in other areas, particularly developing nations with inadequate sanitation (Faruque *et al.* 1998). In non-endemic areas, outbreaks tend to occur when supplies of clean water are disrupted by warfare or natural disasters like hurricanes, earthquakes, and tsunamis (Faruque *et al.* 1998). Moreover, additional areas may be at risk for future disease outbreaks due to climate change and increased global connectivity (Ruiz *et al.* 2000; Harvell *et al.* 2002). Understanding the survival and persistence of *V. cholerae* in aquatic environments is therefore important to human health on a global scale.

Vibrio cholerae is an intriguing organism because it appears to thrive both as a human pathogen and as an environmental heterotroph (Cottingham *et al.* 2003). Heterotrophic bacteria are key components of aquatic food webs because they mineralize relatively unavailable organic nutrients into available inorganic forms (reviewed by Cotner and Biddanda 2002). At present, it is not clear if *V. cholerae* is unique among heterotrophic bacteria, or merely one of many functionally similar species (most of which are not human pathogens). If *V. cholerae* operates similarly to other heterotrophic bacteria, then it should be an ideal model organism for investigating the role of microbes in aquatic ecosystems given the wealth of molecular and genetic tools available for its study (Cottingham *et al.* 2003). Alternatively, if *V. cholerae* is relatively unique among heterotrophic bacteria, then it may be possible to identify ways to manipulate aquatic ecosystems to reduce its abundance and/or transmission to humans—and thereby improve human health.

In this chapter, we consider the community ecology of *V. cholerae* during its time in aquatic ecosystems. We discuss two topics in detail: interactions among strains within the "species" *V. cholerae* and direct interactions between *V. cholerae* and other aquatic organisms (Fig. 8.1). We end by considering briefly how both intraspecific and interspecific interactions may be altered by environmental context. It is important to note that although the

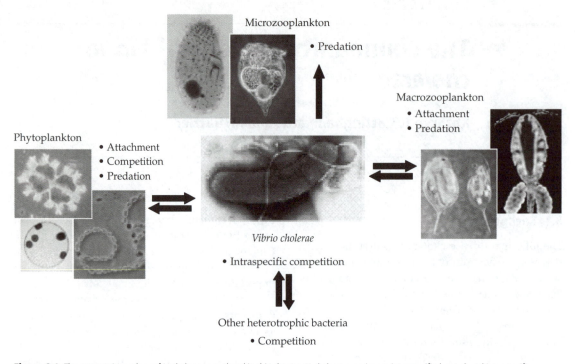

Figure 8.1 The community ecology of *V. cholerae* as explored in this chapter. *V. cholerae* experiences intraspecific (center) and interspecific competition (bottom, left); attaches to phytoplankton (left) and macrozooplankton (right); and is consumed by microzooplankton (top) and macrozooplankton (right). The exact nature of many of these interactions, especially attachment, is as yet undetermined.

microbiology of *V. cholerae* and epidemiology of cholera are well-studied, the ecology of *V. cholerae* is not (Cottingham *et al.* 2003). Thus, this chapter includes a mix of established information, informed hypotheses, and speculation. Our most important take-home message is that the general principles of community ecology provide an excellent framework for understanding both environmental *V. cholerae* and the disease it causes.

8.2 Key behaviors of *V. cholerae*

Cottingham *et al.* (2003) proposed that two behaviors of *V. cholerae* are likely to be important to its ecology: the propensity to attach to both living and nonliving substrates and the ability to utilize a viable-but-nonculturable (VBNC) state to withstand unfavorable environmental conditions. Like many other bacteria, *V. cholerae* can react to changes in environmental conditions by entering a VBNC state (McDougald *et al.* 1998). When bacterial cells enter this state, they lose their flagellum and change to a

smaller, more spherical form (McDougald *et al.* 1998; Huq *et al.* 2000). Importantly, VBNC cells do not reproduce on standard microbiological media, and so can be difficult to detect through conventional plating approaches (Box 8.1). Laboratory experiments indicate that *V. cholerae* can exist in the VBNC state for long periods of time, presumably allowing survival during unfavorable environmental conditions (Huq *et al.* 2000). The VBNC state is of considerable interest to ecosystem ecologists, because such cells can quickly transition back to a metabolically active state in response to changes in environmental conditions, altering processes such as decomposition rates and nutrient cycling (Cole 1999).

Environmental *V. cholerae* also switch between free-living (unattached) and surface-attached forms, and may aggregate into biofilms while attached (Cottingham *et al.* 2003). Interestingly, *V. cholerae* attaches to a wide array of both living (Table 8.1) and nonliving substrates. Attached bacteria survive passage through the gut better than free-living cells

Box 8.1 Techniques for quantifying free-living and attached bacteria

Being able to accurately identify and enumerate attached bacteria is fundamental to advancing our understanding of the ecology of *V. cholerae*. However, despite this obvious need, there is surprisingly little consensus on routine methodology for sampling free-living versus attached environmental bacteria.

General methodologies

Culture methods

This traditional approach to counting bacteria relies on the ability to grow bacteria in or on a laboratory medium. Culture methods can detect very small numbers of cells, and tricks such as formulating the medium to target the growth of specific bacteria while inhibiting others can be implemented for a more sophisticated and specific measure.

However, while straightforward in effort and economically feasible, culture methods have considerable drawbacks. Because the culture method requires growth, measures of species presence and abundance are affected by both the growth environment that is provided and the physiological state of the organisms (e.g. active versus VBNC). In general, culture plates severely underestimate bacterial numbers (Kepner and Pratt 1994). Plate counts also assume that during the process of plating, individual bacteria are separated and will form discrete colonies; if cells are aggregated, there will be further underestimation. Finally, culture methods require an incubation period, and thus cannot be used for immediate detection, which is a problem in the case of pathogens like *V. cholerae*.

Direct microscope counts

The number of cells in a sample can also be counted directly with the aid of a microscope. However, it can be hard to distinguish between bacteria and other small, similarly shaped objects or to differentiate live from dead cells using bright-field or phase contrast microscopy. Consequently, microbiologists frequently use fluorescent techniques to help visualize bacteria, including both conventional fluorochromes such as acridine orange (AO) and 4′,6-diamidino-2-phenylindole (DAPI) that bind to nucleic acids, as well as immunofluorescent dyes developed for particular taxa (e.g. there is a monoclonal antibody stain for *V. cholerae*, Huq *et al*. 1990). Fluorescent dyes can also be combined with fluorochromes designed to assess metabolic activity and cell integrity for more informative analyses.

Fluorescent techniques also have their problems. Choice of stain may influence counts (Suzuki *et al*. 1993), and discrepancies may be related to the type and quality of the sample (Kepner and Pratt 1994). The method also requires the appropriate density of cells in the stained sample to obtain precise counts; too many or too few cells result in poor statistical precision, making it hard to develop reliable protocols in samples of greatly varying densities. Despite these issues, fluorochromes and epifluorescence microscopy are frequently the method of choice for counting bacteria, resulting in better, more accurate counts of total bacterial cells than culture methods.

Molecular techniques

More recently, molecular techniques have grown in prominence, allowing individual species to be identified and sometimes even quantified from environmental samples. These techniques include sequence-based methods, fluorescent *in situ* hybridization (FISH), genetic fingerprinting (e.g. RFLP), and microarrays. Comparative analyses of these techniques with traditional techniques are still in progress, but it is generally believed that they are the wave of the future in environmental microbiology, particularly once reliable approaches to quantifying abundances are more readily available.

Counting attached bacteria

While culture-based, microscopic, and molecular methods are all used to count free-living bacteria, accurate counts of substrate-associated bacteria are difficult, if not impossible, to achieve. For example, visualization of attached bacteria even with the aid of fluorescence may not detect all the bacteria (e.g. those attached to the underside of a substrate). Subsampling can be challenging if the bacteria are not distributed evenly across the substrate. As a result, detachment has become a standard first step in most enumerations of surface-associated bacteria. Several detachment methods have been developed, with different degrees of success (reviewed in Kepner and Pratt 1994). Shaking of the sample does little to detach any significant portion of the associated bacteria, while both homogenization and sonication in combination with pre-incubation agents such as deflocculants, dispersants, and surfactants are more efficient (reviewed in Epstein and Rossel 1995; Griebler *et al*. 2001). Sonication requires determining the correct balance of intensity and duration to

continues

Box 8.1 *continued*

remove the bacteria without disrupting the cell wall (Cottingham *et al*. in preparation). Unfortunately, all of these methods may result in other bacteria-sized particles, thus requiring the use of fluorochromes to highlight bacteria if they are to be viewed microscopically, although even stains like DAPI may result in nonspecific staining in a sample containing substrates (Epstein and Rossel 1995).

Recommendations

Despite the assortment of methodological choices available to a researcher interested in measuring bacteria, the

process is not easy. Although the advantages and disadvantages of many techniques have been acknowledged and explored, comparisons of results are difficult. Even when using the same methodology, small differences in technique can result in large enumeration differences (Jones 1974). Additionally, results from many of these techniques are subject to experimenter bias (Kirchman 1993; Kepner and Pratt 1994). Many of these techniques must be calibrated for each new type of bacteria and sample. We are currently working to develop reliable protocols for enumerating free-living versus attached *V. cholerae* in order to better understand the community ecology of this organism.

Table 8.1 Freshwater (F) and brackish/saltwater (M) organisms to which *V. cholerae* is known to attach (Huq *et al*. 1990; Tamplin *et al*. 1990; Islam *et al*. 1994; Colwell 1996; Cottingham *et al*. 2003)

Organism	Subgroup	Representative species	Approximate size range	Habitat
Phytoplankton	Cyanobacteria	*Anabaena*	mm–cm	F
	Chlorophytes	*Volvox*, desmids, *Rhizoclonium*	μm–mm	F
	Diatoms	*Skeletonema*	μm	F and M
	Dinoflagellates		μm	F and M
Zooplankton	Copepods	*Acartia*	mm	M
		Cyclops, *Diaptomus*	mm	F
	Cladocerans	*Daphnia, Bosmina, Bosminopsis, Ceriodaphnia, Diaphanosoma*	mm	Mostly F
	Rotifers		μm–mm	Mostly F
Macrophytes		*Ulva, Entermorpha, Ceramium, Polysiphonia*	cm–dm	M
		Eichhornia (water hyacinth)	dm	F
		Lemna (duckweed)	cm	F
Benthos	Prawns	*Penaeus, Metapenaeus*	cm	M
		Macrobrachium	up to ~15 cm	F
	Oysters		cm	M
	Crabs		cm–dm	M
	Chironomid egg masses		mm–cm	F
Fish	Sea mullet		up to ~75 cm	M

(Nalin *et al*. 1979; King *et al*. 1991) and survive better when nutrients are limiting (Dawson *et al*. 1981). *V. cholerae* grown with copepods (Huq *et al*. 1983), the cyanobacterium *Anabaena variabilis* (Islam *et al*. 2002), duckweed (Islam *et al*. 1990), and water hyacinth (Spira 1981) survive longer than *V. cholerae*

grown without these substrates. Attachment to plankton could be a commensal relationship, as proposed by Sochard *et al*. (1979), but it also has the potential to be parasitic or mutualistic (see subsection on *Attachment*, below) and to alter relationships with predators (see *Predation*, below).

8.3 Interactions within "*V. cholerae*"

We first consider the community ecology of the diverse group of bacterial strains that are grouped together as the taxonomic entity "*V. cholerae.*" For ecologists accustomed to working with eukaryotic organisms, this probably seems quite silly: how is it possible to ask questions at the community level using a single species? The answer lies in two unique aspects of prokaryotic biology: (1) how "species" are defined and (2) the diversity of mechanisms for exchanging genetic information between individuals.

First, there is considerable genotypic variability within *V. cholerae* (e.g. Beltran *et al.* 1999, Jiang *et al.* 2000). Most ecologists are familiar with the biological species concept for eukaryotic taxa: a species includes all individuals that are actually or potentially interbreeding. However, because prokaryotes are haploid and reproduce asexually, this concept does not work. Instead, prokaryotes are typically classified into species by genetic and genomic similarity, such as a minimum similarity (e.g. 97%) in conservative gene sequences such as 16S ribosomal RNA together with at least 70% homology in DNA sequences (Madigan *et al.* 2003, pp. 345–346). In contrast, eukaryotic species are typically much more similar in both their 18S rRNA sequences and at the genome level; for example, the human and chimpanzee genomes have >98% homology in DNA sequences (e.g. Fujiyama *et al.* 2002). This means that the definition of a species is far broader for microbes than for plants and animals (Oren 2004).

Second, bacterial genomes are much more dynamic than those of eukaryotes due to horizontal gene transfer—the exchange of genes not only among strains within a species, but also among phylogenetically diverse taxa (Madigan *et al.* 2003). This exchange can be achieved by many mechanisms, including plasmids (circular, double-stranded units of DNA that replicate independently of the chromosomal DNA) and bacteriophages (viruses that affect bacteria) (Dale and Park 2004). There are many likely benefits of horizontal gene transfer for bacteria, including increased rates of evolution (Dobrindt and Hacker 2001; Boyd and Brussow 2002) and high genetic diversity within species. For example, horizontal gene transfer via bacteriophages

is thought to play a major role in creating virulent *V. cholerae* from non-virulent environmental strains (Islam *et al.* 1997).

8.3.1 Consequences of within-species diversity

What, if any, are the ecological consequences of the high genotypic diversity within *V. cholerae*? Is the ecology of different genotypes fundamentally different, or do most strains act similarly when faced with changes in the abiotic or biotic environment? As in other systems, questions about the "community genetics" (*sensu* Whitham *et al.* 2003) of *V. cholerae* are just beginning to be addressed.

Epidemiological evidence suggests that the strains known to cause epidemic cholera are not ecologically identical, and that different environmental conditions may favor different strains. For example, although there are > 200 known serogroups of *V. cholerae*, only two—O1 and O139—are known to cause epidemic disease (Faruque *et al.* 1998; Reidl and Klose 2002). Historically, cholera outbreaks were caused by *V. cholerae* O1, which is divided into two biotypes, classical and El Tor, that differ in their hemolytic activity, resistance to bacteriophages, and antibiotic resistance (Manning *et al.* 1994). Classical strains predominated in clinical samples until El Tor was identified in 1961; since then, El Tor strains have gradually displaced classical strains throughout much of the world (Colwell 1996; Faruque *et al.* 1998). Interestingly, the second known virulent serogroup, O139, became the major cause of epidemic cholera in some regions during the 1990s (Faruque *et al.* 1998), but has since waned in importance. O139 is thought to have evolved from O1 El Tor (Huq and Colwell 1996); it has the ability to produce a protective outer capsule and may do better than O1 strains under some environmental conditions (Morris *et al.* 1994).

Researchers are beginning to evaluate whether shifts among the O1 classical, O1 El Tor, and O139 strains are related to environmental fitness, altered virulence, increased transmissibility, or other factors. For example, Spira (1981) reported that the classical biotype is a weaker competitor than the El Tor biotype, and that the two strains seem to peak at different times of the year. O139 may be more resistant to antibiotics than either O1 strain (Calia *et al.* 1994), but whether antibiotic resistance plays a role in aquatic environments is not yet known.

Understanding the relationship between virulent and non-virulent strains of *V. cholerae* is still more difficult. That O1 and O139 strains are relatively uncommon in the environment (Faruque *et al.* 1998) suggests that these bacteria are inferior in some way to nonvirulent strains. For example, O1 strains are more likely to be in a VBNC state than non-O1 strains in aquatic environments, perhaps because O1 strains are more vulnerable to lysis by bacteriophages (Colwell *et al.* 1995). Differential abilities of virulent and non-virulent strains to cope with stress raise a number of interesting and important questions. For example, what (if any) are the costs and benefits of having genes associated with virulence in aquatic environments? Does the presence of virulence genes affect the survival and success of an individual bacterial cell? How does carrying some virulence genes differ from carrying all of them? The answers to these questions are not known at present, but we expect that there might be trade-offs associated with having virulence genes, such that they allow a bacterial strain to multiply quickly inside mammalian intestines but negatively impact performance in aquatic environments. If there are such trade-offs, is an occasional trip through a human (and consequent production of up to 10^{13} bacteria/day, Mintz *et al.* 1994) sufficient to provide selection in favor of the "extra" virulence genes? Studies to evaluate this premise have not yet been conducted.

8.4 Direct interactions with other taxa

Both virulent and non-virulent *V. cholerae* likely interact with other taxa in all of the textbook ways, including competition, predation, parasitism, and mutualism (Fig. 8.1). Because *V. cholerae*'s strongest interactions are likely to be with attachment partners or bacteriophages, we emphasize those two relationships, touching on parasitism and mutualism during those discussions. We also consider competition and predation in less detail.

8.4.1 Interactions with bacteriophages

Most *V. cholerae* strains found in aquatic environments are thought to be incapable of causing epidemic disease because they possess neither the genes for colonizing humans nor those for producing cholera toxin (Faruque *et al.* 1998). The current model suggests that the most critical genes for causing disease are clustered at two places in the bacterial genome: the vibrio pathogenicity island or VPI (Karaolis *et al.* 1998) and the lysogenic bacteriophage CTX-Φ (Waldor and Mekalanos 1996). The VPI encodes a number of genes, including those required to build the structure used to attach to the intestine, the toxin-coregulated pilus (TCP). The CTX-Φ, which harbors the genes needed to produce cholera toxin, uses the TCP to enter only those strains of *V. cholerae* capable of colonizing humans, then integrates its genome into that of the host bacterium (Faruque *et al.* 1998). Thus, a partnership between two organisms, the CTX-Φ and *V. cholerae* expressing TCP, is thought to be required to cause epidemic cholera. Moreover, the acquisition of the VPI and CTX-Φ follows an "assembly rule": the VPI must be acquired first, then the strain must express TCP, and finally the CTX bacteriophage can "parasitize" the strain (Kovach *et al.* 1996; Waldor and Mekalanos 1996).

Although the CTX-Φ and the VPI are thought to be the necessary virulence factors to cause cholera, these genetic elements have been found both together and separately in non-virulent environmental strains (Sarkar *et al.* 2002). Both the mechanism for how these genes were obtained and the function of these genes in non-virulent strains are unknown, but it is clear that environmental strains carrying virulence genes pose a potential source of "new" disease-causing strains in addition to potentially fueling the evolution of existing clinical strains (Banerjee *et al.* 2002). It is important, therefore, for researchers to understand how the VPI and the CTX-Φ are acquired by environmental strains, as well as what happens once these genes are acquired. Are these genes harbored in small numbers, but become advantageous under certain conditions, leading to spread throughout a habitat? Or are these genetic elements introduced or reintroduced into isolated aquatic environments by infected humans? Once the genes are present in one system, does monsoonal flooding facilitate the dispersal of virulent strains to new habitats? There is some evidence that people who use isolated lakes and ponds for their water source are less prone to cholera than those using rivers or canals (Spira 1981). To our knowledge, questions regarding the creation, maintenance, and spread of virulent strains have not been addressed using the perspectives of dispersal ecology and local versus regional dynamics—but clearly such studies would be extremely helpful.

8.4.2 Attachment

As introduced in Section 8.2, above, one of *V. cholerae*'s most striking behaviors is attachment to living substrates (Table 8.1). Whether this interaction represents commensalism, parasitism, or mutualism is at present not well understood. What we do know is that because attachment serves to concentrate *V. cholerae* into sufficiently high densities to cause infection (Box 8.2), it is particularly important that we develop a more complete understanding of *V. cholerae*'s attachment behavior. In this section, we use information gathered from non-virulent heterotrophic bacteria to make predictions about the nature of *V. cholerae*'s attachment behavior. For example, multiple factors appear to influence the prevalence of attachment in aquatic bacteria, including substrate type (e.g. Griebler *et al.* 2001), substrate availability (reviewed in Simon *et al.* 2002), and the physiological state of individual cells (Dawson *et al.* 1981). Laboratory tests show that *V. cholerae* may prefer certain substrates, as well

as particular areas on those substrates (Faruque *et al.* 1998); we believe that the propensity to attach, as well as issues relating to substrate choice, could lend insight to the control of *V. cholerae* populations. We focus here on attachment to pelagic plankton, but note that a better understanding of the processes involving attachment to the benthos is also critical, particularly in estuarine and marine areas where benthic invertebrates are a major source of protein for humans.

From a bacterial perspective, there are interesting differences between phytoplankton versus crustacean zooplankton as hosts, as well as among species within each taxonomic group (Cottingham *et al.* 2003). Phytoplankton, for example, are likely to provide a very nutrient-rich habitat, particularly because of their "leakiness" with regard to fixed carbon and available nutrients (e.g. Fogg 1983). *V. cholerae* also has the potential to derive resources directly from phytoplankton using mucinase, an enzyme that degrades mucin (a common substance of plants, Schneider and Parker 1982); the ability to produce mucinase can prolong survival (Islam *et al.* 2002). We hypothesize that attachment to nitrogen(N)-fixing cyanobacteria like *Anabaena* may be mutualistic, such that *V. cholerae* obtains fixed N while the autotrophic cyanobacterium obtains CO_2 for photosynthesis (cf. Paerl 1982). In support of this hypothesis, Islam *et al.* (1999) found that *V. cholerae* was capable of living within the mucilage of N-fixing *Anabaena* for many months, presumably

---

Box 8.2 Pathogen attachment and transmission

Attachment to water borne particles, plankton, and benthos has long been thought to be a major mechanism for transmission of *V. cholerae* to humans, in part because ~10^4–10^6 *V. cholerae* cells constitute an infectious dose for humans—approximately the same number as may be found on a single copepod (reviewed in Colwell *et al.* 2003). For this reason, Colwell *et al.* (2003) conducted a unique study to determine whether filtration to remove plankton from water would protect people from cholera. This study involved having Bangladeshi households participate in one of three treatments: (1) control (no intervention), (2) use old sari cloth folded to produce eight layers to filter all particles >20 μm from their water before

use, and (3) use 150 μm nylon mesh to filter the water. Results were striking: Filtering water with sari cloth or nylon mesh removed all zooplankton, most of the phytoplankton, and large particles from the water. Cholera incidence was reduced by 52% in households that filtered their water relative to control households. Finally, when cholera did occur in households with filtered water, the disease appeared to be less severe. Thus, Colwell *et al.*'s (2003) results clearly support the hypothesis that *V. cholerae* attached to plankton are a vehicle for infection. Plans are now in development to test the filtration approach on a larger scale (A. Huq, personal communication).

because both partners benefited from the relationship. Similar arguments may hold for *V. cholerae* living in association with large colonial chlorophytes like *Volvox*.

In contrast to phytoplankton, zooplankton may be less "leaky," but they are also more mobile, possibly providing a more effective means of eliminating local nutrient depletion (Threlkeld *et al.* 1993) or of dispersing among areas within a pond through vertical or horizontal migration. *V. cholerae* also has the potential to use chitin from crustacean zooplankton substrates directly through the action of chitinase (Nalin *et al.* 1979). Within the crustaceans, copepods could offer a more stable attachment substrate than cladocerans since copepods have a terminal molt stage, while cladocerans molt throughout their lifetimes. However, studies to date are equivocal regarding whether *V. cholerae* "prefer" to attach to live crustaceans or exuviae (Huq *et al.* 1983; Tamplin *et al.* 1990; Dumontet *et al.* 1996). Tamplin *et al.* (1990) suggested that live copepods have antibacterial defenses, but live plankton are also more likely to move around or to supply readily usable nutrients through excretion or exudates (Islam *et al.* 1994). Moreover, exuviae are likely to sink, providing a one-way trip to the sediments given *V. cholerae*'s size and swimming ability. We speculate that the degree of limitation by carbon versus nutrients could be a factor in altering the choice between live hosts and exuviae: carbon limitation might favor the use of dead hosts (which are likely "undefended" and should be relatively easy to mineralize), while nutrient limitation might favor being near live hosts which release available nutrients. This hypothesis could easily be tested in laboratory experiments manipulating resource availability.

Attached *V. cholerae* are known to form biofilms (Fig. 8.2) under certain conditions (Faruque *et al.* 1998), which may have implications for environmental persistence and transmission to humans. Biofilms are multicell, often structurally complex, associations that can be mutually beneficial to participating cells. For example, a mixed-species biofilm creates physical and chemical heterogeneity that facilitates coexistence (Shapiro 1998) and can physically protect participants from harsh environmental conditions (Costerton *et al.* 1995). In *V. cholerae*, biofilm formation appears to provide protection

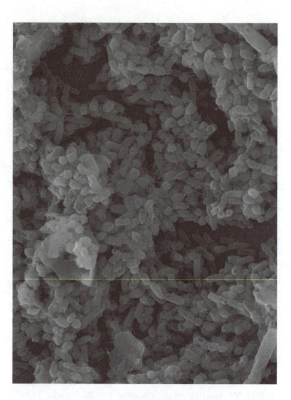

Figure 8.2 Example of an *Escherichia coli* biofilm, magnified 5000 times. Image provided by Daniel Kadouri and George O'Toole, Dartmouth Medical School.

from stomach acids after ingestion (Zhu and Mekalanos 2003) and from the toxic effects of alum and chlorine in water treatment plants (Chowdhury *et al.* 1997). Biofilms may also provide proximity of potential mutualists who may supply one another with a necessary substrate, such as a metabolic product (Madigan *et al.* 2003). At this point, little is known about other species that may form biofilms with *V. cholerae* under field conditions, but this is a topic worthy of further investigation.

Finally, we can link our consideration of attachment back to our discussion above of the potential ecological consequences of the considerable genotypic diversity within the group *V. cholerae*. Are some strains more likely to attach to particles or to living hosts than others? What factors are involved in attachment? For example, does the ability to produce the TCP (and thereby attach to intestines) increase or decrease attachment to plankton? Chiavelli *et al.* (2001) demonstrated that a second pilus, the mannose-sensitive hemagglutinin pilus, is involved in attachment of the O1 El Tor and O139 strains to zooplankton, and suggested that the inability of O1 classical strains to express the genes coding for this pilus might have been a contributing factor to its recent declines. Moreover, mutations in the gene coding for this pilus had stronger effects on O139, for which attachment was blocked completely, than for O1 El Tor, for which attachment was merely suppressed (Chiavelli *et al.* 2001). This suggests that there are some interesting interactions between serotype and attachment behavior worth a closer look from ecologists.

8.4.3 Competition

Vibrio cholerae is likely to compete with other aquatic organisms for both energy and nutrients. To date, the relative competitive abilities of *V. cholerae* and other heterotrophic bacteria have not been well studied, and the few studies that do exist have taken only the first few steps in establishing a competitive hierarchy. For example, experimental microcosms without competing microflora supported *V. cholerae* for longer periods than those that contained bacterial competitors (Spira 1981).

In addition to competing with one another, heterotrophic bacteria are likely to compete with phytoplankton for nutrients, especially phosphorus (P). At present, few general statements about this relationship exist, probably because the winner varies depending on environmental conditions (Wetzel 2001). Free-living bacteria compete directly with phytoplankton for phosphorus when P is limiting (Currie 1990), and bacteria tend to be more effective competitors because of their smaller size (Fuhs *et al.* 1972). However, bacteria may compete less (or not at all) with phytoplankton in a physically close relationship such as attachment. Evidence so far is mixed. Correlational evidence from field studies suggests that phytoplankton blooms encourage *V. cholerae* growth (e.g. Mouriño-Perez *et al.* 2003). However, there were decreases in the number of culturable *V. cholerae* when it was grown with phytoplankton in the laboratory—although it is not clear whether this effect was due to a shift to the VBNC state or to actual inhibition by the phytoplankton (Kogure *et al.* 1980). Clearly, more work is needed in this area.

8.4.4 Predation

Bacterial communities appear to be regulated by both resources and predators (Jürgens and Matz 2002), although the relative importance of each factor likely changes with environmental context. Evidence that bacterivory may be an important influence on bacterial communities comes from two areas: predator feeding selectivity and phenotypic responses by bacteria to predation. Bacterial predators include both microzooplankton (especially protozoans) and macrozooplankton such as the cladocerans *Daphnia* spp. and *Bosmina longirostris* (Sanders *et al.* 1992; Vaque and Pace 1992; Jürgens *et al.* 1997). Moreover, despite the long-held beliefs that copepods are not bacterivores, there is some evidence of copepods grazing upon bacteria (Turner and Tester 1992; Roff *et al.* 1995); this is understudied.

Zooplankton community structure can have strong effects on bacterial communities. Although different zooplankton communities do not have a consistent impact on bacterial abundance or biomass (Jürgens and Jeppesen 2000; Langenheder and Jürgens 2001), they do affect cell morphology, composition, and relative abundance (Jürgens *et al.* 1994; 1997; Jürgens and Jeppesen 2000; Langenheder and Jürgens 2001; Degans *et al.* 2002). For example, in the presence of heterotrophic nanoflagellates (HNFs), bacterial cells tend to shift their morphology to a smaller, grazing-resistant form. Because *Daphnia* have strong negative impacts on HNFs, bacteria tend to maintain their rod and cocci shapes (Jürgens *et al.* 1997) and to shift the balance between free and attached bacterial cells (Langenheder and Jürgens 2001) in *Daphnia*-dominated communities.

Although the effect of bacterivory on *V. cholerae* is unknown, we may predict the response using data from other pelagic bacteria. For example, protistan grazers selectively remove active cells, while cladocerans feed indiscriminately on both active and dormant cells (Pace and Cole 1996; Cole 1999; Langenheder and Jürgens 2001). However, protists can be limited by bacterial size such that cells longer than 2.4 μm are rarely grazed (Pernthaler *et al.* 1996). When active, *V. cholerae* is rod-shaped and measures ~3 μm long by ~1 μm wide; when in the VBNC state, *V. cholerae* is a ~1 μm sphere. Cottingham *et al.* (2003) hypothesized that active *V. cholerae* are highly susceptible to grazing by filter-feeding cladoceran zooplankton like *Daphnia*, but relatively unsusceptible to grazing by protists due to their large size. In contrast, *V. cholerae* in the VBNC state should be vulnerable to grazing by both protists and cladocerans based on size constraints, although protists may not eat them because they are not active. This prediction is quite different from expectations for smaller bacterial species, for which the VBNC state may represent a refuge from predation because the cells are too small to handle (Carman and Dobbs 1997; Baty *et al.* 2000).

It is important to note that the effects of predators on bacteria, including *V. cholerae*, depend on whether ingestion is fatal. Some bacterial species survive passage through the gut of a predator, and may even be stimulated by gut nutrients (King *et al.* 1991). We suspect that bacteria are unlikely to survive gut passage when consumed by ciliates or HNFs, but to our knowledge, no one has examined whether this is true for *V. cholerae* consumed by zooplankton. It is important to begin direct studies of predation on *V. cholerae*, because understanding how predators affect *V. cholerae* and how factors such as attachment and nutrients could mediate these effects is an important step in understanding the regulation of *V. cholerae* populations (Cottingham *et al.* 2003).

8.5 The environmental context for community interactions

The interactions between *V. cholerae* and other taxa just described, as well as interactions within *V. cholerae*, take place against a background of changing abiotic and biotic conditions. Here we highlight a few additional factors that may be particularly important to this organism and its intra- and inter-specific interactions.

How different strains of *V. cholerae* interact with one another and with other species is likely to vary considerably with abiotic factors such as the salinity gradient from marine to estuarine to freshwater systems. For example, *V. cholerae* are least abundant at very low (R. K. Taylor, personal communication) and very high salinities (Jiang 2001; Jiang and Fu 2001;), suggesting that competition between *V. cholerae*, other heterotrophic bacteria, and phytoplankton

could vary with salinity. Stress at extreme salinities could also increase the likelihood of a mutualistic relationship between *V. cholerae* and phytoplankton, if free-living *V. cholerae* fare poorly under these conditions; this may be why there is increased bacterial attachment in freshwaters (Clarke and Joint 1986). The importance of predation could also change with salinity, as dominance by *Daphnia* in freshwater switches over to copepod-domination in salty water (Sommer and Stibor 2002), with consequent effects on lower trophic levels. Understanding how salinity affects *V. cholerae* distribution, abundance, and interactions could be particularly important if salinity regimes are altered by global climate change, for example by increased monsoonal strength.

We also expect *V. cholerae* to be strongly affected by biotic factors such as the structure of aquatic food-webs (Cottingham *et al.* 2003). Specifically, changes in food-web structure may affect predation regimes, the composition and diversity of potential hosts for attached bacteria, or the type of nonliving particles that are available to be colonized. For example, the trophic cascade hypothesis (Carpenter *et al.* 1985) suggests that when piscivorous taxa dominate the fish community, large-bodied zooplankton like *Daphnia* will be abundant, promoting high grazing pressure and relatively small standing stocks of phytoplankton. In contrast, when planktivorous fish dominate (as is true in most South Asian systems, where aquaculture is common), the zooplankton community will be dominated by smaller-bodied, less effective grazers, and phytoplankton will be more abundant. Depending on the preferences of *V. cholerae* for different living hosts (which have not yet been established, see *Attachment* above), changes in the fish community may alter the density and distribution of *V. cholerae* in free-living and attached states, and therefore the potential for transmission to humans (Box 8.2). We are currently engaged in building simulation models to explore the outcomes of different preference functions for *V. cholerae* attachment and transmission, and are planning field and laboratory experiments to test the model's predictions.

Finally, studies from other environmentally mediated diseases suggest that biodiversity may affect the potential for transmission of diseases from the environment to human populations. For example,

Ostfeld *et al.* (chapter 3, this volume) describe how the decline in diversity of potential tick hosts, combined with the increased abundance of a particularly effective disease reservoir, has likely increased the risk of transmission of Lyme disease to humans. Might the same be true for cholera? If we change the potential availability of hosts for attachment, could we change transmission dynamics for the disease? To answer these questions, we must understand the ecology of the communities in which *V. cholerae* is embedded.

8.6 Synthesis

We have described how community interactions such as competition, predation, and mutualism may affect the abundance, behavior, and potential pathogenicity of *V. cholerae*. Understanding the epidemiology of cholera is likely to require understanding the coupling between *V. cholerae* in aquatic environments and human vulnerability to the disease (Collins 2003). We believe that a vital first step toward this improved understanding requires the principles, tools, and techniques of community ecology, as outlined here and elsewhere in this book.

Acknowledgments

We thank the editors for inviting us to contribute to this volume. Megan Donahue participated in several discussions regarding potential topics for inclusion in this review, particularly those involving interactions between *V. cholerae* and potential plankton substrates. Deborah Chiavelli, Ron Taylor, Anwar Huq, and Siraj Islam have provided many insights into the ecology of *V. cholerae* in discussions with KLC over the past 4 years. Amy Dawson, Raquel Martinez, and Elizabeth Wolkovich provided constructive comments on drafts of the manuscript. Our research on *V. cholerae* is supported by an NSF Genome-Enabled Biocomplexity Award (GEO-0120677), as well as the Burke Award for new faculty and the Cramer Fund for graduate student research at Dartmouth College.

References

Banerjee, R., S. Das, K. Mukhopadhyay, S. Nag, A. Chakrabortty, and K. Chaudhuri. (2002). Involvement of in vivo induced cheY-4 gene of *Vibrio cholerae* in motility, early adherence to intestinal epithelial cells and regulation of virulence factors. *FEBS Letters* **532**:221–226.

Baty, A. M., C. C. Eastburn, S. Techkarnjanaruk, A. E. Goodman, and G. G. Geesey. (2000). Spatial and temporal variations in chitinolytic gene expression and bacterial biomass production during chitin degradation. *Applied and Environmental Microbiology* **66**:3574–3585.

Beltran, P., G. Delgado, A. Navarro, F. Trujillo, R. K. Selander, and A. Cravioto. (1999). Genetic diversity and population structure of *Vibrio cholerae*. *Journal of Clinical Microbiology* **37**:581–590.

Boyd, E. F. and H. Brussow. (2002). Common themes among bacteriophage-encoded virulence factors and diversity among the bacteriophages involved. *Trends in Microbiology* **10**:521–529.

Calia, K. E., M. Murtagh, M. J. Ferraro, and S. B. Calderwood. (1994). Comparison of *Vibrio cholerae* O139 with *Vibrio cholerae* O1 classical and El-Tor biotypes. *Infection and Immunity* **62**:1504–1506.

Carman, K. R. and F. C. Dobbs. (1997). Epibiotic microorganisms on copepods and other marine crustaceans. *Microscopy and Research and Technique* **37**:116–135.

Carpenter, S. R., J. F. Kitchell, and J. R. Hodgson. (1985). Cascading trophic interactions and lake productivity. *BioScience* **35**:634–639.

Chiavelli, D. A., J. W. Marsh, and R. K. Taylor. (2001). The mannose-sensitive hemagglutinin of *Vibrio cholerae* promotes adherence to zooplankton. *Applied and Environmental Microbiology* **67**:3220–3225.

Chowdhury, M. A. R., A. Huq, B. Xu, F. J. B. Madeira, and R. R. Colwell. (1997). Effect of alum on free-living and copepod-associated *Vibrio cholerae* O1 and O139. *Applied and Environmental Microbiology* **63**:3323–3326.

Clarke, K. R. and I. R. Joint. (1986). Methodology for estimating numbers of free-living and attached bacteria in estuarine water. *Applied and Environmental Microbiology* **51**:1110–1120.

Cole, J. J. (1999). Aquatic microbiology for ecosystem scientists: new and recycled paradigms in ecological microbiology. *Ecosystems* **2**:215–225.

Collins, A. E. (2003). Vulnerability to coastal cholera ecology. *Social Science and Medicine* **57**:1397–1407.

Colwell, R. R. (1996). Global climate and infectious disease: the cholera paradigm. *Science* **274**:2025–2031.

Colwell, R. R., A. Huq, M. A. R. Chowdhury, P. R. Brayton, and B. Xu. (1995). Serogroup conversion of *Vibrio cholerae*. *Canadian Journal of Microbiology* **41**:946–950.

Colwell, R. R., A. Huq, M. S. Islam, K. M. A. Aziz, M. Yunus, N. H. Khan *et al.* (2003). Reduction of cholera in Bangladeshi villages by simple filtration. *Proceedings of the National Academy of Sciences* **100**:1051–1055.

Costerton, J. W., Z. Lewandowski, D. E. Caldwell, D. R. Korber, and H. M. Lappinscott. (1995). Microbial biofilms. *Annual Review of Microbiology* **49**:711–745.

Cotner, J. B. and B. A. Biddanda. (2002). Small players, large role: microbial influence on biogeochemical processes in pelagic aquatic ecosystems. *Ecosystems* **5**:105–121.

Cottingham, K. L., D. A. Chiavelli, and R. K. Taylor. (2003). Environmental microbe and human pathogen: the ecology and microbiology of *Vibrio cholerae. Frontiers in Ecology and the Environment* **1**:80–86.

Currie, D. J. (1990). Large-scale variability and interactions among phytoplankton, bacterioplankton, and phosphorus. *Limnology and Oceanography* **35**:1437–1455.

Dale J. W. and S. F. Park. (2004). *Molecular Genetics of Bacteria*, 4th edition. John Wiley & Sons, Hoboken, NJ.

Dawson, M. P., B. A. Humphrey, and K. C. Marshall. (1981). Adhesion—a tactic in the survival strategy of a marine *Vibrio* during starvation. *Current Microbiology* **6**:195–199.

Degans, H., E. Zollner, K. Van der Gucht, L. De Meester, and K. Jürgens. (2002). Rapid *Daphnia*-mediated changes in microbial community structure: an experimental study. *FEMS Microbiology Ecology* **42**:137–149.

Dobrindt, U. and J. Hacker. (2001). Whole genome plasticity in pathogenic bacteria. *Current Opinion in Microbiology* **4**:550–557.

Dumontet, S., K. Krovacek, S. B. Baloda, R. Grottoli, V. Pasquale, and S. Vanucci. (1996). Ecological relationship between *Aeromonas* and *Vibrio* spp. and planktonic copepods in the coastal marine environment in southern Italy. *Comparative Immunology Microbiology and Infectious Diseases* **19**:245–254.

Epstein, S. S. and J. Rossel. (1995). Enumeration of sandy sediment bacteria—search for optimal protocol. *Marine Ecology-Progress Series* **117**:289–298.

Faruque, S. M., M. J. Albert, and J. J. Mekalanos. (1998). Epidemiology, genetics, and ecology of toxigenic *Vibrio cholerae. Microbiology and Molecular Biology Reviews* **62**:1301–1314.

Fogg, G. E. (1983). The ecological significance of extracellular products of phytoplankton photosynthesis. *Botanica Marina* **26**:3–14.

Fuhs, G. W., S. D. Demmerle, E. Canelli, and M. Chen. (1972). Characterization of phosphorus-limited plankton algae (with reflections on the limiting-nutrient concept). In G. E. Likens, ed. *Nutrients and Eutrophication: The Limiting-Nutrient Controversy*, pp. 113–133. American Society of Limnology and Oceanography.

Fujiyama, A., H. Watanabe, A. Toyoda, T. D. Taylor, T. Itoh, S. F. Tsai *et al.* (2002). Construction and analysis of a human–chimpanzee comparative clone map. *Science* **295**:131–134.

Griebler, C., B. Mindl, and D. Slezak. (2001). Combining DAPI and SYBR Green II for the enumeration of total bacterial numbers in aquatic sediments. *International Review of Hydrobiology* **86**:453–465.

Harvell, C. D., C. E. Mitchell, J. R. Ward, S. Altizer, A. P. Dobson, R. S. Ostfeld *et al.* (2002). Climate warming and disease risks for terrestrial and marine biota. *Science* **296**:2158–2162.

Huq, A. and R. R. Colwell. (1996). A microbiological paradox: viable but nonculturable bacteria with special reference to *Vibrio cholerae. Journal of Food Protection* **59**:96–101.

Huq, A., R. R. Colwell, R. Rahman, A. Ali, M. A. R. Chowdhury, S. Parveen *et al.* (1990). Detection of *Vibrio cholerae* O1 in the aquatic environment by fluorescent-monoclonal antibody and culture methods. *Applied and Environmental Microbiology* **56**:2370–2373.

Huq, A., I. N. G. Rivera, and R. R. Colwell. (2000). Epidemiological significance of viable but nonculturable microorganisms. In R. R. Colwell and D. J. Grimes, eds. *Nonculturable Microorganisms in the Environment*, pp. 301–323. ASM Press, Washington DC.

Huq, A., E. B. Small, P. A. West, M. I. HUQ, R. Rahman, and R. R. Colwell. (1983). Ecological relationships between *Vibrio cholerae* and planktonic crustacean copepods. *Applied and Environmental Microbiology* **45**:275–283.

Islam, M. S., B. S. Drasar, and D. J. Bradley. (1990). Survival of toxigenic *Vibrio cholerae* O1 with a common duckweed, *Lemna minor*, in artificial aquatic ecosystems. *Transactions of the Royal Society of Tropical Medicine and Hygiene* **84**:422–424.

Islam, M. S., M. J. Alam, and P. K. B. Neogi. (1992). Seasonality and toxigenicity of *Vibrio cholerae* non-O1 isolated from different components of pond ecosystems of Dhaka City, Bangladesh. *World Journal of Microbiology and Biotechnology* **8**:160–163.

Islam, M. S., B. S. Drasar, and R. B. Sack. (1994). The aquatic flora and fauna as reservoirs of *Vibrio cholerae*: a review. *Journal of Diarrhoeal Diseases Research* **12**:87–96.

Islam, M. S., B. S. Drasar, M. J. Albert, R. B. Sack, A. Huq, and R. R. Colwell. (1997). Toxigenic *Vibrio cholerae* in the environment—a minireview. *Tropical Diseases Bulletin* **94**:R1–R11.

Islam, M. S., Z. Rahim, M. J. Alam, S. Begum, S. M. Moniruzzaman, A. Umeda, *et al.* (1999). Association of *Vibrio cholerae* O1 with the cyanobacterium, *Anabaena* sp., elucidated by polymerase chain reaction and transmission electron microscopy. *Transactions of the Royal Society of Tropical Medicine and Hygiene* **93**:36–40.

Islam, M. S., M. M. Goldar, M. G. Morshed, M. N. H. Khan, M. R. Islam, and R. B. Sack. (2002). Involvement of the *hap* gene (mucinase) in the survival of *Vibrio cholerae* O1 in association with the blue-green alga, *Anabaena* sp. *Canadian Journal of Microbiology* **48**:793–800.

Jiang, S. C. (2001). *Vibrio cholerae* in recreational beach waters and tributaries of southern California. *Hydrobiologia* **460**:157–164.

Jiang, S. C. and W. Fu. (2001). Seasonal abundance and distribution of *Vibrio cholerae* in coastal waters quantified by a 16S-23S intergenic spacer probe. *Microbial Ecology* **42**:540–548.

Jiang, S. C., V. Louis, N. Choopun, A. Sharma, A. Huq, and R. R. Colwell. (2000). Genetic diversity of *Vibrio cholerae* in Chesapeake Bay determined by amplified fragment length polymorphism fingerprinting. *Applied and Environmental Microbiology* **66**:140–147.

Jones, J. G. (1974). Some observations on direct counts of freshwater bacteria obtained with a fluorescence microscope. *Limnology and Oceanography* **19**:540–543.

Jürgens, K., H. Arndt, and K. O. Rothhaupt. (1994). Zooplankton-mediated changes of bacterial community structure. *Microbial Ecology* **27**:27–42.

Jürgens, K., H. Arndt, and H. Zimmermann. (1997). Impact of metazoan and protozoan grazers on bacterial biomass distribution in microcosm experiments. *Aquatic Microbial Ecology* **12**:131–138.

Jürgens, K. and E. Jeppesen. (2000). The impact of metazooplankton on the structure of the microbial food web in a shallow, hypertrophic lake. *Journal of Plankton Research* **22**:1047–1070.

Jürgens, K. and C. Matz. (2002). Predation as a shaping force for the phenotypic and genotypic composition of planktonic bacteria. *Antonie Van Leeuwenhoek International Journal of General and Molecular Microbiology* **81**:413–434.

Karaolis, D. K. R., J. A. Johnson, C. C. Bailey, E. C. Boedeker, J. B. Kaper, and P. R. Reeves. (1998). A *Vibrio cholerae* pathogenicity island associated with epidemic and pandemic strains. *Proceedings of the National Academy of Sciences* **95**:3134–3139.

Kepner, R. L. and J. R. Pratt. (1994). Use of fluorochromes for direct enumeration of total bacteria in environmental samples—past and present. *Microbiological Reviews* **58**:603–615.

King, C. H., R. W. Sanders, E. B. Shotts, and K. G. Porter. (1991). Differential survival of bacteria ingested by zooplankton from a stratified eutrophic lake. *Limnology and Oceanography* **36**:829–845.

Kirchman, D. L. (1993). Statistical analysis of direct counts of microbial abundance. In P. F. Kemp, B. F. Sherr, E. B. Sherr, and J. J. Cole, eds. *Handbook of Methods in Aquatic Microbial Ecology*, pp. 117–119. Lewis Publishers, Boca Raton, Fl.

Kogure, K., U. Simidu, and N. Taga. (1980). Effect of phytoplankton and zooplankton on the growth of marine bacteria in filtered seawater. *Bulletin of the Japanese Society of Scientific Fisheries* **46**:323–326.

Kovach, M. E., M. D. Shaffer, and K. M. Peterson. (1996). A putative integrase gene defines the distal end of a large cluster of ToxR-regulated colonization genes in *Vibrio cholerae*. *Microbiology-UK* **142**:2165–2174.

Langenheder, S. and K. Jürgens. (2001). Regulation of bacterial biomass and community structure by metazoan and protozoan predation. *Limnology and Oceanography* **46**:121–134.

Madigan M. T., J. M. Martinko, and J. Parker. (2003). *Brock Biology of Microorganisms*, 10th edition. Prentice Hall, Upper Saddle River, NJ.

Manning, P. A., U. H. Stroeher, and R. Morona. (1994). Molecular basis for O-antigen biosynthesis in *Vibrio cholerae* O1: Ogawa-Inaba switching. In I. K. Wachsmuth, P. A. Blake, and Ø. Olsvik, eds. *Vibrio cholerae and Cholera: Molecular to Global Perspectives*, pp. 77–94. American Society for Microbiology, Washington DC.

McDougald, D., S. A. Rice, D. Weichart, and S. Kjelleberg. (1998). Nonculturability: adaptation or debilitation? *FEMS Microbiology Ecology* **25**:1–9.

Mintz, E. D., T. Popovic, and P. A. Blake. (1994). Transmission of *Vibrio cholerae* O1. In I. K. Wachsmuth, P. A. Blake, and Ø. Olsvik, eds. *Vibrio cholerae and Cholera: Molecular to Global Perspectives*, pp. 345–356. American Society for Microbiology, Washington DC.

Morris, J. G., Jr. and Cholera Laboratory Task Force. (1994). *Vibrio cholerae* O139 Bengal. In I. K. Wachsmuth, P. A. Blake, and Ø. Olsvik, eds. *Vibrio cholerae and Cholera: Molecular to Global Perspectives*, pp. 95–102. American Society for Microbiology, Washington DC.

Mouriño-Perez, R. R., A. Z. Worden, and F. Azam. (2003). Growth of *Vibrio cholerae* O1 in red tide waters off California. *Applied and Environmental Microbiology* **69**:6923–6931.

Nalin, D. R., V. Daya, A. Reid, M. M. Levine, and L. Cisneros. (1979). Adsorption and growth of *Vibrio cholerae* on chitin. *Infection and Immunity* **25**:768–770.

Oren, A. (2004). Prokaryote diversity and taxonomy: current status and future challenges. *Philosophical Transactions of the Royal Society of London Series B-Biological Sciences* **359**:623–638.

Pace, M. L. and J. J. Cole. (1996). Regulation of bacteria by resources and predation tested in whole lake experiments. *Limnology and Oceanography* **41**:1448–1460.

Paerl, H. W. (1982). Interactions with bacteria. In N. G. Carr and B. A. Whitton, eds. *The Biology of Cyanobacteria*, pp. 441–461. University of California Press, Berkeley, CA.

Pernthaler, J., B. Sattler, K. Simek, A. Schwarzenbacher, and R. Psenner. (1996). Top-down effects on the size-biomass distribution of a freshwater bacterioplankton community. *Aquatic Microbial Ecology* **10**:255–263.

Reidl, J. and K. E. Klose. (2002). *Vibrio cholerae* and cholera: out of the water and into the host. *FEMS Microbiology Reviews* **26**:125–139.

Roff, J. C., J. T. Turner, M. K. Webber, and R.R. Hopcroft. (1995). Bacterivory by tropical copepod nauplii—extent and possible significance. *Aquatic Microbial Ecology* **9**:165–175.

Ruiz, G. M., T. K. Rawlings, F. C. Dobbs, L. A. Drake, T. Mullady, A. Huq *et al.* (2000). Global spread of microorganisms by ships. *Nature* **408**:49–50.

Sanders, R. W., D. A. Caron, and U. G. Berninger. (1992). Relationships between bacteria and heterotrophic nanoplankton in marine and fresh waters—an interecosystem comparison. *Marine Ecology-Progress Series* **86**:1–14.

Sarkar, A., R. K. Nandy, G. B. Nair, and A. C. Ghose. (2002). Vibrio pathogenicity island and cholera toxin genetic element-associated virulence genes and their expression in non-O1 non-O139 strains of *Vibrio cholerae. Infection and Immunity* **70**:4735–4742.

Schneider, D.R. and C.D. Parker. (1982). Purification and characterization of the mucinase of *Vibrio cholerae. Journal of Infectious Diseases* **145**:474–482.

Shapiro, J. A. (1998). Thinking about bacterial populations as multicellular organisms. *Annual Review of Microbiology* **52**:81–104.

Simon, M., H. P. Grossart, B. Schweitzer, and H. Ploug. (2002). Microbial ecology of organic aggregates in aquatic ecosystems. *Aquatic Microbial Ecology* **28**:175–211.

Sochard, M. R., D. F. Wilson, B. Austin, and R. R. Colwell. (1979). Bacteria associated with the surface and gut of marine copepods. *Applied and Environmental Microbiology* **37**:750–759.

Sommer, U. and H. Stibor. (2002). Copepoda–Cladocera–Tunicata: the role of three major mesozooplankton groups in pelagic food webs. *Ecological Research* **17**:161–174.

Spira, W. M. (1981). Environmental factors in diarrhea transmission: the ecology of *Vibrio cholerae* O1 and cholera. In T. Holme, M. H. Holmgren, M. H. Merson, and R. Mollby, eds. *Acute Enteric Infections in Children: New Prospects for Treatment and Prevention*, pp. 273–288. Elsevier/North Holland Biomedical Press, Amsterdam, The Netherlands.

Suzuki, M. T., E. B. Sherr, and B. F. Sherr. (1993). DAPI direct counting underestimates bacterial abundances and average cell-size compared to AO direct counting. *Limnology and Oceanography* **38**:1566–1570.

Tamplin, M. L., A. L. Gauzens, A. Huq, D. A. Sack, and R. R. Colwell. (1990). Attachment of *Vibrio cholerae* serogroup O1 to zooplankton and phytoplankton of Bangladesh waters. *Applied and Environmental Microbiology* **56**:1977–1980.

Threlkeld, S. T., D. A. Chiavelli, and R. L. Willey. (1993). The organization of zooplankton epibiont communities. *Trends in Ecology and Evolution* **8**:317–321.

Turner, J. T. and P. A. Tester. (1992). Zooplankton feeding ecology—bacterivory by metazoan microzooplankton. *Journal of Experimental Marine Biology and Ecology* **160**:149–167.

Vaque, D. and M. L. Pace. (1992). Grazing on bacteria by flagellates and cladocerans in lakes of contrasting food-web structure. *Journal of Plankton Research* **14**:307–321.

Waldor, M. K. and J. J. Mekalanos. (1996). Lysogenic conversion by a filamentous phage encoding cholera toxin. *Science* **272**:1910–1914.

Wetzel, R. G. (2001). *Limnology: Lake and River Ecosystems*, 3rd edition. Academic Press, San Diego, CA.

Whitham, T. G., W. P. Young, G. D. Martinsen, C. A. Gehring, J. A. Schweitzer, S. M. Shuster *et al.* (2003). Community and ecosystem genetics: a consequence of the extended phenotype. *Ecology* **84**:559–573.

Zhu, J. and J. J. Mekalanos. (2003). Quorum sensing-dependent biofilms enhance colonization in *Vibrio cholerae. Developmental Cell* **5**:647–656.

CHAPTER 9

Food webs and parasites in a salt marsh ecosystem

Kevin D. Lafferty, Ryan F. Hechinger, Jenny C. Shaw, Kathleen Whitney, and Armand M. Kuris

9.1 Background

Our mothers teach us to grill our meats "well done" and chew them thoroughly. Even if mom did not know why she insisted, both are good precautions against parasites. Parasites may be in our food, but they are not in our food webs. Is it necessary to take the precaution of considering them? In this chapter, we argue that parasites affect important properties of food webs and that it may be difficult to fully understand ecosystems without considering parasites.

Food webs depict trophic interactions among networks of consumers, producers, and non-living material. Units in food webs range from specific life-cycle stages of species to broad taxonomic/ functional groups. At the most basic level, food webs are static diagrams or matrices of who eats whom (topological webs). Some food webs track flows of energy and matter among links (bioenergetic webs). Other food webs denote the strengths of interactions among species (interaction webs). The food-web framework captures much of the current theory on how habitat heterogeneity, species richness, trophic cascades, indirect mutualism, apparent competition, intraguild predation, environmental change, ecosystem stability, nutrient dynamics, and productivity affect community structure (Paine 1988; Winemiller and Polis 1996). Food webs also aid applied research by providing a better understanding of pest control, environmental contamination, bioremediation, and fisheries management (Winemiller and Polis 1996).

Published food webs vary considerably in quality and detail, but nearly all exclude consumers that are not readily detectable, such as endoparasites and other infectious agents (Polis 1991; Cohen *et al.* 1993). Indeed, perhaps because they are difficult to detect, typical parasites have been historically lacking from the bulk of ecological theory. However, parasitism is arguably the most prevalent lifestyle among animals (Price 1980; DeMeeûs and Renaud 2002). As ecologists increasingly consider the role of parasites in ecosystems, it is becoming clear that parasites are embedded in food webs and may need to be considered in food-web theory (Polis 1991; Cohen *et al.* 1993; Marcogliese and Cone 1997; Marcogliese 2003). Incorporating parasites, as we have done here, helps illuminate the role of parasitism in natural communities (Dobson *et al.* 2005), and reveals how changes in community structure may affect rates and patterns of parasitism.

Almost all published food webs describe predator–prey links (e.g. lion–gazelle–grass). Food webs of insect parasitoids and their hosts have also been developed because parasitoids are relatively easy to observe when they emerge from their hosts (Lawton 1989). The full food web in any given community will likely contain predator–prey, parasitoid–host and parasite–host interactions, as well as other trophic interactions described below. However, few community food webs have incorporated more than one of these subwebs. In a key exception, Memmott *et al.* (2000) added a parasitoid–host subweb to a rich web of herbivorous insects, plants and predators. They found that adding parasitoids greatly decreased the web's overall connectance (the average proportion of other species with which each species interacts). This was, in part, due to the relatively high host specificity of parasitoids. Differences between predator–prey and parasitoid–host food webs arise largely because parasitoids are intimate with a single host, while predators have brief interactions with many different prey individuals (Lafferty and Kuris 2002). This comparison illuminates how different types of natural enemies can have different effects on food-web properties.

Analysis of topological predator–prey and parasitoid–host subwebs has led to the discovery of general patterns (Pimm *et al.* 1991). Published webs usually contain three to four trophic levels and an average of less than one predator or parasitoid species per prey or host species. Neither the relative abundance of members in each trophic level, nor the density of linkages varies with the number of species in the web. Finally, omnivory (feeding at more than one trophic level), is less common than would be expected by chance. Such generalizations have received substantial criticism because of the problems concerning data quality associated with the published food webs (Polis 1991).

Rules for assembling topological webs have been inconsistent, and many topological webs seem to reflect authors' conception of what a web should look like rather than direct measurements from nature (Paine 1988; Polis 1991). Studies of interaction webs have generated less contentious predictions, for example, about stability (the ability of a food web to return or maintain equilibrium in the face of disturbance). The stability of a food web is predicted to decrease with (1) diversity, (2) connectance, and (3) the average strength of an interaction (May 1973). With greater species diversity, there are simply more opportunities for instability to arise. Furthermore, strong links allow instability to readily propagate between species. In contrast, many weak interactions may increase ecosystem stability (McCann *et al.* 1998).

Conclusions based on food webs of parasitoids or predators do not necessarily inform us about the role of typical parasites in food webs. At first, the small body size of an individual parasite relative to its host and its generally nonlethal effect implies that a parasite species plays a small role in the flow of energy through a food web. However, parasites have a durable relationship with their host and, unlike predators, their consumption continues over

time. Unlike predators, parasites are very efficient at converting what they consume into reproductive output (Whitlock *et al.* 1966; Ractliffe *et al.* 1969). Even if an individual parasite has a minor impact on the host, when summed over a large population of parasite individuals within the host, the impact may be large. For instance, for lambs with high-intensity infections of *Haemonchus contortus*, the sheep stomach barber-pole worm, the continual export of host energy may result in severe anemia (Ractliffe *et al.* 1969). Such energetic conversion from a host to a parasite infrapopulation (a population of parasites within a host) could profoundly affect food-web dynamics and topography.

Unfortunately, parasite–host links are relatively difficult to elucidate and only a handful of studies have included typical parasites (incorporated as top predators) in food webs (see review in Sukhdeo and Hernandez 2004). In a pioneering study, Huxham *et al.* (1995) incorporated 42 helminth parasites into an 88-species food web for the Ythan Estuary (Aberdeenshire, Scotland). The resulting greater chain lengths and higher proportion of top species were the logically necessary outcomes of affording parasites top-predator status. Also, parasites decreased connectance and increased omnivory (a common food-web statistic) because parasites with complex life cycles usually feed at multiple trophic levels (Huxham *et al.* 1995).

More recently, Thompson *et al.* (2005) explored the role of nine parasite species (as top predators) in a mudflat food web with 67 free-living species and broad categories for basal taxa. In addition to generally supporting the conclusions of Huxham *et al.* (1995), they investigated the effects of each parasite species in the web. They found that parasites only mildly decreased connectance. Only one of the nine parasite species, a trematode, strongly affected the food web, suggesting that generalist parasites with complex life cycles have disproportionate effects on food webs.

Here, we construct a topological food web for an estuary in which we have been studying the role of parasites in ecosystems. We use this food web to help investigate how macroparasites affect community structure. Our goal was to determine how the inclusion of parasites would alter common food-web metrics, such as the number of links, connectance, and vulnerability (the number of enemy species per prey or host). We not only discovered that parasites significantly changed these food-web metrics, but we also uncovered previously unanalyzed classes of food-web interactions. Explicit inclusion of parasitic interactions serves to increase understanding of community structure, and further integrates the impact of infectious diseases into community ecology.

9.2 Methods

9.2.1 Defining the study system

We have investigated the ecology of larval trematode host-parasite interactions in southern California (USA) and Baja California (Mexico) salt marshes for over two decades, and recently began quantifying host distribution and abundance. Our goal was to develop an accurate and comprehensive topological food web for a small estuary, including information on the parasites.

The study site, Carpinteria salt marsh, is a 93-ha wetland and upland habitat located 19 km east of Santa Barbara, CA (34°2′4 N, 119°31′30″ W). The estuary consists of a pickle weed (*Salicornia virginica*) dominated marsh with unvegetated pans, mudflats, and tidal channels that are fed by two seasonal creeks. Although residential and commercial development surrounds the area, the University of California, Santa Barbara Natural Reserve System protects and manages the marsh for scientific research. It serves as the primary site for our long-term studies on ecological parasitology.

Although real food webs may spread over large spatial and temporal scales, topological webs must be constrained by defined limits. We constrained the Carpinteria salt marsh food web to tidally influenced soft sediment and vegetated habitat, excluding several habitats supporting species with trophic links to estuarine species in our web. For example, food and nutrients enter the estuary from streams during the wet season and from the ocean on each incoming tide. Also, many terrestrial birds, mammals, and invertebrates (particularly insects, Cameron 1972) feed along the upland edge of the estuary. Finally, hard substrate at the mouth of the estuary provides habitat for species that are more

characteristic of the open shore. Constraining the food web spatially helped limit the host species pool in the food web to a tractable list.

9.2.2 Naming the players and links

We used species as our preferred taxonomic unit and included known, but unidentified or undescribed "morphospecies." Although we strived to use precise and accurate taxonomy, some members of the food web were grouped into categories (e.g. copepods). We primarily used information from plant transects, bird surveys (R. Hansen, unpublished data), fish seine hauls, and benthic infaunal cores (sieved through either 5 mm or 1 mm mesh) for invertebrates to compile our species lists. For each sampling method, we excluded species that comprised <0.5% of the individuals sampled. We also included species that we knew to be common, but that were not well targeted by our sampling methods. For example, the fish *Mugil cephalus* is abundant in the marsh, yet is notoriously difficult to capture using beach seines. Some top predators that failed the abundance criterion were included because higher trophic levels are relatively important for food webs and species at higher levels are relatively rare.

Topological food webs consist of an $n \times n$ matrix of n species, with predators as columns and prey as rows (Cohen 1978). Binary entries (e.g. 0 or 1) in the matrix indicate whether a predator eats a prey. To add links to the matrix, we consulted published information on diets (Morris *et al.* 1980; Barry *et al.* 1996; Love 1996; CLO 2002). In many cases, the diet descriptions were broad enough (e.g. "fish") to require our discretion in assigning them to particular species. In addition, we incorporated our unpublished data on diet and gut contents, which we often obtained in conjunction with parasitological examinations. We conservatively extrapolated diet information from other locations to the same or analogous food sources found in Carpinteria salt marsh. For some species, we generated diet items of unstudied species from those of similar, well-studied species.

Food webs based on observations are only as complete as the observations are exhaustive. We decided to improve our food web by logically inferring links when specific data were unavailable. Parasites can be useful indicators of host diets (Marcogliese and Cone 1997). For parasites acquired with food, the living parasite stays in the gut far longer than the digested food item, providing a sensitive indicator of host diet (Marcogliese 2003). The opposite logic also applies; a species that serves as an intermediate host for a parasite known to occur in a particular predator is likely to be prey for that predator (Huxham *et al.* 1995; Marcogliese 2003). For this reason, we expanded a host's diet list when a parasite's presence indicated that the host consumed a particular prey item. For example, in our system, the trematode *Cloacitrema michiganensis* parasitizes American coots. These waterfowl forage largely on vegetation. Because the trematode encysts on opercula of the horn snail, *Cerithidea californica*, American coots likely ingest horn snails incidentally while feeding on vegetation. Mallards have similar diets to coots and we assumed that they also ate horn snails. In our results (Appendices 1–4), we distinguish between confirmed and inferred links.

To determine host–parasite links, we used published lists of parasites for the hosts in our study, when such information was available for the region (Russell 1960; Martin 1972; Love and Moser 1983; Huspeni and Lafferty 2004). We also used our unpublished parasite observations. We discuss each of the host–parasite groups in turn, below.

Published reports and our observations indicate that a variety of ecto-and endoparasites commonly infect estuarine fishes. In particular, metacercarial cysts of digenean trematodes frequently infect fishes in Carpinteria salt marsh. Non-digenean trematode parasites recorded from our samples included worms in the gut (camellanid nematodes) and tissue (larval tetraphyllidean and trypanorhynchan cestodes, larval acanthocephalans) and ectoparasites of the skin (dactylogyrid and gyrodactylid monogeneans, ergasilid copepods) mouth (cymothoid isopods), and gills (ciliophoran protozoans and gyrodactylid monogeneans). With the exception of ciliates, we did not include any protozoan, bacterial, or viral parasites of fishes.

For birds, we primarily included intestinal helminth parasites based on published and unpublished dissection data, but we additionally inferred parasitism in birds from diet (see Box 9.1). Birds also serve as hosts for a wide range of viruses, bacteria, and protozoans, as well as a high abundance and diversity of ectoparasitic arthropods. We limited our treatment of these taxa to the assumption that each bird species was infected by one species of *Plasmodium* (avian malaria) (Bennett *et al.* 1993). Vector control efforts have found 10 species of mosquitoes in and around the marsh (Ferren *et al.* 1996); two of these species (*Aedes taeniorhynchus* and *Culex tarsalis*) are common in the marsh and feed on birds. *C. tarsalis* transmits arboviruses and avian malaria to birds. Bird ectoparasites, micropredators, and blood parasites play a more important and diverse role than our food web implies (Janovy 1997).

We also did not consider some potentially important parasites of invertebrates. Although poorly studied, bacteria, viruses, protozoa, and fungi probably parasitize most invertebrates. We included some protozoan parasites of invertebrates, but did not include others we have encountered in similar wetlands. For example, we have evidence from other wetlands that apicomplexan protozoans parasitize clams and crabs. We also did not include symbiotic species for which insufficient information is available to determine whether the symbionts are parasites or commensals. Examples include ciliates that live in the mantle cavity of the high marsh snail, *Assiminea californica*, and two species of copepods that live on the cuticle of thalassinidean ghost shrimp. Some of the trematode metacercariae encyst on the outside of hard-shelled invertebrates. These parasites do not have trophic links with their second intermediate hosts and we did not count them as such. However, we note this association in our table and matrix as they help indicate life cycles and do form predator–parasite links. It is not clear how incomplete parasite information affects our results, but inclusion of parasites that use few hosts (like parasitoids or feather lice) would reduce the linkage density in the parasite–host subweb.

9.2.3 Incorporating parasites into the web

How should parasites be included in food webs? Published food webs usually equate parasites with top predators. This perspective has contributed

---

Box 9.1 Identifying complex life cycles from food webs

So, you want to put parasites in your food web? The best source of information is to dissect samples of the free-living species in the web and identify all parasites to species, or at least to morphospecies. This requires a lot of expertise and effort and it is no surprise that no study has completely accomplished it. In most systems, there will be some published information on parasites from the host species encountered. Because hosts range widely and may pick up parasites from other regions or habitats, one should carefully review host–parasite accounts to be sure that they are likely to occur in the food web under study. The use of hypothetical parasite–host links is often necessary to fully incorporate parasites into food webs (Huxham *et al.* 1995). Even if a comprehensive parasite list is available, one will be forced to guess about some of the links between hosts and parasites, especially for rare or difficult to sample hosts. For example, the trematodes in our system are generalists in birds and it is difficult to obtain birds for parasite analysis. Most of our trematodes have been reported from a wide range of avian final hosts. In addition, experimental infections have repeatedly demonstrated their ability to infect a variety of other hosts, including ducks, pigeons, chickens, and even cats, rats, and mice (Martin 1972).

Thus, the ingestion of intermediate hosts (fish, crustaceans, mollusks, and annelids) should be the primary determinant of parasitism in birds. We therefore assumed that if a bird ate a prey that served as second intermediate host for an avian trematode, the bird could successfully acquire that parasite. For example, the trematode *C. michiganensis* has been reported from nine bird species in our web. This trematode encysts on the shells of burrowing clams and exoskeletons of ghost shrimp, suggesting that the additional eight species of bird that prey on these second intermediate hosts also serve as final hosts for *C. michiganensis*. We did not make such assumptions for non-avian predators. For example, raccoons eat a wide range of prey, but appear to serve as hosts only for a few of the avian trematodes (Lafferty and Dunham, 2005).

We had 64 confirmed instances of trematode–bird links in our system and diet information added an additional 236 probable trematode–bird links. Food webs can greatly aid the development of predicted host–parasite associations, as they reveal what links expose predators to parasites. The specificity of the parasite for the predator host ultimately determines whether exposure leads to transmission.

---

substantial insight to food-web theory, but there are drawbacks. Sometimes food-web theory (cascade and niche models) arranges consumers on a body size axis, and assumes that consumers are larger than prey, a strategy that may provide illogical roles for parasites (Dobson *et al.* 2005). Instead of blending parasites into the predator–prey subweb, we organized the food web into four subwebs. The first was the predator–prey subweb, which corresponded to nearly all published food webs.

The second subweb was the parasite–host subweb. By adding parasites to a subweb, instead of as top predators in the predator–prey web, it was possible to compute statistics for predator–prey interactions that remain comparable to previously published food webs.

The third subweb included predators that feed on parasites, a component missing from all previous food webs. For example, some consumers feed on free-swimming trematode cercariae. We extrapolated limited laboratory observations on fishes to several potential links (we are currently verifying

this aspect of the food web). More importantly, predators unintentionally eat the parasites of their prey, resulting in either parasite transmission or parasite death (Box 9.2). We suspect that in cases where transmission is possible, when a predator eats an infected prey, most of the parasites fail to transmit and the predator digests them. For example, less than 10% of ingested metacercariae establish in a coral reef fish; the rest perish (Aeby 2002). Therefore, we included predation on parasites as independent links in the food web.

The fourth subweb included parasite–parasite trophic interactions, another unrecognized subweb. These were primarily interactions among trematodes that share the same first intermediate host snail species (*C. californica*). Multispecies infections of larval trematodes within an individual snail often result in competitive exclusion through intraguild predation among larval trematodes (Kuris 1990; Sousa 1993; Lafferty *et al.* 1994; Huspeni and Lafferty 2004). There were two other parasite–parasite interactions. A picornavirus infects and

Box 9.2 Parasite transmission and host abundance

A link is just the beginning. It represents a complex consumer–resource interaction that plays out in time and space at individual and population levels. Links, therefore, can be starting points for interesting theoretical and empirical studies. Linkages in food webs can influence directly transmitted diseases as well as those with complex multiple-host life cycles, but links between parasites and hosts are particularly tenuous. This is because links may not be sufficient to maintain transmission if the abundance of hosts is low. If the frequency of contact between infected and susceptible hosts is lower than the death or cure rate of infected hosts, the prevalence of disease will decrease. Such a process eventually dampens epidemics. Infrequent contact between hosts can also prevent initiation of epidemics. Predators can make it difficult for directly transmitted parasites of prey to persist by keeping prey populations at low density, thereby reducing transmission. This is an important consideration as two-thirds of the predator–prey links in the Carpinteria salt marsh food web lead to the death of parasites. For example, Hudson et al. (1992) found that predators limited the abundance of the

parasitic nematode, *Trichostrongylus tenuis*, by feeding on infected grouse. Loss of infected individuals stabilizes grouse populations. Without predators, grouse populations exhibit cyclic fluctuations. These cycles are predominantly caused by a nematode-induced reduction in host fecundity (Hudson et al. 1998). Similarly, predators can keep sea urchin populations at low levels, but where fishing reduces urchin predators, urchins become abundant and bacterial epidemics are more common (Lafferty 2004). Thus, food-web linkages indirectly influence host contact rates, permitting infectious disease to act as a density-dependent mortality source. Sometimes, parasites strengthen trophic links by increasing host susceptibility to predation by other hosts in the life cycle. This reduces the minimum host-threshold density, allowing parasites to exploit less common hosts (Dobson 1988). While exhaustive knowledge of host–parasite links is itself difficult to obtain, this is actually the easy part to tackle. Understanding the dynamics associated with these links requires intensive study and is the key challenge for understanding the role of parasites in communities.

kills the entoniscid isopod that parasitizes shore crabs (Kuris *et al.* 1979) and avian malaria parasites (*Plasmodium* spp.) infect mosquitoes.

Huxham *et al.* (1995) point out that life-cycle stages of parasites differ substantially in their ecology such that each stage could be considered a separate trophic species. We treated different stages of a parasite's life cycle as one species, but coded our results so the different stages could be distinguished in subsequent analyses. Treating each stage as a separate species would decrease linkage density.

9.2.4 Food-web metrics

To assess the effects of parasitism on food-web properties, we calculated several metrics of webs with and without parasites. However, since it was intuitively obvious that including parasites increases food chain length, we did not calculate this property. We did measure vulnerability to predators and parasites, and averaged this within each trophic level of the free-living species. We also calculated several linkage statistics for the complete

web and for each subweb. These were: potential number of links, observed number of links, expected number of links (based on past studies of predator–prey webs), observed connectance and expected connectance (based on past studies of predator–prey webs).

The potential number of links, L_p, in a symmetrical matrix of $S \times S$ species (such as a predator–prey subweb, parasite–parasite subweb, or complete web) is equal to the number of cells in the matrix (S^2). This power relationship causes the potential number of links to increase sharply with species richness. For a subweb comprised of two separate species lists (such as X parasites and Y hosts), the number of cells in the matrix is XY, not S^2, and $L_p = XY$. Only a fraction of the potential links in a food web occurs. The observed number of links, L_o, is simply the sum of the links observed in a web (excluding those few cases, mentioned above, where parasites encyst on the outside of a host and extract no energy). Connectance is a commonly used food-web statistic that indicates linkage density. Observed connectance, C_o, is the proportion of potential links realized, or $C_o = L_o / L_p$.

9.2.5 Assembling the web

For the basal trophic level, one "species" was carrion, two "species" were detritus, and five "species" were functional groupings of plants. We divided the producer component of the food chain into (1) phytoplankton, (2) epipelic fauna (mostly microalgae, foraminiferans, and bacteria), (3) macroalgae (*Ulva* sp., *Enteromorpha* sp., and *Gracilaria* sp.), (4) submergent vascular plants (*Ruppia maritima*), and (5) five common emergent vascular plants (Table 9.1).

Many species feed on bacterial and fungal decomposers. This part of the food web has very high diversity and several trophic levels within the bacterial and phage guilds (Breitbart *et al.* 2004), which we were forced to greatly simplify. Because this part of the food web has no linkage with the parasites in our web, however, simplifying it does not greatly alter our conclusions. We divided the detrital food web into (1) terrestrial and (2) marine "detritus." Isotope studies have found that detritus from vascular plants (e.g. *S. virginica*) contributes to the diet of semiterrestrial detritivores (*Traskorchestia traskiana* and *Melampus olivaceus*), while algal sources supply food for the remaining detritivores that feed in the water (Page 1997). Seventy-five free-living consumers were included in the predator-prey subweb. These were divided into trophic levels, where a predator's trophic level was one level above the highest trophic level of its prey.

Of the 74 invertebrate species reported from the estuary, 8 large invertebrates and 11 small invertebrates met our criteria for abundance and habitat use. We also added 12 species that were common, but inadequately sampled: three crabs, two amphipods, a fly, mosquito larvae, a water boatman, two high intertidal snails, a deep dwelling mud shrimp, and a mussel. Of the 22 reported fish species, five met the criteria for abundance and habitat use. We added two predators (leopard shark and round stingray) and mullet (for reasons noted above). Of the 118 reported bird species, 32 met our criteria for abundance and habitat use. To this list, we added three top predators (Northern harrier, Cooper's hawk and osprey), a scavenger (turkey vulture) and the secretive clapper rail as these species were likely important to the web in a manner disproportionate to their abundance. The other terrestrial

Table 9.1 List of basal food items, including detritus and carrion. L is a taxonomic letter code, # is the rank-order species/item abundance within the letter code, and T is the trophic level (basal taxa are 0). Basal taxa, unlike other taxa, were lumped into broad groups. D = detritus, K = carrion, P = plant

Common name	Details	L	#	T
Marine detritus		D	1	0
Terrestrial detritus	From vascular plants	D	2	0
Carrion		K	1	0
Macroalgae	*Enteromorpha, Ulva, Gracilaria*	P	1	0
Epipellic flora	Mostly diatoms	P	2	0
Pickleweed	*Salicornia virginica*	P	3	0
Jaumea	*Jaumea carnosa*	P	4	0
Salt grass	*Distichilis spicata*	P	5	0
Alkali heath	*Frankenia salina*	P	6	0
Shore grass	*Monanthochloe littoralis*	P	7	0
Submergent vascular	*Ruppia cirrhosa*	P	8	0
Phytoplankton	Undocumented	P	9	0

vertebrate that commonly foraged in the intertidal was the raccoon (*Procyon lotor*).

The binary matrix was too large to present as a single table so we describe the food web in three ways. The first is a set of tables organized taxonomically (Tables 9.1–9.5). These tables provide a common and scientific name for each species, as well as a trophic level and species coding consisting of a letter (taxon specific) and number (rank-order abundance within taxon from most abundant (1) to least abundant). We then broke down the matrix by subweb in Appendices 9.1–9.4. From the tables, we created a traditional web diagram to illustrate the predator–prey subweb (Fig. 9.1). We created Fig. 9.2 by adding the host–parasite subweb to the predator–prey subweb. Here, parasites were oriented along the right vertical axis to better distinguish the parasite–host subweb from the predator–prey subweb.

9.3 Results

The potential number of links (excluding the diagonal) in the 87 × 87 predator–prey subweb was 7569. We observed 505 trophic links (Appendix 9.1). There was an average of 6.7 prey species per predator species. Diet breadth increased and peaked at intermediate trophic levels. This may partly be explained by our grouping of basal taxa, which reduced the number of prey species available for lower trophic levels. As expected, omnivory

Table 9.2 Invertebrates. A = annelid (and a nemertean), C = crustacean, G = gastropod, I = insect, V = bivalve. Other codes as in Table 9.1

Common name	Scientific name	L	#	T
Oligochaete	Unidentified	A	1	1
Polychaete	Capitella capitata	A	2	1
Phoronid	Unidentified	A	3	1
Nemertean	Geonemertes	A	4	2
Spionid	Polydora nuchalis	A	5	1
Polychaete	Eteone lightii	A	6	1
Tube amphipod	Corophium	C	1	1
Copepods	Unidentified harpacticoids	C	2	1
Ostracods	Unidentified	C	3	1
Aquatic amphipod	Anisogammarus confervicolus	C	4	1
Beach hopper	Traskorchestia traskiana	C	5	1
Lined shore crab	Pachygrapsus crassipes	C	6	4
Yellow shore crab	Hemigrapsus oregonensis	C	7	3
Fiddler crab	Uca crenulata	C	8	1
Ghost shrimp	Neotrypaea californiensis	C	9	1
Mud shrimp	Upogebia macginitieorum	C	10	1
Horn snail	Cerithidea californica	G	1	1
Bubble snail	Acteocina inculta	G	2	1
Olive snail	Melampus olivaceus	G	3	1
Assiminea snail	Assiminea californica	G	4	1
Water boatman	Trichocorixia reticulata	I	1	1
Brine fly larva	Ephydra sp.	I	2	1
Brine fly adult	Ephydra sp.	I	3	1
Mosquito larva	See Appendix 9.2, I5–6	I	4	1
Bent-nosed clam	Macoma nasuta	V	1	1
Littleneck clam	Protothaca staminea	V	2	1
Jackknife clam	Tagelus spp.	V	3	1
False Mya	Cryptomya californica	V	4	1
European mussel	Mytilus galloprovincialis	V	5	1

Table 9.3 Fishes. F = fish. Other codes as in Tables 9.1 and 9.2

Common name	Scientific name	L	#	T
Topsmelt	Atherinops affinis	F	1	1
Arrow goby	Clevelandia ios	F	2	2
California killifish	Fundulus parvipinnis	F	3	3
Staghorn sculpin	Leptocottus armatus	F	4	5
Long-jaw mudsucker	Gillichthys mirabilis	F	5	5
Mullet	Mugil cephalus	F	6	1
Round stingray	Urobatis halleri	F	7	5
Leopard shark	Triakis semifasciata	F	8	6

Table 9.4 Mammal and birds. R = raccoon, B = bird. Other codes as in Tables 9.1–9.3

Common name	Scientific name	L	#	T
Raccoon	Procyon lotor	R	1	5
Willet	Catoptrophorus semipalmatus	B	1	5
Black-bellied plover	Pluvialis squatarola	B	2	5
American coot	Fulica americana	B	3	2
Western sandpiper	Calidris mauri	B	4	4
Dunlin	Calidris alpina	B	5	4
Least sandpiper	Calidris minutilla	B	6	4
California gull	Larus californicus	B	7	5
Whimbrel	Numenius phaeopus	B	8	5
Mallard	Anas platyrhynchos	B	9	2
Mew gull	Larus canus	B	10	5
Marbled godwit	Limosa fedoa	B	11	5
Forster's tern	Sterna forsteri	B	12	4
Ring-billed gull	Larus delawarensis	B	13	5
Dowitcher	Limnodromus spp.	B	14	4
Western gull	Larus occidentalis	B	15	5
Bonaparte's gull	Larus philadelphia	B	16	5
Semipalmated plover	Charadrius semipalmatus	B	17	3
Great blue heron	Ardea herodias	B	18	6
Killdeer	Charadrius vociferus	B	19	2
Snowy egret	Egretta thula	B	20	6
Long-billed curlew	Numenius americanus	B	21	5
Greater yellowlegs	Tringa melanoleuca	B	22	3
Black-crowned night heron	Nycticorax nycticorax	B	23	6
Green heron	Butorides virescens	B	24	4
Double-crested cormorant	Phalacrocorax auritus	B	25	6
Great egret	Ardea alba	B	26	6
Surf scoter	Melanitta perspicillata	B	27	5
Pied-billed grebe	Podilymbus podiceps	B	28	6
Belted kingfisher	Ceryle alcyon	B	29	4
Bufflehead	Bucephala albeola	B	30	5
American avocet	Recurvirostra americana	B	31	4
Green-winged teal	Anas crecca	B	32	2
Clapper rail	Rallus longirostris	B	33	6
Turkey vulture	Cathartes aura	B	34	1
Cooper's hawk	Accipiter cooperii	B	35	5
Northern harrier	Circus cyaneus	B	36	5
Osprey	Pandion haliaetus	B	37	6

increased from the first to the sixth trophic level (1.0, 1.5, 2.5, 3.0, 3.6, 4.4 average trophic levels fed on, respectively). Omnivory creates a disparity between the trophic level on which a predator typically fed, and the trophic level to which it was assigned (based on the highest trophic level of its prey). Hence, while the top trophic level of the average species was 3.2, the average trophic level at which a species fed was 2.1. As expected, species at higher trophic levels were preyed on by fewer species than were species at lower trophic levels (by definition species at the top trophic levels have no predators).

Table 9.5 Parasites. C = crustacean, I = insect, L = leech, N = nematode, O = other, T = trematode, W = tapeworm. Other codes as in Tables 9.1–9.4. Note that several free-living crustacean and insect species occur in other tables. No trophic level is defined for parasites in our food web

Common name	Scientific name	L	#
Entoniscid isopod	*Portunion conformis*	C	11
Isopod	*Nerocila californica*	C	12
Bopyrid isopod	*Orthione* sp.	C	13
Copepod	*Ergasilus auritious*	C	14
Mosquito	*Aedes taeniorhynchus*	I	5
Mosquito	*Culex tarsalis*	I	6
Leech	Unidentified glossiphonidae	L	1
Nematode	*Proleptus obtusus*	N	1
Nematode	Unidentified	N	2
Nematode	*Spirocamallanus pereirai*	N	3
Nematode	*Baylisascaris procyonis*	N	4
Acanthocephalan	Unidentified	O	1
Nemertean	*Carcinonemertes epialti*	O	2
Monogene	*Gyrodactylus* sp.	O	3
Ciliate	*Trichodina* sp.	O	4
Gregarine	Eugregarine 1	O	5
Gregarine	Eugregarine 2	O	6
Virus	*Picornavirus*	O	7
Malaria	*Plasmodium* sp.	O	8
Dodder	*Cuscuta salina*	P	10
Bird's beak	*Cordylanthus maritimus*	P	11
Trematode	*Euhaplorchis californiensis*	T	1
Trematode	*Himasthla rhigedana*	T	2
Trematode	*Probolocoryphe uca*	T	3
Trematode	*Himasthla species B*	T	4
Trematode	*Renicola buchanani*	T	5
Trematode	*Acanthoparyphium* spp.	T	6
Trematode	*Catatropis johnstoni*	T	7
Trematode	Unidentified Renicolid	T	8
Trematode	*Parorchis acanthus*	T	9
Trematode	*Austrobilharzia* sp.	T	10
Trematode	*Cloacitrema michiganensis*	T	11
Trematode	*Phocitremoides ovale*	T	12
Trematode	*Renicola cerithidicola*	T	13
Trematode	Unidentified Cyathocotylid	T	14
Trematode	*Stictodora hancocki*	T	15
Trematode	Mesostephanus appendiculatus	T	16
Trematode	*Pygidiopsoides spindalis*	T	17
Trematode	Unidentified microphallid	T	18
Trematode	*Hysterolecitha* sp.	T	19
Trematode	*Parvatrema* sp.	T	20
Trematode	Unidentified Microphallid	T	21
Trematode	*Galactosomum humbargari*	T	22
Cestode	Unidentified Tetraphyllidean	W	1
Cestode	Unidentified Tetraphyllidean	W	2
Cestode	Unidentified Trypanorynch	W	3
Cestode	Unidentified Dilepidid	W	4

The number of species in each trophic level did not conform to the expectation that diversity should decline at top trophic levels (levels 1–6 had 29, 6, 4, 9, 18, and 9 species, respectively, Fig. 9.2). However, for birds, which were the only speciose taxon with data on relative abundance, species feeding at lower trophic levels tended to be more abundant than species feeding at higher trophic levels (correlation between average trophic level at which a species fed and that species' abundance $R = -0.46$, $N = 37$, one–tailed $P = 0.002$).

The frequency of interactions between the predator–prey subweb and parasitism became apparent after considering that 216 of the 321 links between birds and prey and 6 of the 72 links between fish and prey allow the transmission of at least one parasite species from intermediate to final host species.

The parasite–host subweb consisted of 47 parasite species and 87 potential host species (ignoring basal taxa), or 4089 potential links (Appendix 9.2). There were 615 parasite–host links in this subweb, not including the 21 cases where non-feeding parasites encysted on the outside of hosts. The average number of host species per parasite species (14.0) was considerably higher than the average number of prey species per predator species (6.7). The number of parasite species per host species increased with trophic level, with top predators having more parasite species than intermediate species.

The predator–parasite subweb also had 4089 potential links (Appendix 9.3). There were 910 links between predators and parasites driven by the consumption of infected hosts. One-third (338) of these links could lead to parasite transmission. That is, the predator also served as a host for the parasite. In addition, four fishes and three clams had the potential to eat the free-swimming cercarial stage of 19 of the 22 trematode species, providing 139 additional links. Twenty-eight of these were redundant with other predator–parasite links, leading to a total of 1021 predator–parasite links.

The parasite–parasite subweb had 2209 potential links (Appendix 9.4). In addition to the picornavirus–entoniscid and *Plasmodium*–mosquito links, there were 170 intraguild predation links between trematode species, for a total of 172 parasite–parasite links.

There were 2313 links out of the 17,956 potential links in the overall food web (the four combined subwebs).

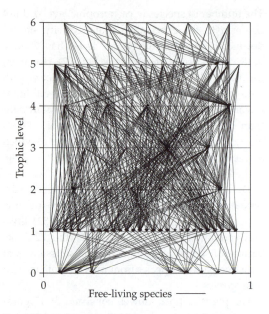

Figure 9.1 Traditional food-web diagram corresponding to the predator–prey subweb. Arrows connect predators to prey (arrow heads located on the prey). Species are arranged vertically by trophic position (basal through 6) and horizontally within a trophic level by the alphanumeric coding in the tables.

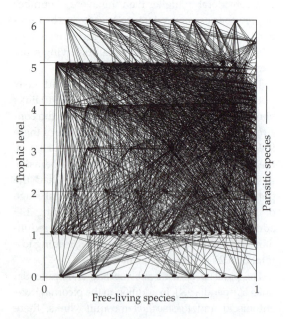

Figure 9.2 Like Fig. 9.1, but including the parasite–host subweb. Parasites aligned on the right vertical axis. Arrows leading from parasites to hosts indicate parasitism.

9.4 Discussion

Including parasites in the Carpinteria salt marsh food web adds new insight to this food web and others. The most general insight is the recognition of three new subwebs that are likely present in all communities. Here, these subwebs contain more than two-thirds of the links.

The inclusion of a parasite–parasite subweb was the greatest departure from previously published webs; our familiarity with larval trematode community structure predisposed us to consider this subweb. For example, the diverse guild of trematodes using the horn snail is characterized by high levels of interspecific competition and intraguild predation (Kuris 1990; Sousa 1993; Lafferty *et al.* 1994). Connectance in parasite–parasite webs will depend on the life-history strategy of the parasites. Typical parasites do not often interact trophically with other parasites. In contrast, parasitic castrators and parasitoids often compete for limited host resources through intraguild predation (Kuris 1974; Lafferty and Kuris 2002). The trematodes that dominate the Carpinteria salt marsh food web affect many aspects of the ecosystem. As parasitic castrators, they reduce snail density (Lafferty 1993a) and size at maturity (Lafferty 1993b). They convert snail reproductive tissue into free-swimming cercariae available to zooplankters and filter feeders. They also increase predation on some second intermediate hosts through behavior modification (Lafferty and Morris 1996).

Many links were a consequence of including a guild of trematodes that have broad final-host specificity. Other types of parasites (e.g. single-host life cycle and host-specific groups such as feather lice) may yield subwebs with less connectance than the predator–prey subweb. This was the case for the parasitoid-host subwebs of Memmott *et al.* (2000), which had low connectance due to high host specificity. Host specificity, therefore, should be the key to determine how parasites affect connectance. The increased diversity and connectance that parasites impart to the Carpinteria salt marsh food web could alter the web's stability, depending on the strengths of the interactions between hosts and parasites. Weak links with long loops characterize trophic interactions of parasites with complex life cycles, and this should increase stability (Dobson *et al.* in press). In addition, infectious diseases tend to disproportionately impact common species, helping to maintain their rarer competitors, thereby promoting coexistence and stability (Dobson *et al.* in press). Interaction webs with parasites will be necessary to fully explore these hypotheses.

Parasites may also alter the interaction strengths in the predator–prey subweb if predators select diseased prey (Packer *et al.* 2003). For instance, experimental removal of helminth parasites in natural populations reveals how easily predators capture parasitized snowshoe hares (Murray *et al.* 1997) and red grouse (Hudson *et al.* 1992), relative to unparasitized conspecifics. Furthermore, many parasites require the ingestion of an intermediate host by a final host to complete their life cycle. Some parasites that achieve transmission via food-web links alter the behavior or appearance of intermediate hosts to increase their risk of being preyed on by final hosts (Lafferty 1999). For example, a common trematode species in snails at Carpinteria salt marsh, *Euhaplorchis californiensis*, uses the third most common fish species, *Fundulus parvipinnis*, as a second intermediate host. Larval *E. californiensis* encyst on the fish's brain and manipulate behavior, rendering infected fish 10–30 times more likely to be eaten by one of the 15 bird species in the Carpinteria salt marsh food web that serve as a final host for the adult worm (Lafferty and Morris 1996).

Similarly, predator–parasite links may alter the interaction strength of parasite–host links. If predators are an important source of parasite mortality in prey, some parasites might have a hard time persisting in predator-rich food webs. This challenge appears to be one explanation for the evolution of complex life cycles. Parasites must be under tremendous pressure to form parasite–host links with the predators of their hosts (Lafferty 1999). When predators strongly prefer parasitized prey (but do not serve as hosts), complex interactions in models of host and parasite populations can result. These include oscillations, alternate stable states, and parasite extinction (Hall *et al.* 2005). However, in more productive environments, predators that do not prefer parasitized prey can cause extinction of hosts followed by extinction of their host-specific parasites (Hall *et al.* 2005).

Some studies show how parasite links can alter food webs. In particular, the invasion and eradication of Rinderpest (a morbillivirus related to measles) in East African ungulates illustrates how one infectious disease strongly affected a food web by altering the density of abundant hosts (Sinclair 1979; Plowright 1982; Dobson 1995; Tompkins *et al.* 2001). Rinderpest arrived with cattle in 1889 and the resulting epidemics caused mass mortality in domestic and wild artiodactyls throughout Africa. This led to reductions in abundance of their predators (Plowright 1982). A vaccine was introduced into cattle and, by 1961, native ungulate populations experienced rapid recovery (Plowright 1982; Spinage 2003). The increased prey base led to increases in lion and hyena populations, which then preyed heavily on gazelles and displaced wild dogs. Canine distemper is currently reducing predator densities in Africa with further resultant alterations to food webs (Roelke-Parker 1996).

The Carpinteria salt marsh food web could be expanded to include meroplanktonic food items in the predator–prey subweb, such as the free-swimming larval stages produced by most of the five annelids, four decapod crustaceans, five bivalves, and six bony fishes in our example. Similarly, trematode life-cycle stages that use mollusks as first intermediate hosts produce many free-swimming cercariae. These motile larvae do not feed while they seek out the next host in the life cycle. The vast majority of cercariae likely fail to infect a host and either become prey or contribute to detritus. Thus, inclusion of cercarial productivity as a planktonic component of food webs strengthens connectance. It is notable that trematodes could comprise half the species richness of the larval zooplankton community in this estuary and biomass could be considerably more than half of the larval zooplankton standing crop (Stevens 1996). It is also possible that increases in the abundance of planktivores could reduce transmission of cercariae.

Food-web structure can also affect what types of parasites can persist (Marcogliese 2002). Parasites that exploit trophic transmission will depend on the presence of trophic linkages among host species (Dobson *et al.* in press). A species-rich, well-connected, predator–prey web will facilitate the completion of more types of complex life cycles. Even simple changes can affect parasite communities if they permit the completion of new life cycles. For instance, when a few pairs of great crested grebes colonized Slapton Ley (Devon, UK) in the early 1980s, a new link (grebe-fish) permitted completion of the life cycles of a cestode linked with copepod, fish and bird hosts, and a trematode linked with snail, fish, and bird hosts (Kennedy and Watt 1994). Both parasites greatly impacted the dominant fish intermediate host and led to significant changes in the fish community (Kennedy and Watt 1994).

Parasites with complex life cycles are good indicators of food-web linkages in an ecosystem. To the extent that food-web linkages indicate ecosystem functionality, parasites can also be good environmental indicators (Lafferty 1997). At our study site, habitat restoration was followed by an increase in the abundance and diversity of the larval trematodes in horn snails, presumably because the improved habitat fostered foraging opportunities for a diverse assemblage of final-host birds (Huspeni and Lafferty 2004).

9.5 Conclusion

The Carpinteria salt marsh food web is far more complicated than a typical predator–prey subweb. Invisibility and small size make it hard to adequately include parasites in food webs, but it seems unwise to completely ignore them. Including parasites strongly affected characteristics of the Carpinteria salt marsh food web. Most notably, in contrast to parasitoid-host subwebs, our parasite subwebs had a large number of links and disproportionately added to food-web connectance. Further incorporation of parasites into food webs will increase our appreciation of their role in ecosystems.

Acknowledgments

We thank T. Huspeni, E. Dunham, C. Boch, L. Mababa, F. Mancini, M. Pickering, A. Kaplan, and members of our research group for their extensive assistance in the field and laboratory. This manuscript has benefited from support received from the National Science Foundation through the NIH/NSF Ecology of Infectious Disease Program (DEB-0224565) and US EPA STAR EaGLe Coastal Initiative through the Pacific Estuarine Ecosystem Indicator Research Consortium, US EPA Agreement EPA/R-82867601. The UCSB Natural Reserve System provided access to field sites.

References

Aeby, G. S. (2002). Trade-offs for the butterflyfish, *Chaetodon multicinctus*, when feeding on coral prey infected with trematode metacercariae. *Behavioral Ecology and Sociobiology* **52**:158–165.

Barry, J. P., M. M. Yoklavich, G. M. Cailliet, D. A. Ambrose, and B. S. Antrim. (1996). Trophic ecology of the dominant fishes in Elkhorn Slough, California, 1974–1980. *Estuaries* **19**:115–138.

Bennett, G. F., M. A. Bishop, and M. A. Pierce. (1993). Checklist of the avian species of *Plasmodium* Marchiafava and Celli, 1885 (Apicomplexa) and their distribution by avian family and Wallacian life zones. *Systematic Parasitology* **26**:171–179.

Breitbart, M., B. Felts, S. Kelley, J. M. Mahaffy, J. Nulton, P. Salamon *et al.* (2004). Diversity and population structure of a near–shore marine-sediment viral community. *Proceedings of the Royal Society of London Series B-Biological Sciences* **271**:565–574.

Cameron, G. N. (1972). Analysis of insect trophic diversity in two salt marsh communities. *Ecology* **53**:58–73.

CLO. (2002). *The Birds of North America Series*. Cornell Lab of Ornithology, Cornell University, Ithaca, NY.

Cohen, J. E. (1978). *Food Webs and Niche Space*. Princeton University Press, Princeton, NJ.

Cohen, J. E., R. A. Beaver, S. H. Cousins, D. L. Deangelis, L. Goldwasser, K. L. Heong, *et al* (1993). Improving food webs. *Ecology* **74**:252–258.

DeMeeûs, T. and F. Renaud. (2002). Parasites within the new phylogeny of eukaryotes. *Trends in Parasitology Today* **18**:247–251.

Dobson, A., K. D. Lafferty, and A. M. Kuris. (2005). Parasites and food webs. *In* M. Pascual, and J. A. Dunne, eds. Ecological Networks: Linking Structure to Dynamics in Food Webs, pp. 119–135. Oxford University Press.

Dobson, A. P. (1988). The population biology of parasite-induced changes in host behavior. *Quarterly Review of Biology* **63**:139–165.

Dobson, A. P. (1995). Rinderpest in the Serengeti ecosystem: the ecology and control of a keystone virus. In R. E. Junge, ed. *Proceedings of a Joint Conference American Association of Zoo Veterinarians*, pp. 518–519. Wildlife Disease Association, and American Association of Wildlife Veterinarians, East Lansing.

Ferren, W. R., Jr., H. M. Page, and P. Saley. (1996). Carpinteria salt marsh: Management plan for a southern California estuary. Draft. Draft Environmental Report No. 5, Prepared for University of California Natural Reserve System, Land Trust for Santa Barbara County, State Coastal Conservancy, City of Carpinteria.

Hall, S. R., M. A. Duffy, and C. E. Caceres. (2005). Selective predation and productivity jointly drive complex behavior in host-parasite systems. *American Naturalist* 165:70–81.

Hudson, P. J., A. P. Dobson, and D. Newborn. (1992). Do parasites make prey vulnerable to predation? Red grouse and parasites. *Journal of Animal Ecology* 61:681–692.

Hudson, P. J., A. P. Dobson, and D. Newborn. (1998). Prevention of population cycles by parasite removal. *Science* 282:2256–2258.

Huspeni, T. C. and K. D. Lafferty. (2004). Using larval trematodes that parasitize snails to evaluate a salt–marsh restoration project. *Ecological Applications* 14:795–804.

Huxham, M., D. Raffaelli, and A. Pike. (1995). Parasites and food–web patterns. *Journal of Animal Ecology* 64:168–176.

Janovy, J. (1997). Protozoa, helminths and arthropods of birds. In D. H. Clayton and J. Moore, eds. *Host–Parasite Evolution: General Principles and Avian Models*, pp. 303–337. Oxford University Press, Oxford.

Kennedy, C. R. and R. J. Watt. (1994). The decline and natural recovery of an unmanaged coarse fishery in relation to changes in land use and attendant eutrophication. *In* I. G. Cowx, ed. *Rehabilitation of Freshwater Fisheries.* pp. 366–375. Blackwell Scientific, Oxford.

Kuris, A. M. (1974). Trophic interactions: similarity of parasitic castrators to parasitoids. *Quarterly Review of Biology* 49:129–148.

Kuris, A. M. (1990). Guild structure of larval trematodes in molluscan hosts: prevalence, dominance and significance of competition. In G. W. Esch, A. O. Bush, and J. M. Aho, eds. *Parasite Communities: Patterns and Processes*, pp. 69–100. Chapman and Hall, London.

Kuris, A. M., G. O. Poinar, R. Hess, and T. J. Morris. (1979). Virus–particles in an internal parasite, *Portunion conformis* (Crustacea, Isopoda, Entoniscidae), and its marine crab host, *Hemigrapsus oregonensis. Journal of Invertebrate Pathology* 34:26–31.

Lafferty, K. D. (1993a). Effects of parasitic castration on growth, reproduction and population dynamics of the marine snail *Cerithidea californica. Marine Ecology Progress Series* 96:229–237.

Lafferty, K. D. (1993b). The marine snail, *Cerithidea californica*, matures at smaller sizes where parasitism is high. *Oikos* 68:3–11.

Lafferty, K. D. (1997). Environmental parasitology: what can parasites tell us about human impacts on the environment? *Parasitology Today* 13:251–255.

Lafferty, K. D. (1999). The evolution of trophic transmission. *Parasitology Today* 15:111–115.

Lafferty, K. D. (2004). Fishing for lobsters indirectly increases epidemics in sea urchins. *Ecological Applications* 14:1566–1573.

Lafferty, K. D. and E. J. Dunham. (2005). Trematodes in snails near raccoon latrines suggest a final host role for this mammal in California salt marshes. *Journal of Parasitology* 91:474–476.

Lafferty, K. D. and A. M. Kuris. (2002). Trophic strategies, animal diversity and body size. *Trends in Ecology and Evolution* 17:507–513.

Lafferty, K. D. and A. K. Morris. (1996). Altered behavior of parasitized killifish increases susceptibility to predation by bird final hosts. *Ecology* 77:1390–1397.

Lafferty, K. D., D. T. Sammond, and A. M. Kuris. (1994). Analysis of larval trematode communities. *Ecology* 75:2275–2285.

Lawton, J. H. (1989). Food webs. In J. M. Cherrett, ed. *Ecological Concepts*, pp. 43–78. Blackwell, Oxford.

Love, M. (1996). *Probably More Than You Want to Know About the Fishes of the Pacific Coast.* Really Big Press, Santa Barbara, CA.

Love, M. S. and M. Moser. (1983). A checklist of parasites of California, Oregon, and Washington Marine and Estuarine Fishes. US Department of Commerce, Washington DC.

Marcogliese, D. (2003). Food webs and biodiversity: are parasites the missing link? *Journal of Parasitology* 82(S):389–399.

Marcogliese, D. J. (2002). Food webs and the transmission of parasites to marine fish. *Parasitology* 124:S83–S99.

Marcogliese, D. J. and D. K. Cone. (1997). Food webs: a plea for parasites. *Trends in Ecology and Evolution* 12:320–325.

Martin, W. E. (1972). An annotated key to the cercariae that develop in the snail *Cerithidea californica. Bulletin of the Southern California Academy of Sciences* 71:39–43.

Martinez, N. (1992). Constant connectance in community food webs. *American Naturalist* 139:1208–1218.

May, R. M. (1973). *Stability and Complexity in Model Ecosystems.* Princeton University Press, Princeton, NJ.

McCann, K., A. Hastings, and G. R. Huxel. (1998). Weak trophic interactions and the balance of nature. *Nature* 395:794–798.

Memmott, J., N. D. Martinez, and J. E. Cohen. (2000). Predators, parasitoids and pathogens: species richness, trophic generality and body sizes in a natural food web. *Journal of Animal Ecology* 69:1–15.

Morris, R. H., D. P. Abbott, and E. C. Haderlie. (1980). *Intertidal Invertebrates of California.* Stanford University Press, Stanford, CA.

Murray, D. L., J. R. Cary, and L. B. Keith. (1997). Interactive effects of sublethal nematodes and nutritional status on snowshoe hare vulnerability to predation. *Journal of Animal Ecology* 66:250–264.

Packer, C., R. D. Holt, P. J. Hudson, K. D. Lafferty, and A. P. Dobson. (2003). Keeping the herds healthy and alert: implications of predator control for infectious disease. *Ecology Letters* 6:797–802.

Page, H. M. (1997). Importance of vascular plant and algal production to macro-invertebrate consumers in a southern California salt marsh. *Estuarine, Coastal and Shelf Science* 45:823–834.

Paine, R. T. (1988). Food webs: road maps of interactions or grist for theoretical development. *Ecology* 69:1648–1654.

Pimm, S. L., J. H. Lawton, and J. E. Cohen. (1991). Food web patterns and their consequences. *Nature* 350:669–674.

Plowright, W. (1982). The effects of rinderpest and rinderpest control on wildlife in Africa. *Symposia of the Zoological Society of London* 50:1–28.

Polis, G. A. (1991). Complex trophic interactions in deserts: an empirical critique of food–web theory. *American Naturalist* 138:123–155.

Price, P. W. (1980). *Evolutionary Biology of Parasites.* Princeton University Press, Princeton, NJ.

Ractliffe, L. H., H. M. Taylor, J. H. Whitlock, and W. R. Lynn. (1969). Systems analysis of a host–parasite interaction. *Parasitology* 59:649–661.

Roelke, Parker, M. E., Munson, L., Packer, C., Kock, R., Cleaveland, S., Carpenter, *et al.* (1996). A canine distemper virus epidemic in Serengeti lions (*Panthera leo*). *Nature* 379:441–445.

Russell, H. T. (1960). Trematodes from shorebirds collected at Morro Bay, California. Ph.D. dissertation. University of California, Los Angeles, CA.

Sinclair, A. R. E. (1979). The eruption of the ruminants. In A. R. E. Sinclair and M. Norton-Griffiths, eds. *Serengeti: Dynamics of an Dcosystem*, pp. 82–103. University of Chicago Press, Chicago, IL.

Sousa, W. P. (1993). Interspecific antagonism and species coexistence in a diverse guild of larval trematode parasites. *Ecological Monographs* 63:103–128.

Spinage, C. A. (2003). *Cattle Plague: A History.* Kluwer, New York.

Stevens, T. (1996). The importance of spatial heterogeneity and recruitment in organisms with complex life cycles: an analysis of digenetic trematodes in a salt marsh community. Ph.D. dissertation. University of California, Santa Barbara, CA.

Sukhdeo, M. V., and A. D. Hernandez. (2004). Food web patterns and the parasite perspective. In F. Thomas, F. Renaud, and J. Guegan, eds. *Parasitism and Ecosystems*, pp. 54–67. Oxford University Press, Oxford.

Thompson, R. M., K. N. Mouritsen, and R. Poulin. (2005). Importance of parasites and their life cycle characteristics in determining the structure of a large marine food web. *Journal of Animal Ecology* 74:77–85.

Thompson, R. M. and C. R. Townsend. (2003). Impacts on stream food webs of native and exotic forest: an intercontinental comparison. *Ecology* 84:145–161.

Tompkins, D. M., A. P. Dobson, P. Arneberg, M. E. Begon, I. M. Cattadori, J. V. Greenman, *et al.* (2001). Parasites and host population dynamics. In P. J. Hudson, A. Rizzoli, B. T. Grenfell, H. Heesterbeek, and A. Dobson, eds. *The Ecology of Wildlife Diseases*, pp. 45–62. University of Oxford Press, Oxford.

Whitlock, J. H., J. R. Georgi, D. S. Robson, and W. T. Federer. (1966). Haemonchosis, an orderly disease. *Cornell Veterinarian* 66:544–554.

Winemiller, K. O. and G. A. Polis. (1996). Introduction. In G. A. Polis and K. O. Winemiller, eds. *Food Webs: Integration of Patterns and Dynamics*, pp. 1–22. Chapman and Hall, New York.

Appendix 9.1

Predator–prey subweb. Interactions for predator trophic levels 1–6 depicted as predator [prey trophic level: prey *i*, prey *j*]. Prey listed in bold = known links. Regular font = putative links. Italics = links inferred from parasitism. Letter codes and numbers correspond to groups and species/item numbers as defined in Tables 9.1–9.5.

First trophic level (all prey in trophic level 0): A1–2,5,6,C1–2[**D1**], A3[**D1, P2, P9**], B34[**K1**], C3[**D1, P2**], C4[**D1, P1–2**], C5[**D2**], C8[**D1, D2, P1–2**], C9–10[**D1, P5**], F1,6[**D1, P1**], G1[D1, **P2**], G2[**D1, P2**], G3[**D2**], G4[D2], I1[**D1, P2**], I2[D1], I3[**D1**, K1], I4[P1–2], V1[**D1, P2, P9**], V2[**P2, P9**], V3–5[**P9**].

Second trophic level: A4[1: A1–3, A5–6, C1–4], B3[0: **P1, P3–4**; 1: C4, *V1*], B9[0: **P1, P3–8**; 1: C4, G2, I2, *V1*], B19[1: C5, I3], B32[0: P3, P9; 1: A1, C4, G2, I2], F2[1: **C1–2**, C3–4, I1].

Third trophic level: B17[1: **A1–2**, A3, A5–6, **C1, I3, V1, V5**; 2: A4], B22[1: **A1**, A2–3, A5–6; 1: *G1*, **I3**; 2: A4, **F2**], C7[0: **D1–2, K1, P1–2, P8**; 1: **A1–3, A5–6**, G2, I2, V1–5; 2: **A4**], F3[1: A1–3, A5–6, C2–4, G2, G4, I1–2, I4; 2: A4].

Fourth trophic level: B4[1: **A1–2**, A3, A5–6, **C1, C3, G1–2, I3**, *V1*, **V4–5**; 2: A4; 3: *C7*], B5[1: A1–3, A5–6, C1, C4–5, *G1*, V1–2; 2: A4; 3: *F3*], B6[1: **A1–2**, A3, **A5–6, C2–5**, *G1*, **I2–3**, *V1*; 2: A4; 3: *F3*], B12[1: F1; 2: F2; 3: F3], B14[1: **A1–2**, A3, **A5–6, C1, C3–4, G1–3, I2, V1–3**; 2: A4, **F2**; 3: *C7*, *F3*], B24[1: F1; 2: F2; 3: **F3**], B29[1: F1; 3: *F3*], B31[1: A1–3, A5–6, **C3**, *G1*, **I1**, I3; 2: A4, F2; 3: *F3*], C6[0: **D1–2, K1, P1–3, P8**; 1: **A1–3, A5–6**, C4, C8, **G1–2**, G3, I2, V1–5; 2: **A4**; 3: C7].

Fifth trophic level: B1[A1–2, A3–6, **C1, C3**, C4, **C5, C8–10**, *G1*, *I2*, 14, **V1–3**, V4, **V5**; 2: A4, **F2**; 3: *C7*; 4: **C6**], B2[1: **A1–2**, A3, **A5–6, C1, C4–5**, C8, **G1, I3, V1–2, V4–5**; 2: **A4, F2**; 3: *C7*; 4: C6], B7[0: K1; 1: F1, V1–3, V5; 3: C7, *F3*; 4: C6], B8[1: C8, **G3**; 3: C7; 4: **C6**], B10[0: K1; 1: **F1**, V1–3, **V5**; 3: **C7**; 4: **C6**], B11[1: **A1–2**, A3, A5–6, **C1, C3–5**, C8, **G3, V1–2**; 2: A4, *F2*; 3: *C7*; 4: **C6**], B13,16[0: K1; 1: F1, V1–3, V5; 3: C7; 4: C6], B15[0: **K1**;

1: **F1**, V1–3, **V5**; 3: **C7**; 4: **C6**], B21[1: **C8–10**, V3, **V4**; 2: **F2**; 3: **C7**; 4: **C6**], B27[1: C4, C8–10, G1, V1, **V2**, V3, **V5**; 3: C7; 4: C6], B30[1: C4, C8, **G1–2**, **V1–2**, **V5**; 3: C7; 4: C6], B33[1: C8, *G1*, G3; 3: C7; 4: C6], B35[4: B4–6], B36[4: B4–6, B14], F4[1: **C1**, C3, **C4**, C5, C8, **C9–10**; 2: **F2**; 3: **C7**, **F3**; 4: C6], F5[1: C2–4, **C5**, C8–10; 2: **F2**; 3: **C7**, **F3**; 4: **C6**], F7[1: C8–10, V1–3; 2: F2; 3: C7; 4: C6], R1[0: **K1**, 1: C8, F1; 2: B3, B9, B19; 3: **C7**; 4: **C6**; 5: B33].

Sixth trophic level: B18[1: **F1**, F6; 2: F2; 3: **F3**; 5: F4–5], B20[1: **C8**, **F1**, I3; 2: F2; 3: **C7**, **F3**; 4: **C6**; 5: F4–5], B23[1: **C8**, F1; 2: F2; 3: C7, **F3**; 4: **C6**; 5: **F4–5**], B25[1: F1, F6; 2: F2; 3: F3; 5: F4–5], B26[1: F1, F6; 2: F2; 3: **F3**; 5: F4–5], B28[1: C4, C8, F1; 2: F2; 3: C7, F3; 4: C6; 5: F4–5], B37[1: F1, **F6**; 3: F3; 5: F4–5], F8[1: C8–10,, F1, V1–3; 2: F2; 3: **C7**, F3; 4: C6; 5: F4

Appendix 9.2

Parasite–host subweb. Superscripts denote the following: 1 = parasite-1st intermediate host link; 2 = parasite-2nd intermediate host link; 3 = parasite-final host link. The superscript 2' indicates a metacercaria that excysts on the outside of the host and does not feed on the host. These are not counted as links in the parasite–host food web but are presented to illustrate life cycles (although they are included in the predator–parasite subweb). Excluded from the table are: (1) the two adult mosquitoes (I5–6) whom we assume feed on raccoons and all the birds, and (2) *Plasmodium* (avian malaria) which we assume infects all bird species and uses the mosquito *C. tarsalis* as a vector. Other codes as in Appendix 9.1.

Trophically transmitted parasites: N2[1: **V3**^{1}; 5: F7^3; 6: F8^3], N3[1: **C2**^{1}, **F1**^{3}, **F6**^{3}; 2: **F2**^{3}; 3: **F3**^{3}; 5: **F4–5**^{3}], N4[6: **R1**], O1[2: **B19**^{3}; 3: **B17**^{3}; 4: **B14**^{3}; 5: **B1**^{3}], T19[1: C2^2, G2^1; 5: **F5**^{3}], T20[1: **V3**^{2}; 4: B14^3; 5: B1^3, B7^3, B10^3, B13^3, B15–16^3, B21^3, B27^3], T21[1: **G4**^{1}, 4: C6^2; 5: B1^1, B22^1, B7–8^1, B10–11^1, B13^1, B15–16^1, B21^1, B27^1, B30^1, B33^1], T22[1:**F1**^{2}], W1[1: **V3**^{2}; 5: F7^3; 6:F8^3], W2[5: F7^3; 6:F8^3], W3[3: F3^2; 5: F4^2; 6:F8^3], W4[3: F3^2; 4: B5–6^3, B12^3, B14^3, B24^3, B29^3, B31^3, C6^3; 6: B18^3, B20^3, B23^3, B25–6^3, B28^3, B37^3].

Trematodes that use *C. californica* as a 1st intermediate host: T1[1: **G1**^{1}; 3: **F3**^{2}; 4: B5–6^3, B12^3, B14^3, B24^3, B29^3, **B31**^{3}; 5: B7^3, B18^3, B20^3, B23^3, B25–6^3, B28^3, B37^3], T2[1: **C8**$^{2'}$, **C10**$^{2'}$, **G1**^{1}, **G1**$^{2'}$; 3: C7$^{2'}$; 4:

B4^3, **B14**^{3}, **C6**$^{2'}$; 5: **B1–2**^{3}, B7–8^3, B10–11^3, B13^3, B15–16^3, **B21**^{3}, B27^3, B30^3, B33^3; 6: B20^3, B23^3, B28^3], T3[1: **C8**^{2}, **G1**^{1}; 3: **C7**^{2}; 4: B4^3, B14^3, **C6**^{2}; 5: **B1–2**^{3}, B7–8^3, B10–11^3, B13^3, B15–16^3, B21^3, B27^3, B30^3, **B33**^{3}; 6: B20^3, B23^3, B28^3], T4[1: **A5**^{2}, **G1**^{1}, **G2**^{2}; 2: B32^3; 3: **B17**^{3}, **B22**^{3}; 4: B4–5^3, **B6**^{3}, **B14**^{3}, B31^3; 5: B1–2^3, B11^3, B30^3], T5[1: **G1**^{1}; 3: **F3**^{2}; 4: **B5–6**^{3}, **B14**^{3}, B24^3, B29^3, B31^3; 5: **B7**^{3}, **F5**^{3}; 6: B18^3, B23^3, B25–6^3, B28^3, B37^3], T6[1: **A2**^{2}, **A5**^{2}, **G1**^{1}, **G2**^{2}, **V1–4**^{2}; 2: B3^3, 3: B17^3, **B22**^{3}; 4: **B4**^{3}, B5–6^3, **B14**^{3}, **B31**^{3}; 5: B1–2^3, B7^3, B10–11^3, B13^3, B15–16^3, B21^3, B27^3, B30^3, B33^3], T7[1:**G1**^{1}, **G1**$^{2'}$; 3: B22^3; 4: **B4–5**^{3}, B6^3, **B31**^{3}; 5: **B1–2**^{3}, B27^3, B33^3], T8[1: **A2**^{2}, **A5–6**^{2}, **G1**^{1}; 3: B17^3, B22^3; 4: B4–6^3, B14^3, B31^3; 5: B1–2^3, B11^3], T9[1: **C8**$^{2'}$, **C9**$^{2'}$, **G1**^{1}, **G1**$^{2'}$, **V1**$^{2'}$, **V3**$^{2'}$; 3: B17^3, **B22**^{3}, C7$^{2'}$; 4: **B4–6**^{3}, **B14**^{3}, B31^3, **C6**$^{2'}$; 5: **B1**–2^3, **B7**^{3}, *B8*^{3}, B10–**11**^{3}, B13^3, **B15**–16^3, B21^3, B27^3, B30^3, **B33**^{3}; 6: *B20*^{3}, *B23*^{3}, *B28*^{3}], T10[1: **G1**^{1}; 4: **B4–5**^{3}, B12^3, **B14**^{3}, **B31**^{3}; 5: **B1–2**^{3}, B13^3, B15^3], T11[1: **C8**$^{2'}$, **C9**$^{2'}$, **G1**^{1}, **G1**$^{2'}$, **V1**$^{2'}$, **V3**$^{2'}$; 3: B17^3, **B22**^{3}, C7$^{2'}$; 4: **B4–6**^{3}, **B14**^{3}, B31^3, **C6**$^{2'}$; 5: **B1–2**^{3}, B7^3, *B8*^{3}, B10–11^3, B13^3, **B15**–16^3, B21^3, B27^3, B30^3, **B33**^{3}; 6: *B20*^{3}, *B23*^{3}, *B28*^{3}], T12[1: **G1**^{1}; 3: B22^3, **F3**^{2}; 4: B5–6^3, **B12**^{3}, B14^3, B24^3, B29^3, B31^3; 5: B1–2^3, B7^3, B10–11^3, **B13**^{3}, **B15**–16^3, B21^3, **F5**^{2}; 6: B18^3, B20^3, B23^3, B25–6^3, B28^3, B37^3], T13[1: **G1**^{1}; 3: **F3**^{2}; 4: **B5–6**^{3}, B12^3, **B14**^{3}, B24^3, B29^3, B31^3; 5: **B7**, **F5**^{2}; 6: B18^3, B23^3, B25–6^3, B28^3, B37^3], T14[1: **G1**^{1}; 3: B22^3, **F3**^{2}; 4: B5–6^3, B12^3, B14^3, B24^3, B29^3, B31^3; 5: B1–2^3, B7^3, B10–11^3, B13^3, B15–16^3, B21^3, **F5**^{2}; 6: B18^3, B20^3, B23^3, B25–6^3, B28^3, B37^3], T15[1: **G1**^{1}; 2: B3^3; 3: **B22**^{3}, **F3**^{2}; 4: B5–6^3, B12^3, B14^3, B24^3, B29^3, B31^3; 5: **B1–2**^{3}, B7^3, B10–**11**^{3}, B13^3, B15–16^3, B21^3, **F5**^{2}, R1^3; 6: B18^3, B20^3, B23^3, B25–6^3, B28^3, B37^3], T16[1: **G1**^{1}; 3: B22^3; 4: B12^3, B14^3, B24^3, B29^3, B31^3; 5: B1–2^3, B7^3, B10–11^3, B13^3, B15–16^3, B21^3, **F5**^{2}, **R1**^{3}; 6: B18^3, B20^3, **B23**^{3}, B25–6^3, B28^3, B37^3], T17[1: **G1**^{1}; 3: B22^3, **F3**^{2}; 4: B5–6^3, B12^3, B14^3, B24^3, B29^3, B31^3; 5: B1–2^3, B7^3, B10–11^3, B13^3, B15–16^3, B21^3, **F5**^{2}; 6: B18^3, B20^3, **B23**^{3}, B25–6^3, B28^3, B37^3], T18[1: C4^2, **G1**^{1}; 4: B4^3, B14^3, C6^2; 5: B1–2^3, B7^3, B8^3, B10–11^3, B13^3, B15–16^3, B21^3, B27^3, B30^3, B33^3; 6: B20^3, B23^3, B28^3].

Nontrophically transmitted parasites depicted as parasite[host trophic level: host]. C11[3: **C7**^{3}], C12[1: **F1**^{3}, **F6**^{3}; 6: **F8**^{3}], C13[1: **C10**^{1}], C14[1: **F1**^{3}, F6^3; 2: **F2**^{3}; 3: F3^3; 5: **F4–5**^{3}], L1[5: **F4–5**^{3}], N1[1: **C9**^{1}; 5: F7^3; 6: F8^3], O2[3: **C7**^{3}], O3–4[1: F1^3, F6^3; 2: F2^3; 3: F3^3; 5: F4^3, F5^3], O5[1: **A2**^{3}], O7[4: **C6**^{3}].

Parasitic plants. P10[O: P3–P7], P11[O: P3,P5]

Appendix 9.3

Predator-parasite subweb. Superscripts denote the following: 5 = cercarial (water column) feeding; 6 = vector feeding; 7 = predation by a non-host (no parasite transmission); 8 = predation with parasite transmission. Other codes and notations as in Appendices 9.1 and 9.2.

First trophic level: V1–V3[T1–19^5].

Second trophic level: A4[O5^7, N3^7, T4^7, T6^7, T8^7, T18–19^7], B3[T6^8, T9^8, T11^7, T18^8], B9[T18^8, T19^7], B32[T18^8, T19^7], F2[N3^8, T1–19^5, T19^7].

Third trophic level: B17[O5^7, T4^7, T6^8, T8–9^8, T11^8], B22[C14^7, O3–5, N3^7, T1–5^7, T6–8^8, T9–11^7, T12^8, T13^7, T14^8, T15^7, T17–18^8], C7[O5^7, N2^7, T4^7, T6^7, T8–9^7, T11^7, T19–20^7, W1^7], F3[C14^7, O5^7, N3^8, T1–19^5, T4^7, T6^7, T8^7, T19^7].

Fourth trophic level: B4[O7^7, O2^7, O5^7, T1–2^7, T3–4^8, T5–7^7, T8^8, T9–17^7, T19^7], B5[O3–5^7, N3^7, T1^8, T2–3^7, T4, T5^7, T6^8, T7^7, T8^8, T9–11^7, T12^8, T13^7, T14–15^8, T16^7, T17–18^8], B6[O3–5^7, N3^7, T1^8, T2–6^7, T7–8^8, T9–11^7, T12^8, T13^7, T14–15^8, T16^7, T17–18^8, T19^7], B12[C12^7, C14^7, O3–4^7, N3^7, T1^8, T5^8, T12^7, T13–17^8, T22^7, W3^7, W4^8], B14[O7^7, C14^7, O2–5^7, N2–3^7, T1^8, T2^7, T3^8, T4–7^7, T8^8, T9–11^7, T12^8, T13^7, T14–18^8, T19^7, T20^8, W1^7, W3^7, W4^8], B24[C7^7, C14^7, O3–4^7, N3^7, T1^7, T5^8, T12–17^8, T22^7, W3^7, W4^8], B29[C7^7, C14^7, O3–4^7, N3^7, T1^7, T5^8, T12–17^8, T22^7, W3^7, W4^8], B31[C14^7, O3–5^7, N3^7, T1–3^7, T4–5^8, T6–7^7, T8–9^8, T10–11^7, T12–17^8, W3^7, W4^8], C6[C11^7, O7^7, O2^7, O5^7, O8^7, T1–20^7, W1^7].

Fifth trophic level: B1[C11^7, O7^7, C13–14^7, O1–6^7, N2–3^7, T1–18^8, T20^7, T21^8, W1^7], B2[C11^7, O7^7, C14^7, O2–6^7, N3^7, T1^7, T2–4^8, T5–7^7, T8–9^8, T10–11^7, T12^8, T13^7, T14–18^8, T21^8], B7[O7^7, C12^7, C14^7, O2–4^7, O6^7, N2–3^7, T1–3^8, T5–6^8, T9^8, T11–17^8, T20^8, T21^8, T22^7, W1^7], B8[C11^7, O7^7, O2^7, O6^7, T2^7, T3^8, T9^7, T11^7, T18^7, T21^8], B10[O7^7, C12^7, C14^7, O2–4^7, O6^7, N2–3^7, T2–3^8, T6^8, T9^8, T11–12^8, T14–18^8, T20–21^8, T22^7, W1^7], B11[C11^7, O7^7, C14^7, O2–6^7, N3^7, T2–4^8, T6^8, T8^8, T9^7, T11^7, T12^8, T14^8, T15^7, T16–18^8, T21^8], B13[O7^7, C12^7, C14^7, O2–4^7, O6^7, N2–3^7, T2–3^8, T6^8, T9^8, T11^8, T12^7, T14–T18^8, T20–21^8, T22^7, W1^7], B15[O7^7, C12^7, C14^7, O2–4^7, O6^7, N2–3^7, T2–3^8, T6^8, T9^7, T11^8, T12^7, T14–T18^8, T20–21^8, T22^7, W1^7], B16[O7^7, C12^7, C14^7, O2–4^7, O6^7, N2–3^7, T2–3^8, T6^8, T9^8, T11^8, T12^8, T14–T18^8, T20–21^8, T22^7, W1^7], B21[C11^7, O7^7, C12^7, C13–14^7, N1^7, O2–4^7, O6^7, N2–3^7, T2–3^8, T6^8, T9^8, T11^8, T12^8, T14–T18^8, T20–21^8, W1^7], B27[C12^7, C13^7, N1^7, O2^7, O6^7, N2^7, T1^7, T2–3^8, T4–5^7, T6–7^8, T8^7, T9^8, T10^7, T11^8, T12–17^7, T18^8, T20–21^8, W1^7], B30[C11^7, O7^7, C14^7, O2^7, O6^7, T1^7, T2–4^8, T5^7, T6^8, T7–8^7, T9^8, T10^7, T11^8, T12–17^7, T18^8, T19^8, T21^8], B33[C11^7, O7^7, C14^7, O2–4^7, O6^7, N3^7, T1–7^8, T9^8, T12–18^8, T19^7, T21^8, W3^7, W4^8], B35[O8^7, T1–15^7, T17^7, W4^8], B36[O8^7, O1^7, T1–17^7, T20^7, W4^8], F4[C11^7, O7^7, C13–14^7, N1^7, O2–4^7, O6^7, N3^7, T1–3^7, T1–19^5, T5^7, T9^7, T11–18^7, T21^7, W3–4^7], F5[C11^7, O7^7, C13–14^7, N1^7, O2–4^7, O6^7, N3^7, T1–3^7, T1–19^5, T5^7, T9^7, T11–18^7, T19^8, T21^7, W3–4^7], F7[C11^7, O7^7, C13–14^7, N1^8, O2–4^7, O6^7, N2^8, N3^7, T2–3^7, T6^7, T9^7, T11–12^7, T14–18^7, T20–21^7, W1^8], R1[C11^7, O7^7, C12^7, C14^7, O2–4^7, O6^7, N3, T2–3, T6^7, T9^7, T11–12^7, T14–15^7, T16^8, T17–18^7, T21–22^7].

Sixth trophic level: B18,25–26,37[C12^7, C14^7, L1^7, O3–4^7, N3^7, T1^8, T5^8, T12–18^8, T19^7, T22^7, W3^7, W4^8], B20[C11^7, O7^7, C12^7, C14^7, L1^7, O2–4^7, O6^7, N3^7, T1–3^8, T5^7, T9^8, T11–12^8, T13^7, T14–18^8, T19^7, T21^8, T22^7, W3^7, W4^8], B23[C11^7, O7^7, C12^7, C14^7, L1^7, O2–4^7, O6^7, N3^7, T1–3^8, T5^8, T9^8, T11–18^8, T19^7, T21^8, T22^7, W3^7, W4^8], B28[C11^7, O7^7, C12^7, C14^7, L1^7, O2–4^7, O6^7, N3^7, T1–3^8, T5^8, T9^8, T11–18^8, T19^7, T21^8, T22^7, W3^7, W4^8], F8[C11^7, O7^7, C12^7, C13–14^7, L1^7, N1^8, O2–4^7, O6^7, N2^8, N3^7, T1–3^7, T5^7, T9^7, T11–18^7, T20–22^7, W1^8, W3^8, W4^7].

Appendix 9.4

Parasite–parasite subweb. Most species interact via intraguild predation (as described in Kuris and Lafferty 1994). Other codes and notations as in Appendices 9.1–9.3.

Trematode–trematode interactions: T1[**T3**, **T5**, **T7–8**, **T12–17**, T18], T2[**T1**, **T3–8**, **T11–17**, T18], T3[**T5**, **T7**, **T13**, **T16**, T18], T4[**T1**, **T3**, **T5–9**, **T11–17**, T18], T5[**T3**, **T8**, **T13–14**, **T16**, 18], T6[**T1**, **T3**, **T5**, **T7–8**, **T11–17**, T18], T7[**T3**, **T5**, **T8**, **T13–14**, **T16**, T18], T8[**T3**, **T5**, **T7**, **T13–14**, **T16**], T9[**T1–8**, **T11–17**, T18], T11[**T1**, **T3**, **T5–8**, **T12–17**, T18], T12[**T1**, **T3**, **T5**, **T7–8**, **T13–17**, T18], T13[**T3**, **T5**, **T8**, **T14**, **T16**, T18], T14[**T3**, **T5**, **T7–8**, **T13**, **T16**, T18], T15[**T1**, **T3**, **T5**, **T7–8**, **T12–14**, **T16–17**, T18], T16[**T1**, **T3**, **T5**, **T7–8**, **T12–15**, **T17**, T18], T17[**T1**, **T3**, **T5**, **T7–8**, **T12–16**, T18], T18[**T3**, **T5**, **T7**, **T13**, **T16**].

Other parasite–parasite interactions: O7[6: **C11**^{3}], O8[6: *I6*^{3}].

CHAPTER 10

Shifting roles of abiotic and biotic regulation of a multi-host parasite following disturbance

Mary F. Poteet

10.1 Background

Impacts of macroparasitic diseases can scale from the individual host to the community (Anderson and May 1978; Holmes 1982; Scott 1988; Scott and Dobson 1989), however our knowledge of the community-level mechanisms that drive macroparasite dynamics in wildlife is still limited. Even more limited is empirical evidence that shows how parasites of wildlife respond to anthropogenic disturbances. Many of the current emergent and resurgent parasitic diseases in wildlife appear to be associated with anthropogenic activities (Schrag and Wiener 1995; Harvell *et al.* 1999; Daszak *et al.* 2000), but the paucity of rigorous data on wildlife diseases in general and their ecological aspects in particular limit our ability to assess causality. There are cases in which causality can be assigned, but these generally are limited to zoonoses (e.g. Lyme disease, Spielman 1994; LoGiudice *et al.* 2003; Wasserberg *et al.* 2003) and introduced pathogens of endangered or charismatic species (e.g. malaria in Hawaiian birds (Van Riper *et al.* 1986), whirling disease in trout (Hedrick *et al.* 1998), distemper in black-footed ferrets (Thorne and Williams 1988), upper respiratory disease in desert tortoises (Jacobson *et al.* 1991)). To date, few studies rigorously test for the impacts of anthropogenic disturbances, such as habitat loss, change, and degradation, on macroparasitic diseases in wildlife.

The evidence needed to link disturbance with diseases is often anecdotal, even for well-studied human diseases (McSweegan 1996). Recent work provides clues to the importance of anthropogenic disturbance in macroparasitic diseases with complex life cycles (Wasserberg *et al.* 2003). For example, overfishing in Lake Malawi is hypothesized to increase densities of the intermediate host snail of schistosomiasis and lead to increased prevalence in humans (Stauffer *et al.* 1997). Although this is a compelling argument, the authors acknowledge that their data are anecdotal and more study is necessary to test their hypothesis. A recent paper also suggested that eutrophication could alter food webs in a cascading effect from snail hosts to parasite abundance to limb deformities in amphibians (Johnson and Chase 2004). Again, this is a compelling hypothesis that deserves further testing but the data that support the links between eutrophication, snails, and infection in amphibians is generated from different studies in different sites over different years (see Skelly *et al.*, chapter 11, this volume for a systematic study of urbanization effects on trematode infection in amphibians).

Due to the extent and severity of anthropogenic disturbances and the likelihood that they will significantly alter parasite–host dynamics, it is essential to rigorously measure the response of different types of parasites and pathogens to disturbances and then apply this knowledge in ecological restoration and conservation efforts. This chapter focuses primarily on macroparasites that are especially sensitive to disturbance due to the diversity of hosts and transmission stages necessary to complete their life cycles. In addition to their inherent sensitivity to disturbance, macroparasites can have significant, but difficult to detect effects on their host populations. Indeed, recent work demonstrates that nematode parasites can cause population cycles in grouse (Hudson *et al.* 1998). Thus, a change in macroparasitism in response to disturbance could greatly affect host populations, and the dynamics between hosts and parasites (May and Anderson 1979).

One of the main limitations in assessing impacts of anthropogenic disturbances on parasite populations in wildlife is the inability to replicate these disturbances. Natural disturbances play a strong role in structuring patterns of species diversity and distribution (Sousa 1984, 2001; Pickett and White 1985). The effects of natural disturbances are often measured through replicated experimental manipulations within a designated temporal and/or spatial regime (Levin and Paine 1974; Sousa 1979; Hobbs and Mooney 1991). The effects of large-scale, single-point anthropogenic disturbances, such as oil spills, can be difficult to assess as they are often generated by events that are unreplicated through time or space (for review see Schmitt and Osenberg 1996). As long as care is taken in site selection, some anthropogenic disturbances, such as habitat fragmentation and road building, can be used for natural experiments; however these are the exception to the rule. In addition, understanding the effects of disturbance on epidemiology can be made more difficult due to dispersal of infected individuals, parasite stages, or vectors away from or into the site of disturbance. Parasites with complex life cycles often infect hosts that cross ecosystem boundaries, such as schistosomes in humans, or migrate long distances, such as *Nanophyetus* in salmon. The difficulty is in assessing not only the patterns of infection, but also whether and how they are affected by anthropogenic impacts.

In this chapter, I report results of a study designed to measure the effects of three levels of anthropogenic disturbance on each host and parasite stage of a macroparasite that occurs in stream communities of the Pacific Northwest, USA. The disturbance of interest is clearcut logging: a prevalent, replicated, large-scale disturbance in the northwestern United States. I chose a "closed" parasite–host system in which none of the hosts regularly disperses or migrates outside of the local

watershed. This eliminates the need to estimate parasite loss due to host movement. I carefully selected 18 creeks in watersheds exposed to three levels of disturbance associated with clearcut logging. They include streams located in old growth forests without anthropogenic disturbances, streams in clearcut forests, and streams in clearcut forests that experienced severe winter flooding (debris flow) that was exacerbated by logging. I measured the effects of disturbance level on the density of each obligate host and on the prevalence, intensity, and density of each stage of the parasite. I then assessed whether disturbance alters the strength or direction of the relationship between host and parasite densities and explored the implications of these changes to parasite transmission. I interpret these results in the context of general Anderson and May (1978, 1979) models for macroparasites. These models assume mass-action transmission that results in a positive relationship between host and parasite densities with or without an upper threshold. These models are commonly used to predict the response of parasites to environmental disturbances (e.g. Lafferty and Holt 2003). Finally, I test whether disturbance shifts the role of environmental and biotic factors in the host–parasite populations.

10.2 The parasite-host system

The trematode parasite, *Cephalouterina dicamptodoni*, obligately and sequentially infects three stream-dwelling species: the Pacific giant salamander, *Dicamptodon tenebrosus*, an abundant snail, *Juga silicula*, and the stonefly, *Calineuria californica* (Fig. 10.1) (Senger and Macy 1953; Schell 1985). Adult parasites live and sexually reproduce in the intestines of their salamander hosts. Parasite eggs are released into the environment with the host's feces where they are consumed by snails and subsequently hatch into miracidia. The miracidia migrate to the snail's gonads and transform into a series of sporocyst stages. Each of these sporocysts asexually produces thousands of cercariae that are then released into the aquatic environment. To continue the life cycle, these cercariae search for the next obligate host species which is a nymphal stonefly, *C. californica*. Once found, the cercaria

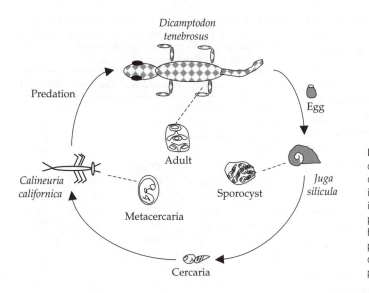

Figure 10.1 Life cycle diagram of *Cephalouterina dicamptodoni*, a trematode parasite that infects the definitive host, *Dicamptodon tenebrosus*, the first intermediate host, *Juga silicula*, and the second intermediate host, *Calineuria californica*. Free-living parasite stages transmit to the snail and stonefly host. Parasites transmit to the salamander via predation of an infected stonefly. Arrows indicate direction of transmission for each stage of the parasite between hosts.

pierces the stonefly with a scalpel-like stylet and penetrates the exoskeleton through the incision. Cercariae encyst as metacercariae in the muscle tissues of the stonefly. The life cycle of the parasite is completed when a salamander preys upon an infected stonefly and the metacercaria excysts and grows to sexual maturity.

Each host of *C. dicamptodoni* is an important component of the aquatic food web in small streams in the Cascade Mountains of Oregon. Larvae of *D. tenebrosus* often comprise the greatest vertebrate biomass in small streams throughout western Oregon and California and are voracious predators (Murphy and Hall 1981; Corn and Bury 1989). *Dicamptodon* larvae eat a wide variety of aquatic and terrestrial prey, with aquatic macroinvertebrates comprising the most significant prey base (Parker 1992). Salamander larvae of different size classes overlap significantly in the prey they consume with preference toward certain macroinvertebrates, including *Calineura* spp. During their aquatic stage, *D. tenebrosus* are territorial and cannibalistic. With the exception of neotenic individuals, larval salamanders reside in streams for 2–3 years until metamorphosis to the terrestrial adult stage (Nussbaum and Clothier 1973).

Juga silicula is an abundant aquatic snail inhabiting mid-elevation streams from northern California north to southern Washington (Burch 1982). This species often comprises the majority of total

invertebrate biomass in streams, reaching densities of 1500 m^2, thus making them strong competitors with macroinvertebrate grazers, particularly Diptera (Hawkins and Furnish 1987).

Calineuria californica, the second intermediate host, is distributed from central California north through British Columbia and east to Montana (Stewart and Stark 1993). In the central Cascades, stonefly nymphs are semivoltine. *Calineuria* prey dominantly on larval Diptera and Ephemeroptera (Sheldon 1969; Peckarsky 1984).

10.3 Methods

10.3.1 Host censuses

To measure the effects of anthropogenic disturbance on patterns of parasite and host abundance, I surveyed each host species from 18 streams located in the McKenzie and Fall creek watersheds, Oregon. The streams were located in small watersheds (4–16 km^2) that had experienced one of three levels of anthropogenic disturbance associated with logging. The three categories of disturbance were: no disturbance (ND), intermediate disturbance (ID), and severe disturbance (SD). ND streams ($n = 7$) were located in watersheds covered by mature forests that were at least 80 years old. ID streams ($n = 7$) were in watersheds with at least 50% clearcuts. SD streams ($n = 4$) were in watersheds with predominantly clearcut forests that experienced major flooding and debris flows (as defined in Leopold *et al.* 1964) 2 years prior to the survey. Clearcut watersheds were defined as having ≤ 20-year-old clearcuts covering at least 50% of the area of the watershed. Each watershed was selected to minimize differences in logging-independent geomorphology such as stream gradient, elevation, and watershed size. Streams were randomly sampled with respect to date from June 13 through July 30, 1998.

Each stream was sampled over a 2-day period. Macroinvertebrates and physical data were collected on the first day and salamanders were collected on the second day. Streams were sampled in a stratified random manner and samples were collected every 5 m along a 150 m transect for a total of 30 surber samples per stream. *D. tenebrosus* larvae and neotenes were collected from each stream along the 150 m transect using a fish electroshocker. Seine nets were placed at least every 50 m along the transect to block individuals from escaping. All *D. tenebrosus* were counted, measured, and weighed in the field. A representative sample of larvae was euthanized, dissected (Table 10.1), and all intestinal parasites were counted and preserved.

Snails, stoneflies, and other macroinvertebrates were collected from a 30 × 30 cm quadrat using a surber sampler. All snails greater than 5 mm were dissected for sporocyst presence. Counting sporocysts was time-prohibitive so intensity of this stage was estimated based on a regression of percentage of gonad infected and gonad length (Poteet 2001). Snails smaller than 5 mm were not included in these data since prior dissections revealed that small snails were never infected (Poteet 2001). All encysted metacercariae were counted in each stonefly. To count all the metacercariae, each stonefly was digested in an HCl and pepsin bath that dissolved stonefly muscles, but not parasite cysts (Ash and Orihel 1991).

Prevalence, intensity, and density of each parasite stage were calculated following Bush *et al.* (1997). Prevalence was calculated as the proportion of hosts in the population that were infected by one parasite stage. Mean parasite intensity was measured as the number of parasites of a single

Table 10.1 Number of *D. tenebrosus* larvae captured and dissected along a 150 m transect within each creek. All captured larvae were weighed and measured in the field. Larvae that were not dissected were released in the creek from where they were captured.

Creek	Date	Disturbance	Captured	Dissected
CONE	17 June	ND	42	18
JONES	21 June	ND	74	23
SLICK	24 June	ND	12	10
SFGATE	28 June	SD	24	10
HOLDEN	1 July	ID	4	3
OSBORNE	3 July	ID	43	20
RITCHIE	6 July	ID	46	21
FINN	8 July	ID	14	10
WFNFGATE	10 July	SD	31	17
HAGAN	11 July	ND	100	30
EFNFGATE	15 July	SD	48	19
SIMMONDS	17 July	ND	38	17
ELK	19 July	ND	24	11
WFDEER	21 July	ID	46	23
EFDEER	23 July	ID	42	19
NFNFGATE	25 July	SD	21	11
MONA	28 July	ND	45	22
STURDY	31 July	ID	8	5

Disturbance levels are ND = no disturbance, ID = intermediate disturbance, SD = severe disturbance.

stage averaged across all infected hosts in the population. Mean parasite density was calculated as the number of parasites of a single stage averaged across all hosts per square meter. For parasites in snails and stoneflies, each metric was averaged per quadrat. Stream averages were calculated as the grand mean for all quadrat means. Means for prevalence, intensity, and density of the adult parasites were averaged across all dissected salamanders and then divided by total creek area sampled. The total creek area sampled was the product of the transect distance of 150 m and the mean wetted width of the creek.

10.3.2 Disturbance, environmental variables, and parasitism

Logging leads to increased stream temperatures, altered stream velocity, and decreased habitat heterogeneity. Clearcuts in the Cascade mountains are associated with high rates of hillslope erosion and increased storm peak discharge (Jones and Grant 1996) that affect stream channel morphology, particle size, and discharge. Each of these variables can significantly affect the success of parasite transmission (Chernin and Perlstein 1969; Upatham 1974; Anderson *et al.* 1982; Jewsbury 1985; Woolhouse and Chandiwana 1989; Shostak and Esch 1990; Sousa and Grosholz 1991; McKindsey and McLaughlin 1994). Along each 150 m transect, I measured a series of environmental attributes associated with logging and used these measures to correlate parasitism with disturbance-related environmental variables. These attributes included dominant substrate particle size, thalweg depth, thalweg velocity, percent channel morphology (pool, riffle, run, or cascade), and percentage of canopy cover. I also measured substrate embeddedness, or the extent to which fine sediments filled the interstitial spaces around larger substrates (Bovee 1982; Gordon *et al.* 1992). The interstitial spaces formed within creek substrates are important habitat for salamanders, stoneflies, and other stream biota. Thus, as embeddedness increases, habitat availability and biotic productivity decreases.

To standardize host and parasite density measurements across creeks, I measured bank-full width and depth and wetted-channel width. Air temperature was measured in the morning, and minimum and maximum diurnal water temperatures were measured over the 48-h sampling period. Watershed area was calculated from USGS 7.5′ topographic maps.

10.3.3 Statistical analyses

I tested for differences in host density and parasite prevalence, intensity and density across forest disturbance levels with analysis of variance (ANOVA) followed by adjusted Tukey post hoc comparisons. I regressed parasite density on host density for each host–parasite pair to test model assumptions that parasite transmission leads to positive correlation between host and parasite densities (May and Anderson 1979). All variables were transformed where necessary to meet the assumptions of homogeneity of variance and normality.

I tested for the responses of parasite density to abiotic and biotic variables with principal components analysis (PCA) followed by analysis of covariance (ANCOVA). Seven correlated abiotic variables were transformed into their principal components (Selvin 1998; S-Plus 2000). Variables used in the PCA included maximum water temperature, thalweg velocity, pool/riffle ratio, percentage canopy cover, channel shape (measured as width/depth ratio), embeddedness (Brusven Index, Gordon *et al.* 1992), and mean substrate particle size (Dunne and Leopold 1978). These variables were chosen for their high probability of affecting host or parasite populations. Before conducting the analysis, the data were transformed where necessary to meet the assumptions of normality and homogeneity of variance and all variables were standardized to a mean of 0 and unit variance to account for differing scales of measurement.

Biotic variables considered for the ANCOVA included host length, host density, parasite density and, in the case of metacercarial transmission, salamander diet (i.e. the mean number of stoneflies found in salamander stomachs per treatment, see Fig. 10.1). Abiotic variables considered for the ANCOVA included the first three principal components. Because the number of possible explanatory variables for the ANCOVA was greater than the number of replicate streams, I chose leaps and bounds analyses to select the best-fit models for each host–parasite pair (Furnival and Wilson 1974; S-Plus 2000). Leaps and bounds analysis is similar to model selection analyses that evaluate the best fit models from the full set of explanatory variables. However, unlike other model selection analyses leaps and bounds uses an algorithm developed by Furnival and Wilson (1974) that identifies the best fit by testing all possible models. The resulting best-fit models of donor-target pairs had at least four explanatory variables and thus I was unable to divide the forests into all three disturbance levels for the analyses due to low replication. The final best-fit models lumped ID with SD into a single "disturbed" category.

10.4 Results

10.4.1 Responses of host density and parasite prevalence, intensity, and density to environmental disturbance

Densities of each host species were significantly lower in logged creeks, but patterns differed by

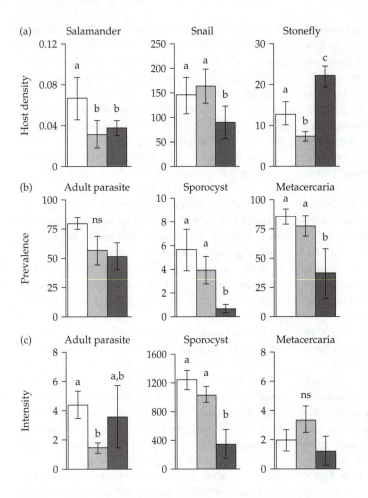

Figure 10.2 Host density, parasite prevalence, and parasite intensity for 18 streams of three disturbance intensities. (A) Host density is the mean number of hosts/m². (B) Prevalence is the mean proportion of hosts infected. (C) Parasite intensity is the mean number of parasites averaged across all infected hosts. Small letters denote statistical significance at the $p < 0.05$ level. Error bars are ± 1 SE. White bars = no disturbance (ND) sites, grey bars = intermediate disturbance (ID) sites, and black bars = severe disturbance (SD) sites.

host species and level of disturbance (Fig. 10.2(a)). Salamander density was similar across ID and SD creeks, but snail densities were lower only in creeks with the most severe disturbances. Stonefly densities differed across disturbance levels such that the lowest stonefly densities were found in ID streams and the highest densities were found in SD streams.

Prevalence and intensity of each parasite stage was generally lower in logged sites but did not track host density (Fig. 10.2(b) and (c)). Interestingly, adult parasite intensity recovered somewhat in severely disturbed streams even though salamander densities remained low (Fig. 10.2(a) and (c)). At the same time, prevalence of adult parasites remained constant across disturbance (Fig. 10.2(b)) leading to a recovery in the density of adult parasites in SD streams as compared to ID streams

(Fig. 10.3(a)). These results run counter to many population models of macroparasite population dynamics (e.g. May and Anderson 1979) and to predictions that parasite densities will decrease following disturbances that cause decreased host densities (Lafferty and Holt 2003). This anomaly is likely explained by an increase in the rate of parasite transmission from stoneflies to salamanders that result from the predation-dependent transmission of this parasite stage (Box 10.1).

Of all stages, the sporocysts were most affected by disturbance, with significant declines in prevalence and intensity in ID and SD creeks. This density-dependent effect is partially explained by the sharp decline in snail host density in the sites with severe disturbance, but is also associated with changing abiotic conditions (see *Principal Components Analyses*, below). Intensity of metacercariae was not

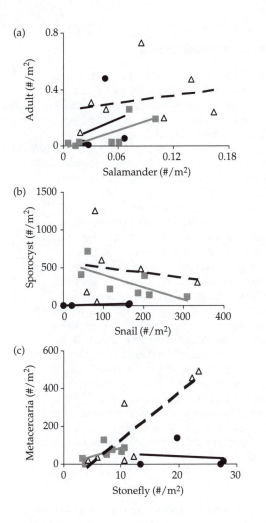

(a)

(b)

(c)

Figure 10.3 Regressions between each host and parasite pair at three levels of disturbance. Common models for macroparasite populations assume a positive correlation between parasite and host densities. These regressions demonstrate that this assumption is not valid for most of the parasite stages in areas with environmental disturbances. (a) Adult parasite in salamanders, (b) sporocyts in snails, (c) metacercariae in stoneflies. Open triangles with dashed lines = no disturbance (ND) sites, gray squares with solid gray lines = intermediate disturbance (ID) sites, and filled circles with solid black lines = severe disturbance (SD) sites.

statistically different across the disturbance gradient (Fig. 10.2(c)), but metacercarial density was lower in SD than ND sites (Fig. 10.3(c)). The low metacercarial density in SD sites was somewhat surprising since stonefly densities in these sites were the highest of the three stream types. The low density of metacercariae in SD sites was probably due to

low recruitment of cercariae from small snail populations at these severely disturbed sites.

10.4.2 Environmental disturbance and model assumptions

If the assumption of mass-action transmission is correct in the general macroparasite models (May and Anderson 1979), then regressions of parasite density on host density should have positive slopes. Significantly positive regressions between parasite and host densities were found in only two cases (Fig. 10.3(a) and (c)): between salamanders and adult parasites in ID ($R^2 = 0.5584$, $F_{1,5} = 6.321$, $p = 0.054$) and between stoneflies and metacercariae in ND ($R^2 = 0.6153$, $F_{1,5} = 7.999$, $p = 0.037$). In general, the regression slope between adult parasites and salamanders trended toward positive across all disturbance levels (Box 10.1). This is not the case for the two other parasite stages. In fact, the regression between snails and sporocyst densities was significantly negative across ID sites ($R^2 = 0.6096$, $F_{1,5} = 7.806$, $p = 0.038$) and was not significantly different from 0 at ND and SD sites (Fig. 10.3(b)).

10.4.3 Physical attributes of streams: univariate analyses

When selecting streams to test for effects of environmental disturbance on parasite populations, I controlled for geographic location, watershed area, elevation, and stream gradient to minimize differences among watersheds that were not caused by disturbance. All but three streams were located in the McKenzie River watershed. The remaining three streams, Jones, Slick, and Sturdy, were in the Little Fall creek watershed, which is the drainage immediately south of the McKenzie River watershed. There were no differences in watershed area, elevation or stream gradient among streams in different forest types (basin area: $F_{2,15} = 0.271$, $p = 0.766$; elevation: $F_{2,15} = 1.743$, $p=0.208$; gradient: $F_{2,15} = 0.052$, $p = 0.949$).

Undisturbed streams had significantly higher pool to riffle ratios (30%) than ID (11%) or SD (2%) streams. Thalweg velocity and substrate embeddedness (Brusven Index) were higher in streams at logged sites (velocity: $F_{2,15} = 28.276$, $p = <0.001$;

Box 10.1 Transmission through predation of an obligate, intermediate host

Predicting how changes in salamander density will affect parasite dynamics is not straightforward since salamanders acquire infections by consuming infected stoneflies. Thus, transmission of metacercariae will depend upon the predator–prey functional response curve between salamanders and stoneflies. May and Anderson (1979) suggest that transmission completed through a trophic link is extremely efficient and that the threshold density of predators, in this case salamanders, required to maintain the adult parasite population is low (May and Anderson 1979). So even at extremely low salamander densities, metacercarial transmission should be successful. However, the rate of transmission will vary with the predator–prey functional response, which will depend upon the density of salamanders and stoneflies. Pacific giant salamander larvae prey disproportionately on mayflies and large predaceous insects, including stoneflies (Parker 1994). The proportion of stoneflies relative to the other prey items preferred by salamanders is not constant across forest type (M. Poteet, unpublished data). This suggests that the functional response curve is likely to be nonlinear with disturbance, either Type II or Type III, which would lead to nonlinear parasite transmission and not the linear transmission function assumed by mass-action models (e.g. Crofton 1971; Anderson and May 1978). In addition, since the salamander must eat an infected stonefly to become infected, the rate of transmission will not only be affected by the functional response of the predator, but also by the proportion of stoneflies that are infected. Thus, a transmission term that is dependent upon prevalence of infection in stoneflies would provide a better description of metacercarial transmission than would mass-action transmission. This is reminiscent of frequency-dependent models in which infection of the vector is dependent upon the frequency of infected nonvector hosts (Getz and Pickering 1983; Thrall et al. 1995; McCallum et al. 2001). One interesting outcome of frequency-dependent transmission is the lack of a host threshold, since transmission depends upon proportional infection. By this model, even if stonefly and salamander densities are extremely low, parasites should still be able to establish in salamanders. That seems to be the case in this system, where even at high levels of disturbance and low metacercarial densities (Fig. 10.3(c)) adult parasite density almost recovers to undisturbed levels (Fig. 10.3(a)). In either transmission model, decreased salamander density should result in decreased metacercarial transmission and this is the case here. At each level of disturbance, regardless of salamander density, there is a direct correlation between salamander densities and adult parasites. This is not the case for the free-living transmission stages (sporocysts and metacercariae), whose densities are affected by both environmental stressors and host density.

embeddedness: $F_{2,15} = 5.391$, $p = 0.005$). The only abiotic factor that was significantly lower at logged sites was canopy cover ($F_{2,15} = 20.770$, $p < 0.001$). The decreased canopy cover in ID and SD streams corresponded to slightly increased air temperature and maximum water temperature, though neither differed significantly with disturbance level (air temperature: $F_{2,15} = 2.667$, $p = 0.102$; water temperature: $F_{2,15} = 0.648$, $p = 0.537$).

10.4.4 Physical attributes of streams: principal components analyses

Each of the principal components described some aspect of the physical responses of streams to logging. Logging increased sediment load delivered to the creeks, increased peak storm flows (Jones and Grant 1996), and decreased canopy cover. These changes altered channel shape, increased stream velocity, and decreased streambed particle size. Each of these features is described by at least one principal component, with channel shape a significant feature in each principal component.

The first principal component (PC1) described channel shape and was composed of positive correlations between stream velocity and the ratio of bank full width to bank full depth (width/depth). This reflected higher stream velocities and wider, shallower channels following logging. The second principal component (PC2) described stream channel pool/riffle morphology. Logging increased the proportion of riffle habitat which led to greater mean channel width. Pool/riffle ratio was inversely proportional to width/depth ratio and stream temperature. The third principal component (PC3) described streambed particle size

Table 10.2 Results of ANCOVA testing for the effects of disturbance on the biotic and abiotic variables that best explain variation in each stage in the life cycle of the parasite. Best fit models were selected with the leaps and bounds method (see text for explanation)

Adult

	C	t	p
ND	-0.504	-0.949	0.361
D	-0.469	-0.883	0.394
Salamander #/m² (ND)	0.236	2.224	0.046
Salamander #/m² (D)	0.179	3.554	0.004
Salamander SVL (ND)	0.274	1.912	0.080
Salamander SVL (D)	0.113	2.575	0.024

Sporocyst

	C	t	p
ND	-31.663	-2.25	0.059
D	-20.61	-1.464	0.186
Snail #/m² (ND)	8.797	2.726	0.03
Snail #/m² (D)	0.905	1.224	0.26
PC3 (ND)	-4.02	-1.267	0.246
PC3 (D)	0.494	0.831	0.434
PC1 (ND)	7.525	2.464	0.043
PC1 (D)	-0.946	-2.943	0.022

Metacercaria

	C	t	p
ND	-0.987	-0.455	0.663
D	-3.476	-1.601	0.153
Stonefly #/m² (ND)	3.407	3.907	0.006
Stonefly #/m² (D)	0.858	0.946	0.376
PC1 (ND)	1.468	1.578	0.159
PC1 (D)	-0.217	-0.705	0.503
Snail #/m² (ND)	2.828	2.086	0.075
Snail #/m² (D)	1.74	4.109	0.004

ND = no disturbance, or watersheds in old growth forests; D = disturbance, or watersheds in clearcut forests with and without debris flows; SVL = salamander length measured from the snout to the vent in mm; P1 = principal component 1; P3 = principal component 3; C = regression coefficients. The first two coefficients in the 'C' column are regression intercepts for the ND or D sites respectively. The remaining coefficients are regression slopes for each variable for the ND or D sites respectively.

as a function of channel shape and was composed of the pebble count, maximum water temperature, and width/depth ratio. Width to depth ratio and pebble count were positively correlated with each other and inversely related to the maximum water temperature. The first three principal components among all streams explained 76% of the variation in abiotic variables. The significant components were based on variables with loadings greater than 0.40 or less than -0.40 (Hair *et al.* 1987; McGarigal *et al.* 2000).

10.4.5 Disturbance shifts the importance of biotic and abiotic variables

Because host density did not explain significant amounts of variability in abundance for most of the parasite stages, I expanded the regression analyses to include host density and the first three principal components. Leaps and bounds analyses selected the following explanatory variables for each parasite stage to minimize the Mallow's Cp:

- adult parasite density: salamander density and salamander length;
- sporocyst density: snail density, PC3, and PC1;
- metacercarial density: stonefly density, PC1, and snail density.

The models were analyzed with ANCOVA using forest type as a covariate. Since there were only four replicates of SD streams, I combined the ID and SD forests into a "disturbed" category (D).

In all but the adult parasite stage, disturbance switched the dominant variable that best explained parasite density (Table 10.2). Although disturbances had significant effects on the overall density of adult parasites, they did not alter the positive correlation between the parasite and its salamander host. For example, adult parasite density was positively and significantly correlated with salamander density in both logged and unlogged streams, and significantly correlated with salamander size in logged streams (Table 10.2). Adult parasite densities could not be explained by variation in abiotic variables for either logged or unlogged streams.

Unlike adult parasites, disturbance caused a significant shift in the type of variables that controlled sporocyst density. Both abiotic and biotic variables correlated with sporocyst density in unlogged streams, but only abiotic variables affected sporocyst density in logged streams. Specifically, sporocyst density was significantly and *positively* correlated with snail density and the channel shape/velocity principal component (PC1). However, in streams with disturbance, sporocyst density was significantly and *negatively* correlated with PC1 and not correlated with snail density (Table 10.2).

Disturbance caused a shift in the biotic variables controlling metacercarial densities, but as with adult parasite density, abiotic variables were not associated with metacercarial densities in logged or unlogged streams. In unlogged streams, stonefly density explained the majority of variation in metacercarial density. Disturbance shifted control over metacercarial density from stonefly hosts to snail hosts in logged streams (Table 10.2).

10.5 Discussion

Land use change and resource use by humans increasingly force species to cope with fragmented and degraded habitats that can alter infection dynamics of diseases and parasites (e.g. Dobson and Carper 1992; Lafferty and Holt 2003; LoGiudice *et al.* 2003, this volume). Although several reviews report that diseases and parasites of wildlife respond to anthropogenic disturbances (Schrag and Wiener 1995; Lafferty 1997; Daszak *et al.* 2000), most of the studies cited are either anecdotal or are not sufficiently replicated, which limits our ability to interpret them (but see Wasserberg *et al.* 2003). By measuring each stage of a macroparasite and its host species across replicated environmental disturbances, this study measures the response of parasite infection levels to disturbance and also explores the mechanisms that drive these changes.

Disturbances caused by logging led to significant declines in host density and in the prevalence, intensity, and density of infection by trematodes in these three host species. Regressions between parasite and host densities were also affected by disturbance, suggesting that disturbance affected the success or functional form of parasite transmission. Disturbance could act directly on parasite transmission by changing abiotic factors that impact the free-living stages of the parasite, or indirectly by affecting host abundance or distribution (in space or time) (Sousa and Grosholz 1991; Sapp and Esch 1994; Marín *et al*. 1998). For example, changes in abiotic factors such as temperature and velocity can directly affect reproduction and survival of parasite transmission stages (Anderson *et al*. 1982; Evans 1985; Jewsbury 1985). Higher temperatures lead to increased reproductive rate of parasites, often at the expense of survivorship of the free-living stages (Anderson *et al*. 1982). On the other hand, increases in stream velocity result in damage to and decreased transmission success of parasite infective stages (Upatham 1974; Jewsbury 1985). Transmission of free-living stages can also be directly affected by changes in geomorphology and microhabitat heterogeneity (Chernin and Perlstein 1969, for review see Sousa and Grosholz 1991), features of streams that are often affected by logging (Dunne and Leopold 1978; Beschta *et al*. 1987; Bisson *et al*. 1987; Everest *et al*. 1987).

Indirect effects of logging on parasitism are just as likely to occur as direct effects, and will be manifest through changes in host population features including host density and size structure. Logging did have a strong effect on density of each of the three host species. In high gradient streams similar to those I censused, larval salamander and nymphal stonefly densities generally increase while snail densities generally decrease after logging (Murphy and Hall 1981; Hawkins *et al*. 1982, 1983, but Corn and Bury 1989 found decreased salamander density in logged creeks). In this study, host density responded strongly to logging both with and without debris flows but the strength and direction of the effect was dependent upon host species and severity of logging. Salamander density decreased following logging, regardless of debris flows whereas snail density did not change following logging unless it was coupled with debris flows. Stoneflies were the most sensitive to logging disturbance. Their population density decreased in logged creeks but rebounded above unlogged levels in streams with severe disturbances (debris flows). The increased abundance of stoneflies following debris flows is

most likely due to the decrease in canopy cover and subsequent increase in light penetration to the stream. Increased sunlight penetration in streams leads to increased algal production (e.g. Gregory 1980; Hill and Harvey 1990), which translates into more herbivorous prey for the predaceous stoneflies (Power 1992; Hill *et al*. 1995).

The response in host densities to disturbance was not mirrored by the parasites. Different disturbance levels led to complex, noncorrelated responses among the suite of parasite stages and their hosts. This suggests that the decline in parasite infections in disturbed streams was accompanied by changes in transmission dynamics of the parasites. The simple mass-action transmission that is often used in models of parasite population dynamics assumes that the rate of transmission is directly proportional to the densities of uninfected and infected hosts or parasitic stages (e.g. Crofton 1971; Anderson and May 1978, 1979; May and Anderson 1979). These linear transmission models generally predict a threshold host density below which parasites cannot persist and a stable equilibrium in which the disease is maintained. Logging-induced disturbances in this study generated complex patterns among parasite stages and their hosts that suggest nonlinear transmission. For example, the correlations between snail and sporocyst densities in ND and ID sites (Fig. 10.3(b)) show decreasing sporocysts with increasing snail densities, suggesting density-dependent transmission. In SD sites for this same host–parasite pair, there was no significant correlation.

Unlike sporocyst–snail pairs, correlations between salamander densities and adult parasites suggest a maximum threshold of infection, possibly limited by recruitment from stoneflies (Fig. 10.3(a)). Although the salamander–adult parasite pair seems to fit the mass-action model, it also has the characteristics of frequency-dependent transmission (Box 10.1). The sporocyst–snail and metacercaria–stonefly pairs are more likely to fit models that assume nonlinear transmission and that exhibit more complex behaviors including unstable host–parasite equilibrium points, multiple stable equilibrium points, lack of host thresholds in some cases, and limit cycles (May and Anderson 1979; Gabriel *et al*. 1981; Getz and Pickering 1983; Liu *et al.* 1986; Hochberg 1991; Briggs and Godfray 1995; Dwyer *et al.* 1997; McCallum *et al.* 2001).

The sensitivity of models to transmission functions has implications for maintenance, epidemics, and invasion of disease and parasitism. Since transmission is a function of the densities of susceptible hosts and infected hosts or parasite stages, anthropogenic disturbances that alter the availability of either host or parasite will inevitably affect transmission. That is certainly the case here. Transmission dynamics can be teased apart through careful experiments to test for shifts in the functional form of transmission due to changes in the donor (infected) and target (susceptible) host species and to determine how to model these parasite dynamics to predict the effects of different disturbance levels on parasite population dynamics (Box 10.2).

Box 10.2 *In-situ* **manipulations of host and parasite density to test responses of transmission to disturbance**

Because the success of parasites hinges on transmission from one host to the next, disturbance-induced changes in density of infected or susceptible hosts are likely to significantly affect the rate or functional response of transmission (May 1977; May and Anderson 1979; Schwartz 1985; Hochberg 1991; Woolhouse *et al.* 1991; Anderson and May 1992; Gubbins and Gilligan 1997; Hudson and Dobson 1997). The direction and strength of these effects will depend on characteristics of the particular host–parasite association. Transmission between hosts can be accomplished by free-living stages of the parasite, consumption of parasite eggs or cysts by susceptible hosts, or through consumption of infected prey by susceptible hosts. Thus one parasite with at least three hosts could employ each mode of transmission during its life cycle. The parasite species, *C. dicamptodoni*, which I discuss in this chapter, is a good example of this. Elucidating the form of transmission is essential for building models of parasite–host dynamics and for predicting at which life-history stage and in which direction will parasites respond to disturbances.

Transmission of parasites by a free-living stage combines the processes of reproduction in and dispersal away from the infected or "donor" host, and location of and recruitment into the subsequent or "target" host. Changes in density of the donor host could thus alter reproduction of parasite recruits, whereas changes in the density of target hosts could affect the probability of locating and recruiting to a host. Parasites that transmit through predator–prey interactions will also respond to altered host densities if the trophic functional response is altered as a result of disturbance (see Box 10.1).

McCallum (2000) and McCallum *et al.* (2001) provide short reviews of empirical and analytical methods to estimate parasite transmission rates and force of infection. The following methods specifically refer to field experiments that test for the effects of disturbance on the functional form of transmission in macroparasites. The form of transmission can be measured empirically by simultaneously manipulating donor (reproduction) and target (recruitment) host densities in a fully factorial, replicated experiment (Fig. 10.4). Host densities should span the range of densities found in all sites across the disturbance gradient. Experiments should

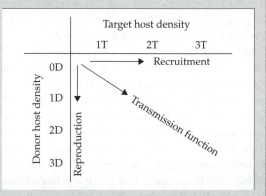

Figure 10.4 Factorial design for experimental estimation of the transmission function as it is affected by disturbance-induced changes in host densities. The response variable is parasite density in target hosts. Densities of donor (D) and target (T) hosts are selected to span the range of host densities found across the disturbance gradient. This diagram shows three densities of target hosts and four densities of donor hosts. The 0 donor host treatment is included to control for background levels of parasite reproduction in the environment. Density gradients in donor hosts with target host density held constant test for density-dependence in parasite reproduction. Density gradients in target hosts with donor host density held constant test for density dependence in parasite recruitment. The form of transmission can be estimated when donor and target host densities are manipulated simultaneously to determine the final parasite density in target hosts.

continues

Box 10.2 *continued*

last just long enough for the parasites to recruit and mature, but not long enough for asexual reproduction to occur, if present in the parasite species. Host age or size should be standardized as appropriate. The response variable is the density of parasites that successfully recruit into the target hosts. Density of infective parasite stages can be assessed from dissections of donor hosts at the end of the experiments. While holding target host density constant, regressions of the response variable on infective parasite density provides an estimate of parasite transmission that is dependent on reproduction. While holding donor host density constant, regressions of the response variable on target host density provides an estimate of parasite transmission that is dependent on recruitment. Simultaneous analysis of the response variable across densities of infective parasites and target hosts provides a three-dimensional functional response plane for transmission across varying target and host densities. To date, I am aware of only one study that has accomplished this for all transmission stages of a single macroparasite in the field (Poteet 2001).

Experimental tests of the response of parasite transmission to changes in host density are more straightforward for parasites of small, nonmigratory hosts such as those reported in this chapter (closed system). They become more difficult for parasites that infect large, migratory, or highly mobile species such as large mammals, salmon, or birds (open system). It is feasible to cage small hosts by scaling the cage size to the organism and maintaining a gradient in natural host densities while also taking care not to alter dispersal or behavior of parasite stages or hosts (e.g. in aquatic systems, measure flow through the cage to test for changes in flow velocity). For "open" systems, the density of highly mobile donor hosts can be manipulated by placing an "attractant" within the research area. The attractant

could be, for example, a scent, recorded call, food, or enhanced refugia (e.g. bird houses). For these types of manipulations, estimates of donor host density could be quite difficult and would have to be developed for each species. In addition, instead of measuring density of infectives within the donor host, it is more likely that density of infectives would be measured as number of "transmitting" parasites (e.g. through counts of eggs in feces, or number of cercariae in the environment if possible).

Robust interpretation of the data in these experiments depends on researcher acknowledgment of underlying assumptions. Assumptions inherent in these experiments include:

1. Increased donor host density correlates significantly and linearly with the number of recruits produced. This might not be the case for territorial or aggressive host species whose behavior changes at higher host densities.
2. Target hosts have equal susceptibility to hosts naturally infected in the wild. If uninfected hosts are collected from wild populations, then there could be bias toward collecting hosts that are predisposed to repel infections (see McCallum 2000 for discussion). This could underestimate transmission, but if hosts are well-mixed across replicates, it is unlikely to alter the functional form of transmission.
3. Behavior of hosts or parasites does not change with caging.
4. No parasite deaths occur in the donor host for the duration of the experiments. If deaths occur, then calculations of transmission could increase estimates of transmission per infective parasite. To solve this problem, estimate the deaths of infective parasites by subsampling parasites from a representative sample of donor hosts before and after the experiments.

In addition to the apparent nonlinearities in transmission, the relative roles of abiotic and biotic variables in this parasite–host system were disturbance-dependent. Explanatory variables for sporocyst densities switched from a positive correlation with snail densities, stream velocity, and width/depth ratio in unlogged streams (Fig. 10.5(a)) to a negative correlation with velocity and width/depth ratio (Fig. 10.5(b)). Transmission of free-living aquatic trematodes increases with

velocity up to a maximum threshold. Beyond this threshold, stream velocity can result in damage to and decreased transmission success of parasite infective stages (Upatham 1974; Jewsbury 1985). Logging disturbance increased the proportion of riffle and run habitats which led to higher average stream velocities. In streams with high pool/riffle ratios and low average velocity, parasite transmission was enhanced by snail densities and stream velocity. However, in streams with low pool/riffle

(a) Unlogged   (b) Logged

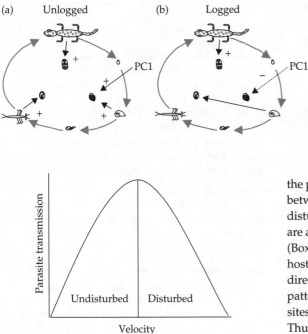

Figure 10.5 Diagram that depicts ANCOVA results of effects of disturbance on the relationship between parasite stages and the biotic and abiotic variables associated with logging. Abiotic and biotic variables that explain the majority of variation in each parasite stage differ between (a) unlogged and (b) logged sites. Gray lines show the direction of parasite transmission. Solid lines represent positive correlations. Dashed lines represent negative correlations. PC1 = principal component 1 and is composed of stream velocity and the stream width/depth ratio.

Figure 10.6 Conceptual diagram relating parasite transmission to stream velocity in undisturbed and disturbed sites.

ratios and high average stream velocity, parasite transmission was harmed by increasing stream velocity (Fig. 10.6).

As with sporocyst parasites, the explanatory variables for metacercariae switched with disturbance. In undisturbed streams metacercarial density was positively correlated with stonefly hosts (Fig. 10.5(a)), but disturbance switched the explanatory variable to snail host density (Fig. 10.5(b)). Stonefly density was high in streams that experienced the most severe disturbance and mass-action models suggest that metacercarial recruitment would respond positively to this increase. However, in SD streams snail density was at its lowest and thus snails limited the recruitment of cercariae to stoneflies and led to low metacercarial density.

The dynamics of this parasite–host system are clearly context-dependent. Parasite abundance and transmission depend on the level of disturbance and its effects on host density, stream velocity, and channel morphology. In undisturbed sites, the mass-action transmission model seems to apply. This suggests a threshold host density below which

the parasite cannot persist, and a stable equilibrium between the parasite and host species. However, in disturbed sites, this model does not apply. Parasites are able to persist and transmit at low host densities (Box 10.1) and correlations among parasite stages, host densities, and abiotic variables shift in direction and strength with disturbance. The patterns and correlations in the data from these sites suggest some form of nonlinear transmission. Thus, this parasite–host system may shift from one transmission function to another based on the disturbance regime.

10.6 Conclusion

In addition to affecting the patterns of infection in each host, logging-induced disturbance changed the relationships between the parasite stages, host densities, and environmental features in the streams. Patterns in parasite infections differed with severity of disturbance and parasite stage and these differences were explained in part by transmission, host densities, and abiotic variables. But biological interactions apart from those between a parasite and its hosts are very likely to influence the response of parasites to disturbance. Each of these hosts is linked by a single parasite, but each host also interacts within the stream community through competition, predation, or herbivory. Changes in stream community composition following disturbance lead to altered relative abundance of each host species within the stream community. This in turn feeds back into changes in trophic and competitive interactions which could affect transmission of the parasite. For parasites with multiple life-history stages, complex community-level effects on parasite–host dynamics could obscure the results of parasite population studies that consider only a single host and parasite stage. Thus, empirical examination of community-level influences on a parasite and its multiple hosts could help tease apart the mechanisms that drive complex parasite–host interactions.

An example of one scenario where community processes could affect parasite transmission is in streams that experienced logging and debris flows such that snail populations were decimated to the point of local extinction. Because snails are competitively dominant grazers, the decline in snail populations may release macroinvertebrate grazers from competition. Since many of these macroinvertebrates are eaten by stoneflies, this competitive release could increase the prey available to *C. californica*, the second intermediate stonefly host of the parasite. Stonefly densities increased significantly in creeks with severe disturbances; this suggests that the mechanism of competitive release of macroinvertebrates could be occurring. It is probably the high density of stoneflies that increases the probability that the cercariae, which are at low densities in areas with severe disturbance, will find a host. Thus, this cascading trophic effect from algae to stoneflies could ultimately influence the probability of parasite transmission.

Acknowledgments

S. Collinge and C. Ray provided helpful comments on this manuscript. I thank W. Sousa, M. Power, E. Hadly, V. Resh, and C. Bell for their discussions and support while conducting this study. Weyerhaeuser Industries and E. Arnett provided generous and unlimited access to private timberlands in the McKenzie and Fall creek watersheds, Oregon. The McKenzie Ranger District provided access to public lands and logistical support. Many thanks to D. Anderson, C. Nerney, R. Wildman, S. Gregory, and the Andersons for their help and support during field work and D. Sanver, K. Rothwangl, and A. Talianchich for laboratory work. The H. J. Andrews Experimental Forest and LTER in Blue River, Oregon and the Brackenridge Field Laboratory in Austin, TX generously provided laboratory space. This research was supported by NSF dissertation grant DEB-9701128, the ARCS foundation, Inc., and the H. J. Andrews LTER.

References

Anderson, R. M. and R. M. May. (1978). Regulation and stability of host–parasite interactions. I. Regulatory processes. *Journal of Animal Ecology* **47**:219–247.

Anderson, R. M. and R. M. May. (1979). Population biology of infectious diseases: Part I. *Nature* **280**:361–367.

Anderson, R. M. and R. M. May. (1992). *Infectious Diseases of Humans: Dynamics and Control*. Oxford Science Publications, Oxford University Press, New York, 757 pp.

Anderson, R. M., J. G. Mercer, R. A. Wilson, and N. P. Carter. (1982). Transmission of *Schistosoma mansoni* from man to snail: experimental studies of miracidial survival and infectivity in relation to larval age, water temperature, host size and host age. *Parasitology* **85**:339–360.

Ash, L. R. and R. C. Orihel. (1991). *Parasites: A Guide to Laboratory Procedures and Identification*. ASCP Press, Chicago, IL.

Beschta, R. L., R. E. Bilby, G. W. Brown, L. B. Holtby, and T. D. Hofstra. (1987). Stream temperature and aquatic habitat: fisheries and forestry interactions. In E.O. Salo and T. W. Cundy, eds. *Streamside Management: Forestry and Fishery Interactions*, pp. 191–232. Forestry Resources Contribution no. 57, University of Washington, Seattle, WA.

Bisson, P. A., R. E. Bilby, M. D. Bryant, C. D. Andrew, G. B. Grette, R. A. House, *et al.* (1987). Large woody debris in forested streams in the Pacific Northwest: past, present and future. In E. O. Salo and T. W. Cundy, eds. *Streamside Management: Forestry and Fishery Interactions*, pp. 143–190. Forestry Resources Contribution no. 57, University of Washington, Seattle, WA.

Bovee, K. D. (1982). A guide to stream habitat analysis using the Instream Flow Incremental Methodology. Instream Flow information Paper 12, FWS/OBS-82/86, Co-operative Instream Flow Group, US Fish and Wildlife Service, Office of Biological Services.

Briggs, C. J. and H. C. J. Godfray. (1995). The dynamics of insect–pathogen interactions in stage-structured populations. *American Naturalist* **145**:855–887.

Burch, J. B. (1982). Freshwater snails (Mollusca: Gastropoda) of North America. US Environmental Protection Agency Publication. EPA-600/3-82-026.

Bush, A. O., K. D. Lafferty, J. M. Lotz, and A. W. Shostak. (1997). Parasitology meets ecology on its own terms: Margolis *et al.* revisited. *Journal of Parasitology* **83**:575–583.

Chernin, E. and J. M. Perlstein. (1969). Further studies on interference with the host-finding capacity of *Schistosoma mansoni* miracidia. *Journal of Parasitology* **55**:500–508.

Corn, P. S. and R. B. Bury. (1989). Logging in western Oregon: responses of headwater habitats and stream amphibians. *Forest Ecology and Management* **29**:39–57.

Crofton, H. D. (1971). A model of host–parasite relationships. *Parasitology* **63**:343–364.

Daszak, P., A. A. Cunningham, and A. D. Hyatt. (2000). Emerging infectious diseases of wildlife—threats to biodiversity and human health. *Science* **287**:443–449.

Dobson, A. P. and R. Carper. (1992). Global warming and potential changes in host–parasite and disease–vector relationships. In R. L. Peters and T. E. Lovejoy, eds. *Global Warming and Biological Diversity*, pp. 201–217. Yale University Press, New Haven, CT.

Dunne, T. and L. B. Leopold. (1978). *Water in Environmental Planning*. W.H. Freeman & Co., San Francisco, CA.

Dwyer, G., J. S. Elkinton, and J. P. Buonaccorsi. (1997). Host heterogeneity in susceptibility and disease dynamics: tests of a mathematical model. *American Naturalist* **150**:685–707.

Evans, N. A. (1985). The influence of environmental temperature upon the transmission of *Echinostoma liei* (Digenea: Echinostomatidae). *Parasitology* **90**:269–275.

Everest, F. H., R. L. Beschta, J. C. Scrivener, K. V. Koski, J. R. Sedell, and C. J. Cederholm. (1987). Fine sediment and salmonid production: a paradox. In E. O. Salo and T. W. Cundy, eds. *Streamside Management: Forestry and Fishery Interactions*, pp. 98–142. Forestry Resources Contribution no. 57, University of Washington, Seattle, WA.

Furnival, G. M. and Wilson, R. W. Jr. (1974). Regressions by Leaps and Bounds. *Technometrics* **16**:499–511.

Gabriel, J. P., H. Hanisch, and W. M. Hirsch. (1981). Dynamic equilibria of helminthic infections? In D. G. Chapman and V. F. Gallucci, eds. *Quantitative Population Dynamics*, pp. 83–104. Statistical Ecology Series, vol. 13. International Co-operative Publishing House, Fairland, MD.

Getz, W.M. and J. Pickering. (1983). Epidemic models: thresholds and population regulation. *American Naturalist* **121**:892–898.

Gordon, N. D., T. A. McMahon, and B. L. Finlayson. (1992). Stream hydrology: an introduction for ecologists. John Wiley & Sons, New York.

Gregory, S. V. (1980). Effects of light, nutrients, and grazing on periphyton communities in streams. Ph.D. dissertation. Oregon State University, Corvallis, Oregon, USA.

Gubbins, S. and C. A. Gilligan. (1997). Persistence of host–parasite interactions in a disturbed environment. *Journal of Theoretical Biology* **188**:241–258.

Hair, J. F., Jr., R. E. Anderson, and R.L. Tatham. (1987). *Multivariate Data Analysis with Readings*, 2nd edition, Macmillan, New York.

Harvell, C. D., K. K. Kim, J. M. Burkholder, R. R. Colwell, P. R. Epstein, D. J. Grimes, *et al.* (1999). Emerging marine diseases—climate links and anthropogenic factors. *Science* **285**:1505–1510.

Hawkins, C. P. and J. K. Furnish. (1987). Are snails important competitors in stream ecosystems? *Oikos* **49**:209–220.

Hawkins, C. P., M. L. Murphy, and N. H. Anderson. (1982). Effects of canopy, substrate composition, and gradient on the structure of macroinvertebrate communities in Cascade Range streams of Oregon. *Ecology* **63**: 1840–1856.

Hawkins, C. P., M. L. Murphy, N. H. Anderson, and M. A. Wilzbach. (1983). Density of fish and salamanders in relation to riparian canopy and physical habitat in streams of the Northwestern United States. *Canadian Journal of Fisheries and Aquatic Sciences* **40**:1173–1185.

Hedrick, R. P., M. El-Matbouli, M. A. Adkison, and E. MaConnell. (1998). Whirling disease: re-emergence among wild trout. *Immunological Reviews* **166**:365–376.

Hill, W. R. and B. C. Harvey. (1990). Periphyton responses to higher trophic levels and light in a shaded stream. *Canadian Journal of Fisheries and Aquatic Sciences* **47**:2307–2314.

Hill, W. R., M. G. Ryon, and E. M. Schilling. (1995). Light limitation in a stream ecosystem—responses by primary producers and consumers. *Ecology* **76**: 1297–1309.

Hobbs, R. J. and H. A. Mooney. (1991). Effects of rainfall variability and gopher disturbance on serpentine annual grassland dynamics. *Ecology* **72**:59–68.

Hochberg, M. E. (1991). Non-linear transmission rates and the dynamics of infectious disease. *Journal of Theoretical Biology* **153**:301–321.

Holmes, J. C. (1982). Impact of infectious disease agents on the population growth and geographical distribution of animals. In R. M. Anderson and R. M. May, eds. *Population Biology of Infectious Diseases*, pp. 37–51. Dahlem Konferenzen, Springer-Verlag, Berlin.

Hudson, P. J. and A. P. Dobson. (1997). Transmission dynamics and host–parasite interactions of *Trichostrongylus tenuis* in Red Grouse (*Lagopus lagopus scoticus*). *Journal of Parasitology* **83**:194–202.

Hudson, P. J., A. P. Dobson, and D. Newborn. (1998). Prevention of population cycles by parasite removal. *Science* **282**:2256–2258.

Jacobson, E. R., J. M. Gaskin, M. B. Brown, R. K. Harris, C. H. Gardiner, J. L. LaPointe, *et al.* (1991). Chronic upper respiratory tract disease of free-ranging desert tortoises (*Xerobates agassizii*). *Journal of Wildlife Diseases* **27**:296–316.

Jewsbury, J. M. (1985). Effects of water velocity on snails and cercariae. *Parasitology Today* **1**:116–117.

Johnson, P. T. J. and J. M. Chase. (2004). Parasites in the food web: linking amphibian malformations and aquatic eutrophication. *Ecology Letters* **7**:521–526.

Jones, J. A. and G. E. Grant. (1996). Peak flow responses to clear-cutting and roads in small and large basins, western Cascades, Oregon. *Water Resources Research* **32**:959–974.

Lafferty, K. D. (1997). Environmental parasitology: what can parasites tell us about human impacts on the environment? *Parasitology Today* **13**:251–255.

Lafferty, K. D. and R. D. Holt. (2003). How should environmental stress affect the population dynamics of disease? *Ecology Letters* **6**:654–664.

Leopold, L. B., M. G. Wolman, and J. P. Miller. (1964). Fluvial processes in geomorphology. W. H. Freeman & Co., San Francisco, CA.

Levin, S. A. and R. T. Paine. (1974). Disturbance, patch formation, and community structure. *Proceedings of the National Academy of Sciences* **71**:2744–2747.

Liu, W.-M., S. A. Levin, and Y. Iwasa. (1986). Influence of nonlinear incidence rates upon the behavior of SIRS epidemiological models. *Journal of Mathematical Biology* **23**:187–204.

LoGiudice, K., R. S. Ostfeld, K. A. Schmidt, and F. Keesing. (2003). The ecology of infectious disease: effects of host diversity and community composition on Lyme disease risk. *Proceedings of the National Academy of Sciences* **100**:567–571.

Marín, S. L., W. E. Grant, and N. O. Dronen. (1998). Simulation of population dynamics of the parasite *Haematoloechus coloradensis* in its three host species: effects of environmental temperature and precipitation. *Ecological Modeling* **105**:185–211.

May, R. M. (1977). Dynamical aspects of host–parasite associations: Crofton's model revisited. *Parasitology* **75**:259–276.

May, R. M. and R. M. Anderson. (1979). Population biology of infectious diseases: Part II. *Nature* **280**: 455–461.

McCallum, H. (2000). Population parameters: estimation for ecological models. Blackwell Science Ltd., Oxford, UK.

McCallum, H., N. Barlow, and J. Hone. (2001). How should pathogen transmission be modeled? *Trends in Ecology and Evolution* **16**:295–300.

McGarigal, K., S. Cushman, and S. Stafford. (2000). *Multivariate Statistics for Wildlife and Ecology Research*. Springer-Verlag, New York.

McKindsey, C. W. and J. D. McLaughlin. (1994). Transmission of *Cycloceolum mutabile* (Digenea) to

snails: the influence of temperature on the egg and miracidium. *Canadian Journal of Zoology* **72**: 1745–1751.

McSweegan, E. (1996). The infectious diseases impact statement: a mechanism for addressing emerging diseases. *Emerging Infectious Diseases* **2**:103–108.

Murphy, M. L. and J. D. Hall. (1981). Varied effects of clear-cut logging on predators and their habitat in small streams of the Cascade Mountains, Oregon. *Canadian Journal of Fisheries and Aquatic Sciences* **38**: 137–145.

Nussbaum, R. A. and G. W. Clothier. (1973). Population structure, growth, and size of larval *Dicamptodon ensatus* (Eschscholtz). *Northwest Science* **47**:218–227.

Parker, M. S. (1992). Feeding ecology of larvae of the Pacific giant salamander (*Dicamptodon tenebrosus*) and their role as top predator in a headwater stream benthic community. Ph.D. dissertation University of California at Davis, Davis, CA, 131pp.

Parker, M. S. (1994). Feeding ecology of stream-dwelling Pacific giant salamander larvae (*Dicamptodon tenebrosus*). *Copeia* **1994**:705–718.

Peckarsky, B. L. (1984). Predator–prey interactions among aquatic insects. In V. H. Resh and D. M. Rosenberg, eds. *The Ecology of Aquatic Insects*, pp. 196–254. Praeger Publishers, New York.

Pickett, S. T. A. and P. S. White, eds. (1985). *The Ecology of Natural Disturbance and Patch Dynamics*. Academic Press, Orlando, FL.

Poteet, M. F. (2001). Effects of disturbance on host–parasite interactions: a case study involving the Pacific giant salamander. Ph.D. thesis, University of California at Berkeley, Berkeley, CA, 209pp.

Power, M. E. (1992). Top-down and bottom-up forces in food webs: do plants have primacy? *Ecology* **73**:733–746.

Sapp, K. K. and G. E. Esch. (1994). The effects of spatial and temporal heterogeneity as structuring forces for parasite communities in *Helisoma anceps* and *Physa gyrina*. *American Midland Naturalist* **132**:91–103.

Schell, S. C. (1985). Handbook of trematodes of North America north of Mexico. University Press of Idaho, Moscow, Idaho.

Schmitt, R. J. and C. W. Osenberg, eds. (1996). Detecting ecological impacts: concepts and applications in coastal habitats. Academic Press, San Diego, CA.

Schrag, S. J. and P. Wiener. (1995). Emerging infectious disease: what are the relative roles of ecology and evolution? *Trends in Ecology and Evolution* **10**:319–324.

Schwartz, I. B. (1985). Multiple recurrent outbreaks and predictability in seasonally forced non-linear epidemic models. *Journal of Mathematical Biology* **12**:347–361.

Scott, M. E. (1988). The impact of infection and disease on animal populations: implications for conservation biology. *Conservation Biology* 2:40–56.

Scott, M. E. and A. Dobson. (1989). The role of parasites in the regulation of host abundance. *Parasitology Today* 5:176–183.

Selvin, S. (1998). *Modern Applied Biostatistical Methods Using S-Plus*. Monographs in epidemiology and biostatistics, vol. 28. Oxford University Press, New York.

Senger, C. W. and R. W. Macy. (1953). A new digenetic trematode (*Cephalouterina dicamptodoni* n.g., n.sp., Pleurogenetinae) from the Pacific giant salamander. *Journal of Parasitology* 39:352–355.

Sheldon, A. L. (1969). Size relationships of *Acroneuria californica* (Perlidae, Plecoptera) and its prey. *Hydrobiologia* 34:85–94.

Shostak, A. W. and G. W. Esch. (1990). Temperature effects on survival and excystment of cercariae of *Halipegus occidualis* (Trematoda). *International Journal of Parasitology* 20:95–99.

Sousa, W. P. (1979). Experimental investigations of disturbance and ecological succession in a rocky intertidal algal community. *Ecological Monographs* 49:227–254.

Sousa, W. P. (1984). The role of disturbance in natural communities. *Annual Review of Ecology and Systematics* 15:353–391.

Sousa, W. P. (2001). Natural disturbance and the dynamics of marine benthic communities. In M. D. Bertness, S. D. Gaines, and M. E. Hay, eds. *Marine Community Ecology*, pp. 85–130. Sinauer Associates, Sunderland, MA.

Sousa, W. P. and E. D. Grosholz. (1991). The influence of habitat structure on the transmission of parasites. In S. S. Bell, E. D. McCoy, and H. R. Mushinsky, eds. *Habitat Structure: The Physical Arrangement of Objects in Space*, pp. 301–324. Chapman and Hall, New York.

Spielman, A. (1994). The emergence of Lyme disease and human Babesiosis in a changing environment. In M. E. Wilson, R. Levins, and A. Spielman, eds. *Disease in Evolution: Global Changes and Emergence of Infectious Diseases*, pp. 146–156. Annals of the New York Academy of Sciences, vol. 740. New York Academy of Sciences, New York.

S-Plus 2000. (1999). Data analysis products division, Mathsoft, Inc. Seattle, WA.

Stauffer, J. R., M. E. Arnegard, M. Cetron, J. J. Sullivan, L. A. Chitsulo, G. F. Turner, *et al.* (1997). Controlling vectors and hosts of parasitic diseases using fishes. *Bioscience* 47:41–49.

Stewart, K. W. and B. P. Stark. (1993). Nymphs of North American stonefly genera (Plecoptera). University of North Texas Press, Denton, TX.

Thorne, E. R. and E.S. Williams. (1988). Disease and endangered species: the black-footed ferret as a recent example. *Conservation Biology* 2:66–74.

Thrall, P. H., A. Biere, and M. K. Uyenoyama. (1995). Frequency-dependent disease transmission and the dynamics of the *Silene-Ustilago* host–pathogen system. *American Naturalist* 145:43–62.

Upatham, E. S. (1974). Dispersion of St. Lucian *Schistosoma mansoni* cercariae in natural standing and running waters determined by cercaria counts and mouse exposure. *Annals of Tropical Medicine and Parasitology* 68:343–352.

Van Riper III, C., S. G. Van Riper, M. L. Goff, and M. Laird. (1986). The epizootiology and ecological significance of malaria in Hawaiian land birds. *Ecological Monographs* 56:327–344.

Wasserberg, G., Z. Abramsky, B. P. Kotler, R. S. Ostfeld, I. Yarom, and A. Warburg. (2003). Anthropogenic disturbances enhance occurrence of cutaneous Leishmaniasis in Israel deserts: patterns and mechanisms. *Ecological Applications* 13:868–881.

Woolhouse, M. E. J. and S. K. Chandiwana. (1989). Spatial and temporal heterogeneity in the population dynamics of *Bulinus globosus* and *Biomphalaria pfeifferi* and in the epidemiology of their infection with schistosomes. *Parasitology* 98:21–34.

Woolhouse, M. E. J., C. H. Watts, and S. K. Chandiwana. (1991). Heterogeneities in transmission rates and the epidemiology of schistosome infection. *Proceedings of the Royal Society of London B* 245:109–114.

CHAPTER 11

Urbanization and disease in amphibians

David K. Skelly, Susan R. Bolden, Manja P. Holland, L. Kealoha Freidenburg, Nicole A. Freidenfelds, and Trent R. Malcolm

11.1 Background

Growth of the human population and accelerating urbanization are leading to unprecedented rates of landscape alteration (McKinney 2002). As this transformation continues, urban regions are becoming a significant component of the landscape, now roughly equivalent to the area characterized as wilderness in the United States (United Nations 2001). Because urbanized areas are growing, and because associated landscape changes are likely to be persistent, it is critical to understand biotic responses to urbanization. Among the possible consequences, impacts on infectious disease are of particular concern.

The influence of urbanization on infectious disease has been a subject of concern for at least the past decade (Morse 1993, 1995; Schrag and Wiener 1995; Gratz 1999). Spurred by reports of increasing infectious disease in humans, epidemiologists have hypothesized that anthropogenic influences on the environment can lead to the emergence or resurgence of infectious disease. Subsequent consideration of wildlife host species has revealed similar phenomena (Daszak *et al.* 2001; Epstein *et al.* 2003; Johnson *et al.* 2003; Williams *et al.* 2003). Disease can emerge in urban contexts because human alterations to ecosystems may foster increased rates of transmission (Williams *et al.* 2003), or decreased resistance to infection (Gendron *et al.* 2003). In addition, increased movement of people, livestock, and freight can lead to "pathogen pollution," when parasites and pathogens are unintentionally transited from one part of the globe to another (Berger *et al.* 1998).

Community ecologists and conservation biologists have considered the effects of urbanization as well. Although parasites and pathogens are not usually an explicit focus, consistent generalizations are evident in this literature. Urbanization causes loss of habitat and, consequently, may lead to species extinctions (Thompson and Jones 1999; McKinney 2002; Turner *et al.* 2004). Because species are often dependent on one another, initial species losses may propagate further extinctions (Ebenman *et al.* 2004). Through these means, and also because urbanization can alter fluxes of nutrients within ecosystems (e.g. Paul and Meyer 2001), impoverishment of biodiversity is expected to be a signature of urbanization (Turner *et al.* 2004). In support of these and similar claims, many studies have found that urbanized areas tend to be biologically depauperate (Richter and Azous 1995, Gibbs 1998, Thompson and Jones 1999, Marzluff 2001). Other studies have noted that extinctions associated with urbanization are not random. As an example, specialized species (such as host-specific parasites) are expected to be particularly vulnerable (Aizen *et al.* 2002).

These contrasting perspectives on the effects of urbanization prompted us to review studies estimating the association between urbanization and macroparasite infection. Three important patterns emerge from this review (Table 11.1). First, the total number of studies is small. Second, most studies have focused on human hosts. Third, and most critical here, is that there is no consistent association between urbanization and macroparasite infection. Both increases and decreases in infection responses

Table 11.1 Published studies examining the effects of urbanization-associated gradients on macroparasite infection responses (prevalence or intensity)

Macroparasite	Host	Urbanization gradient	Infection response +	0	−	Reference
Wildlife Studies						
Cestoda						
Dipylidium caninum	*Vulpes vulpes*	Human density	X			Richards *et al.* 1995
Echinococcus multilocularis	*V. vulpes*	Human density			X	Hofer *et al.* 2000
Taenia hydatigena	*V. vulpes*	Human density		X		Richards *et al.* 1995
Taenia pisiformis	*V. vulpes*	Human density			X	Richards *et al.* 1995
Nematoda						
Toxocara canis	*Canis familiaris*	Human density			X	Habluetzel *et al.* 2003
T. canis	*V. vulpes*	Human density		X		Hofer *et al.* 2000
Toxocaris leonina	*V. vulpes*	Human density		X		Richards *et al.* 1995
Uncinaria stenocephala	*V. vulpes*	Human density		X		Hofer *et al.* 2000
Nematomorpha						
Gordiidae	*Physa gyrina*	Human density		X		Hanelt *et al.* 2001
Trematoda						
Brachylaima recurva	*V. vulpes*	Human density	X			Richards *et al.* 1995
Cryptocotyle lingua	*Littorina saxatilis*	Land use intensity	X			Bustnes and Galaktionov 1999
C. lingua	*V. vulpes*	Human density	X			Richards *et al.* 1995
Microphallus piriformes	*L. saxatilis*	Land use Intensity	X			Bustnes and Galaktionov 1999
M. piriformes	*L. obtusata*	Land use Intensity		X		Bustnes and Galaktionov 1999
M. similis	*L. saxatilis*	Land use Intensity	X			Bustnes and Galaktionov 1999
M. similes	*L. obtusata*	Land use Intensity	X			Bustnes and Galaktionov 1999
M. pygmaeus	*L. saxatilis*	Land use Intensity		X		Bustnes and Galaktionov 1999
M. pygmaeus	*L. obtusata*	Land use Intensity		X		Bustnes and Galaktionov 1999
Ribeiroia ondatrae	*Hyla regilla*	Eutrophication	X			Johnson and Chase 2004
Human studies						
Cestoda						
Hymenolepis nana	*Homo sapiens*	Human density	X			Mason and Patterson 1994
Nematoda						
Ascaris lumbricoides	*H. sapiens*	Human density	X			Nyan *et al.* 2001
A. lumbricoides	*H. sapiens*	Human density			X	Azazy and Al-Tiar 1999
A. lumbricoides	*H. sapiens*	Human density			X	Dagoye *et al.* 2003
A. lumbricoides	*H. sapiens*	Human density			X	Roche and Benito 1999
A. lumbricoides	*H. sapiens*	Human density	X			Carneri *et al.* 1992
A. lumbricoides	*H. sapiens*	Human density	X			Phiri *et al.* 2000
A. lumbricoides	*H. sapiens*	Human density			X	Mngomezulu *et al.* 2002
Necator americanus	*H. sapiens*	Human density			X	Dagoye *et al.* 2003
N. americanus	*H. sapiens*	Human density	X			Nyan *et al.* 2001
Trichuris trichiura	*H. sapiens*	Human density	X			Dagoye *et al.* 2003
T. trichiura	*H. sapiens*	Human density	X			Roche and Benito 1999
T. trichiura	*H. sapiens*	Human density			X	Mngomezulu *et al.* 2002
Trematoda						
Schistosoma haematobium	*H. sapiens*	Human density			X	Mngomezulu *et al.* 2002
S. mansoni	*H. sapiens*	Human density			X	Mngomezulu *et al.* 2002
S. mansoni	*H. sapiens*	Human density			X	Amorin *et al.* 1997
S. mansoni	*H. sapiens*	Human density			X	Azazy and Al-Tiar 1999

Studies of human and wildlife hosts are listed separately. Responses are categorized as increasing (+), unchanged (0), or decreasing (−) with increasing urbanization. Studies were uncovered using a keyword search in ISI Web of Science (urban* and parasit*). The search was completed on October 18, 2004 and included articles published since 1970. Infection responses denoted as + or − were reported as statistically significant associations in the original papers.

have been reported with roughly equal frequency, and many studies report no response to urbanization. Of equal interest, predominant patterns appear to differ between human and wildlife hosts. Outcomes in human studies are divided between increased and decreased infection with urbanization; no studies in Table 11.1 reported a lack of response. By contrast, increasing infection and no response to urbanization are the predominant patterns among wildlife. There are just three studies showing declines in infection with urbanization. Taken together, these studies show that we can expect a diversity of responses to urbanization, and that wildlife hosts may reveal different patterns than human hosts.

Based on our review (Table 11.1), it appears that the emphasis by epidemiologists on urbanization-mediated disease emergence does not reflect the entire pattern of responses observed in prior studies. It is equally clear that the perspective adopted by ecologists and conservation biologists on biodiversity loss with urbanization does not adequately capture responses by macroparasites. We suggest that additional work is needed, particularly on nonhuman hosts and with a focus on factors that may suggest mechanisms for contingent responses to urbanization. With these issues in mind, our goal was to evaluate the effects of urbanization on macroparasite infection of amphibians.

Amphibians are noteworthy both because infectious disease has been implicated in worldwide declines and deformity outbreaks (Johnson *et al.* 1999), and because relatively few large-scale studies have examined macroparasite infection patterns in nature (see Johnson *et al.* 2002 for an exception). Patterns of infection across an urbanization gradient can be sorted into the following three categories, each suggesting an alternate hypothesis for prevalence or intensity of infection.

1. *Emerging Disease:* Because of inadvertent parasite movement and because urban environments may compromise host immune responses, we might expect infectious disease to become more common and infections to become more intense in urbanized environments. Even where focal host biology is not significantly influenced by urbanization, anthropogenic changes in the environment may lead to increases in intermediate host density and subsequent focal host infections. For example, control

of human infection by snail-borne trematodes in the genus *Schistosoma* requires snail reduction through water quality programs as well as molluscicide application (World Health Organization 1993, Brown 1994).

2. *Safe zone:* Because macroparasites may suffer from alteration of their environment, or decline due to the loss of host species, urbanization may lead to reductions in prevalence or infection intensity (Sprent 1992, Bush and Kennedy 1994). This "safe zone" hypothesis has been used to describe the protective effect on prey or host species that can survive in urbanized contexts where their predator or parasites are excluded (Gering and Blair 1999).

3. *No response:* The null expectation is that infection patterns will be unresponsive to urbanization. Many macroparasite taxa with complex life cycles are fairly generalized in their host requirements. Even if host species composition shifts with anthropogenic influences, these macroparasites may be able to persist by using different hosts, which themselves may be weedy species associated with urban contexts (Marzluff 2001). Parasites may also be somewhat insulated from the direct impacts of altered environments because much of their life is spent in host tissues that buffer environmental variation (Pietrock and Marcogliese 2003).

To evaluate competing hypotheses regarding the distribution and abundance of macroparasites in relation to urbanization, we focus on two parasite taxa, echinostomes and *Megalodiscus,* and two amphibian hosts, the green frog (*Rana clamitans*), and the spring peeper (*Pseudacris crucifer*). Both macroparasites are trematodes with complex life cycles in which one or more stages are resident within larval/metamorphic amphibians and at least one stage is dependent on freshwater snails (Box 11.1).

11.2 Methods

11.2.1 Study sites

We studied patterns of trematode infection in amphibians from 60 wetlands in northeastern Connecticut, USA (Fig. 11.2). Sampled wetlands represented a subset of those appearing on US Geological Survey National Wetland Inventory

Box 11.1 Community structure and the life cycle of echinostome trematodes

Adult echinostomes inhabit the intestines and bile ducts of a range of vertebrate hosts including aquatic birds, such as ducks (Fig. 11.1). Most echinostome species exhibit a lack of definitive host specificity (Huffman and Fried 1990; Kanev *et al.* 1995). Echinostome eggs are released when the infected definitive host defecates in the water, and develop into miracidia upon hatching. Miracidia swim through the water column and penetrate their first intermediate host, a freshwater snail of the genus *Planorbella*, *Helisoma*, or *Physa*. Host snails occupy a variety of habitats, ranging from small temporary ponds to more permanent larger ponds. Typically, each echinostome species is capable of infecting a small number of host snail species (Christensen *et al.* 1980; Fried *et al.* 1987; Huffman and Fried 1990). Upon penetration, miracidia transform into sporocysts and then rediae, often undergoing prodigious asexual reproduction. During the late spring or early summer, snails shed free-swimming cercariae. Cercariae can penetrate a broad range of second intermediate hosts, including snails, tadpoles, and fish (Beaver 1937; Anderson and Fried 1987, Huffman and Fried

1990, Martin and Conn 1990). Following penetration of the second intermediate host, cercariae migrate to the kidneys, where they encyst (Huffman and Fried 1990; Fried et al. 1997). The echinostome life cycle is completed when a definitive host such as a bird feeds on an infected second intermediate host. Echinostomes reproduce sexually in their definitive host.

In this study, we evaluate factors that may affect the prevalence and abundance of infection in larval amphibian hosts across an urbanization gradient. We evaluated the relationship between snail density and tadpole infection patterns. Several factors, including increased nutrient levels and light, may contribute to the observed elevated density of the host snails in urban areas. The densities of the first intermediate host snails may have strong effects on transmission of echinostomes to tadpoles. Finally, the absence of fish predators may result in increased survival of both snails and tadpoles, thereby indirectly benefiting the echinostome parasite and facilitating transmission to the definitive host. Figure modified from Haas *et al.* (1995).

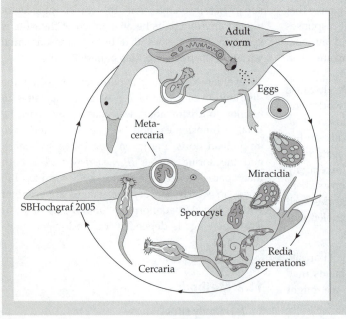

Figure 11.1 A trematode life cycle: echinostomes.

maps for three regions: the Yale-Myers Forest (undeveloped), the municipalities of Tolland (intermediate), and Manchester (urban). Yale-Myers Forest (38 km²) is undeveloped, subject to a low

level of disturbance from timber extraction (< 30 ha per year) and research activities related to forestry and ecology; there are no full-time human inhabitants within the boundary of the forest (shown on

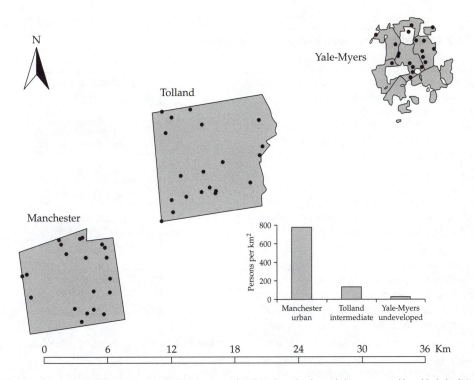

Figure 11.2 Map of study sites within three regions in NE Connecticut (USA). Each wetland sampled is represented by a black dot (20 per region). Manchester is an urban region, Tolland is intermediate, and the Yale-Myers Forest is undeveloped. A histogram shows the number of humans per square kilometer according to the 2000 US Census.

Fig. 11.2) and a low density of humans in the areas adjacent to Yale-Myers Forest. Tolland (104 km^2) is a town with a human density of 134 individuals km^{-2}. Manchester (70 km^2) is a city with a human density of 799 individuals km^{-2}. We selected, at random, an initial list of 20 wetlands from each region. Upon visiting the wetland for the first time it was retained for sampling if it contained any evidence of amphibian reproduction (chorusing, eggs, or larvae). Only those wetlands without amphibian activity were discarded from the sample and replaced with an additional wetland randomly selected from all of those within the region. In general, discarded wetlands were extremely small and often without standing water.

11.2.2 Wetland sampling

Each wetland was sampled during three periods in 2001: May, June, and "metamorphic" sampling periods. May and June sampling periods each lasted less than 2 weeks. During these periods, each wetland was visited once for "pipe" and dipnet sampling of snails and the aquatic stages of amphibians. Pipe samplers (Skelly 1996) were constructed of wide (36 cm diameter × 91 cm tall) aluminum ducting. Each pipe sampled 0.1 m^2 of the sediments and associated water column. Each sample was taken by quietly approaching an area and quickly thrusting the pipe through the water column and into the sediments to seal the sample area, leaving the top of the pipe above the water surface. With the pipe held in place, nets (22 × 27 cm^2; 1 × 2 mm^2 mesh size) were swept within the pipe to remove all amphibians from the sampled water column and the first few centimeters of the sediments. We collected a number of pipe samples scaled to the surface area of the wetland. In the smallest wetlands (< 300 m^2) we collected 10 pipe samples. In intermediate-sized wetlands we collected 20 (300–1000 m^2) or 30 (1000–1500 m^2) pipe samples. In all larger wetlands (> 1500 m^2) we collected 40 pipe samples. Each pipe sample was separated at least 2 m from the nearest

Box 11.2 Estimating trematode infection in amphibians

The primary goal of our study is to estimate infection patterns across an urbanization gradient. We were careful to use methods of study site selection and sample collection that ensured meaningful estimation of infection responses (Fig 11.3). We selected 60 wetlands at random based on National Wetlands Inventory Maps for three regions ranging from undeveloped to heavily urbanized.

In each wetland we collected up to 100 metamorphs (Gosner Stages 40–46) of our target amphibian host species. At some sites this was possible in only one visit due to the abundance of metamorphosing frogs, while other sites took several visits to reach our goal.

In the laboratory, host amphibians were randomly selected from specimen jars for parasite analysis. During dissection, the entire alimentary canal and both kidneys were removed. The organs were systematically teased apart and searched for parasites under a dissecting microscope, removed, and vialed by taxon.

Preliminary identification based on host-tissue origin and morphology (e.g. Prudhoe and Bray 1982; Schell 1985) was used to place recovered parasites in morphotaxonomic categories. Vouchers of each morphotaxon were sent to a trematode specialist for verification using molecular methods.

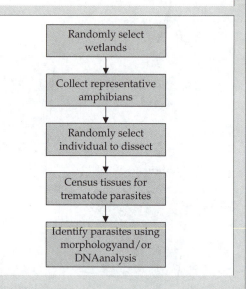

Figure 11.3 Methods for quantifying trematode infection in amphibians.

---

sample and we included representative habitat types in the sampling.

During May and June, we also dipnetted each wetland for a duration matching person-minutes of effort to the number of pipe samples collected (dipnet dimensions: 25×18 cm²). For example, we dipnetted for 20 person-minutes in wetlands where we collected 20 pipe samples. Individuals collected during dipnetting were preserved separately (in 70% ethanol) from those collected in pipe samples. If, at the end of the dipnetting period, we had recovered small numbers of the focal amphibian species (< 20 individuals), we spent additional time dipnetting and kept these targeted samples of individuals from focal species separate from pipe and dipnetting samples.

The metamorphic sampling period was defined by the developmental progress of the resident species discovered in each wetland during May and June samples. We revisited these ponds between one and seven times in July and August to capture metamorphs of our target species. We used a combination of dipnetting, hand capture, and seining to recover metamorphic individuals (defined as being between Gosner Stages 40 and 46; Gosner 1960). Preserved snails were identified to species and measured by shell diameter (e.g. planospiral snails, *Planorbella*) or shell height (e.g. spiral snails, *Physa*). Preserved amphibians were identified to species, measured (snout-vent length), and staged (according to Gosner (1960). We focused our analyses on two amphibian species: the green frog (*R. clamitans*) and the spring peeper (*P. crucifer*). Both species were relatively common across the urbanization gradient, allowing examination of adequate numbers of populations (16 populations of the green frog, 15 of the spring peeper).

11.2.3 Parasite assays

For each amphibian species, we dissected up to 10 metamorphs per wetland (mean = 8) to estimate patterns of infection by trematodes (Box 11.2). Specifically, we were interested in infection prevalence (fraction of individuals infected with a trematode taxon), infection intensity (average number of trematode individuals recovered from infected hosts), and infection abundance (average number of trematode individuals recovered from each examined host, including uninfected hosts). Within each host individual we examined the digestive tract and kidneys. These tissues are common sites for parasitic trematodes, and the trematode taxa infecting these tissues are relatively well known (Smyth and Smyth 1980, Prudhoe and Bray 1982, McAlpine and Burt 1998, Huffman and Fried 1990, Graczyk and Fried 1998, Fried 2001).

Tissues to be examined were removed from the body cavity. After being isolated, host tissues were systematically fragmented into small pieces which were then thoroughly examined under a microscope (at 25–50 ×) for metacercarial cysts, mesocercariae, and adult worms. In some specimens, cyst counts within kidneys were extremely high (> 800 metacercarial cysts per kidney). In such specimens, we dissected and counted the left kidney only. Infection intensity was estimated by doubling the cyst count from the single examined kidney. This estimate is likely to be conservative as the cyst counts in left kidneys tend to be lower possibly due to asymmetries in the development of left versus right kidneys (Thiemann and Wassersug 2000; this study). All recovered trematodes were identified as far as visual examination would allow, assigned to a tentative taxonomic identification, and counted. Vouchers for each taxon were sent to Dr. Vasyl Tkach at the University of North Dakota for identification using molecular methods (Tkach and Pawlowski 1999; Tkach et al. 2000).

11.2.4 Wetland attributes

In each sampled wetland we estimated a number of characteristics: dissolved oxygen (DO), water temperature, pH, conductivity, canopy cover, total phosphorous (P), and total nitrogen (N) concentrations. Temperature, DO, pH, and conductivity were estimated using electronic meters during each of up to two visits to each wetland. Total P and N were estimated during May and June visits. Water samples

were collected in clean Nalgene bottles, placed on ice and then frozen after returning from the field. Samples for estimation of total N were processed using the Cadmium reduction method (EPA Method # 353.2). Samples for total P were processed using the ascorbic acid method (EPA Method # 365.2). Canopy cover was estimated once during the summer months while deciduous trees were leafed out, and a second time when leaves were absent, using a spherical densiometer at four points along the shoreline. In smaller wetlands, these points were spaced along the shoreline at the four cardinal compass points. In large wetlands the points were spaced evenly around the sampled portion of the wetland. In all cases, multiple measurements of the same variable were averaged for analyses to represent a single estimate for each wetland.

11.3 Results

11.3.1 Wetland attributes

We used principal components analysis to reduce dimensionality of data on physicochemical attributes of 59 Connecticut wetlands; one of the 60 selected wetlands dried early and was dropped from the analyses. We retained two principal components for analysis based on nine raw variables; together these components explained 53% of the variation in the data. The first principal component sorted wetlands along an axis dominated by distinctions among pH, DO and depth, and forest canopy cover. The second component distinguished wetlands with high nutrients (N, P) and conductivity and those with dense canopy and high DO. Wetland attributes varied characteristically with urbanization; that is, scores from the two principal components varied among undeveloped, intermediate and urban regions (MANOVA, Wilks' Lambda = 0.786, $F_{2,110}$ = 3.52, P = 0.010).

11.3.2 Amphibian host distribution

Amphibian host species were chosen for study based on their broad distribution across the three regions. Spring peepers were detected in 29 wetlands, and green frogs were detected in 34 wetlands. Among these, 16 populations of green frogs and 15 populations of spring peepers were selected for parasite analysis (selected populations included those with adequate numbers of metamorphs available for dissection). For neither species did the frequency of presence vary among regions (Discriminant Analysis: $P > 0.05$ in both cases). Green frog density did vary with wetland attributes (PC 1: linear regression, $F_{1,57} = 4.26$, $P = 0.044$). Spring peeper density was independent of wetland attributes (linear regressions: $P > 0.05$), but only two wetlands within the city of Manchester held sufficient densities to be included in parasite analyses of spring peepers.

11.3.3 Echinostome infection patterns

Echinostomes were entirely absent from the sample of 132 spring peeper metamorphs. Here we focus exclusively on echinostome infection within green frogs. Of 131 green frogs examined, 50 (38%) were infected with echinostome metacercariae. Among infected individuals, intensities ranged from 1 to 1648 cysts (mean = 245 cysts, median = 33). Prevalence of infection (Fig. 11.4(a)) averaged 37% and ranged from 0% to 100% across the 16 wetlands examined. Echinostomes were not detected in 4 of the 16 wetlands. There was no evidence that prevalence varied among undeveloped, intermediate, and urban regions (ANOVA: mean square = 0.305,

$F_{2,13} = 0.836$, $P = 0.455$). Neither infection abundance (ANOVA: mean square = 1.051, $F_{2,13} = 0.574$, $P = 0.577$) nor infection intensity (ANOVA: mean square = 0.462, $F_{2,8} = 0.519$, $P = 0.614$) varied among regions. In part, results regarding infection abundance and intensity stem from the sharp inequality in the distribution of infection among wetlands (Fig. 11.4(b)). More than 99% (of over 12,000) recovered cysts came from just three wetlands (two in the urban region and one in the intermediate region).

Echinostome infections were discovered only within wetlands where we detected snail taxa (*Helisoma anceps, Physa vernalis, Physella* spp., and *Planorbella* spp.) known to serve as intermediate hosts for echinostomes. Host snail density was related to wetland attributes described by principal components (linear regression: $F_{2,56} = 3.57$, $P = 0.035$) and varied among regions (Fig. 11.5; ANOVA: mean square = 2.52, $F_{2,57} = 3.56$, $P = 0.035$). Host snails were five times more abundant in the most urban region (Manchester) than in the undeveloped Yale-Myers Forest (Scheffe test: $P < 0.05$). Although the abundance of host snails was intermediate in the region of intermediate development (the town of Tolland), contrasts involving this region were not significant. Infection abundance within green frog hosts was a strong function of host snail density (Fig. 11.6; linear regression: $F_{1,14} = 53.638$, $P < 0.001$).

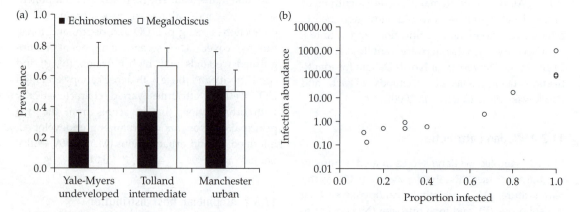

Figure 11.4 (a) Proportion of green frog (*R. clamitans*) hosts infected in wetlands from three regions along an urbanization gradient. Infection prevalence is presented for echinostome and *Megalodiscus* trematodes. Bars represent mean prevalence + 1 SE. Data are presented for 16 wetlands: Yale-Myers (*n* = 6 wetlands); Tolland (*n* = 5 wetlands); and Manchester (*n* = 5 wetlands). (b) Relationship between echinostome infection abundance and prevalence of infection in green frogs (*R. clamitans*). Responses are shown for 12 of 16 wetlands examined. The remaining four wetlands showed no evidence of echinostome infection.

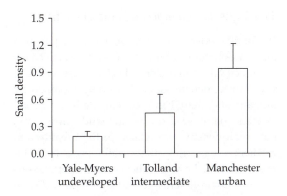

Figure 11.5 Variation in the density of host snails in 59 wetlands along an urbanization gradient. See Fig. 11.2 for location details. Snail densities were estimated using time-constrained dipnet sampling conducted twice in each wetland (May, June). Host-snail taxa included members of the following genera: *Helisoma*, *Physa*, *Physella*, and *Planorbella*.

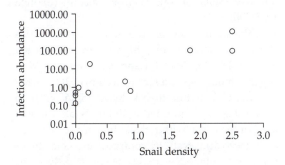

Figure 11.6 Relationship between the density of host snails and echinostome infection abundance within kidneys of the green frog, *R. clamitans*. Snails included all individuals of the genera *Helisoma* and *Planorbella*. Snail density was measured as the number of individuals recovered per person-minute of dipnetting. Infection abundance is plotted on a logarithmic scale and measured as the number of cysts recovered from both kidneys. Responses are plotted for 12 of 16 wetlands examined. The remaining four wetlands yielded no evidence of echinostome infection.

11.3.4 *Megalodiscus* infection patterns

Megalodiscus were recovered from 11 of 132 spring peeper metamorphs (8%) and infected metamorphs were collected from 5 of the 15 wetlands. Prevalence of infection ranged from 0% to 40%. Infected spring peepers had either one or two worms within their digestive tracts (mean intensity = 1.3). *Megalodiscus* were recovered from both undeveloped and inter-mediate (Yale-Myers and Tolland) wetlands but were absent from urban (Manchester) wetlands.

However, it should be noted that just two urban wetlands afforded sufficient spring peeper samples for analysis. Because of their scarcity, we did not further analyze *Megalodiscus* infection patterns within spring peepers.

Megalodiscus were recovered from the digestive tracts of 86 of the 131 green frogs examined (66%). Among infected individuals, intensities ranged from 1 to 94 worms (mean = 12, median = 4). Prevalence of infection averaged 61% and ranged from 0% to 100% across the 16 wetlands examined; worms were recovered from all but one of the wetlands sampled. There was no evidence that prevalence varied among regions (Fig. 11.4(a), ANOVA: mean square = 0.115, $F_{2,13} = 0.540$, $P = 0.593$). Neither infection abundance (ANOVA: mean square = 85.6, $F_{2,13} = 0.800$, $P = 0.469$) nor infection intensity (ANOVA: mean square = 206.8, $F_{2,8} = 1.11$, $P = 0.364$) varied among regions.

Within individual hosts, infection intensity of *Megalodiscus* was inversely related to green frog developmental stage (linear regression: $F_{1,129} = 88.51$, $P < 0.001$). Hosts in early stages of metamorphosis often had high infection intensities (> 10 worms, usually of small body size). Individuals nearing the end of the metamorphic period (Gosner Stage 46) typically had just one to a few worms, often of larger body size.

There was some indication that infection abundance is positively related to the density of snails that can serve as prior intermediate hosts of *Megalodiscus* (linear regression: $F_{1,14} = 6.57$, $P = 0.02$). In addition, the infection response in metamorphic green frogs may be influenced by the density of amphibians that can serve as prior hosts; for example, second-year larvae of green frogs, bullfrogs (*R. catesbeiana*), and adult newts (*Notophthalmus viridescens*). Even after correcting for the influence of Gosner Stage, infection intensity tended to be higher at lower amphibian host densities (ANCOVA: mean square = 411.6, $F = 3.04$, $P = 0.003$).

11.4 Discussion

Within the next three decades, the number of humans living in urbanized environments will surpass the number living in non-urbanized environments (United Nations 2001). This condition is historically unprecedented and is expected to rapidly disappear into the rear view mirror; an ever-greater fraction of humanity will be urban, and this trend will continue at ever-increasing rates for the foreseeable future. Even though it is of great significance to humans, it has been customary for ecologists to place a low relative priority on urbanization as a threat to species. Until recently, urban zones covered a small fraction of terrestrial environments, and the direct effects of urbanization were thought to be similarly restricted in geographic scope. These attitudes are changing (Thompson and Jones 1999; Johnson and Collinge 2004). As the fraction of the land surface dedicated to dense human settlement begins to rival that of wilderness, it is appropriate to explore the consequences.

Of all hypothesized impacts, the potential for urbanization to enhance the spread of infectious disease may be of particular concern (e.g. Williams et al. 2003). Much prior work has focused on the phenomenon of disease emergence and its consequences for host species (e.g. Daszak et al. 2003). Based on these findings, we are now in a stronger position to begin asking how often pathogens and parasites emerge and to explore context dependence that may explain the observed variety in responses to urbanization (Table 11.1).

In this regard, the pattern of macroparasite infection in amphibians that we uncovered is instructive. Across two parasite taxa and two host species, there was no evidence that prevalence of infection varied with urbanization. Broadly speaking, trematodes were widely distributed among wetlands and prevalence was relatively unresponsive to massive changes in the structure of surrounding landscapes. In one sense, this may not be surprising. Both parasite taxa are presumed to be native to the study region, and we selected amphibian host species for study that remained common across the urbanization gradient. Previous epidemiological studies have noted that parasites often emerge outside their native host and geographic ranges (e.g. zoonotic diseases, Daszak et al. 2003); a corollary might be that native taxa are less likely to emerge. Nevertheless, while prevalence was unresponsive to urbanization, we do have evidence that parasite emergence occurred within one of the hosts. Echinostomes within green frog hosts reached extreme infection intensities in three of the sampled wetlands.

11.4.1 Disease emergence in the green frog

We found evidence of severe echinostome infection intensities within 3 of the 16 wetlands for which we examined infection patterns. Each of these wetlands was surrounded by uplands heavily modified by humans and shared in common the highest snail densities discovered during the study. In general, host snail density was related to the urbanization gradient, suggesting that snails used by echinostomes may be weedy hosts whose populations grow in environments altered by humans (Dillon 2000; Johnson and Chase 2004). The specific wetland attributes critical to host snails will require further study; we note that the three extreme infection wetlands had the highest conductivities measured. Prior studies have concluded that snail distributions can be limited by the availability of ions such as calcium (Jokinen 1983; Dillon 2000).

Echinostome infection intensities recorded in this study are among the highest ever recorded (see Beasley et al. 2004 for another example). Wild-caught green frogs can harbor well over 1000 metacercarial cysts within their kidneys (Fig. 11.4(b)). In the most severely infected individuals, almost one-third of the tissue within the kidney was comprised of metacercarial cysts. By contrast, amphibian hosts from undeveloped wetlands were as likely to be infected, but the infections were uniformly of low intensity. Although the appearance of heavily infected kidneys is remarkable, the influence of echinostomes on amphibians in nature is not known. In the laboratory, even modest infection intensities (exposure to as few as 20 cercariae) are associated with mortality at early stages of tadpole development (Schotthoefer et al. 2003). Because we examined metamorphs, our host individuals had survived their entire larval period in spite of severe infection. We have no evidence from our study that infection compromises growth or survival. However, we did record the presence of severe edema of the hind limbs and abdomen among individuals collected from the three wetlands with the highest echinostome infection intensities; edema was largely absent from other wetlands. Edema may be symptomatic of compromised kidney function.

11.4.2 Interspecific host comparison

We studied two host amphibians, green frogs and spring peepers, with the hope of comparing infection patterns between species. In general, spring peepers were infected less often than their green frog counterparts. Echinostomes were never found in spring peepers in spite of their documented host association (Najarian 1954). Prevalence of infection by *Megalodiscus* was much lower in spring peepers (8%) compared with green frogs (66%). Several factors may contribute to these distinctions. One is the potential time for transmission (Tinsley 1995). At the time of capture, green frog metamorphs were 12–15 months old. A green frog metamorph has endured two growing seasons offering a much greater opportunity for infection. Spring peepers hatched from eggs 2–3 months before capture. Parasites have a short time window within a single year during which to infect spring peeper hosts. Further, green frogs and spring peepers may represent host opportunities of differing quality. Spring peeper larvae are among the smallest amphibian larvae in our study area while green frogs are among the largest. For echinostomes, the diameter of the cloaca and nephric duct may provide cues to, or constrain, free-swimming cercariae (Thiemann and Wassersug 2000). Among *Megalodiscus* worms, the relatively small gut of spring peepers could limit the number of individuals that can grow and survive regardless of the inoculation size. We never recovered more than two *Megalodiscus* worms from a spring peeper compared with as many as 94 in a single green frog. This dramatic disparity may reflect differences in body size and gut volumes of the two species at metamorphosis.

11.4.3 Urbanization as a mechanism underlying disease emergence

The etiology of echinostome emergence in our study can be related to that observed for schistosomes (*Schistosoma*), a well-studied genus of snail-borne trematodes responsible for schistosomiasis. Endemic in 74 nations of Africa, Asia, and South America, schistosomiasis affects an estimated 200 million people worldwide (World Health Organization 1993). Similar to the pattern of echinostome emergence described here, transmission of schistosomiasis is closely associated with human-mediated alteration of landscapes (Patz *et al.* 2000). However, increases in schistosome density and distribution appear to be fostered primarily through the creation of new wetland habitats suitable for intermediate host snails (Brown 1994). For this reason, water resource development projects featuring damming and irrigation are frequently implicated in the emergence of schistosomiasis (e.g. Picquet *et al.* 1996), and transmission control strategies have historically incorporated snail control through molluscicide application or habitat modification (World Health Organization 1993; Brown 1994).

As in this study, emergence of schistosomiasis in urban and peri-urban settings has been considered in the context of species introductions of the snail host, parasite vector, or both (Mott *et al.* 1990). The impact of urbanization on light, temperature, and salinity regimes in existing wetlands may also exert a strong influence on the distribution and abundance of pulmonate snails and schistosomes (Appleton 1978; Brown 1994). More recently, a comparable scenario has been proposed for emergence of trematode infections linked with amphibian limb deformities (Johnson and Chase 2004). These authors relate nutrient concentrations to increases in density of the host snail species (*Planorbella trivolvis*), and then to increases in infection by *Ribeiroia ondatrae* in amphibian hosts.

Collectively, the patterns of wetland variation and infection responses uncovered in this study support strong roles for both abiotic and biotic factors (see Poteet, chapter 10, this volume). Extremely dense snail populations associated with echinostome emergence are only possible where snails have adequate resources and are not persecuted by efficient predators such as fish (Dillon 2000). By greatly increasing the concentration of nutrients such as nitrogen, phosphorous, and calcium, humans may inadvertently create conditions in which snail food resources, such as periphyton, thrive and where the creation and maintenance of shell is fostered. The three wetlands in which echinostomes emerged also lack fish predators that might otherwise reduce snail densities (Dillon 2000). These conditions, coincidentally, are ideal for many larval amphibians, including both spring peepers and green frogs (Skelly 1996; Wellborn *et al.* 1996). In spite of any effects of disease, green frog densities were high in wetlands with high infection intensities. It is possible that the means by which urbanization promotes disease emergence may be linked with conditions that maintain dense populations of both snail and amphibian hosts. However, it is worth noting that, overall, urban wetlands have lower amphibian species richness than undeveloped or intermediate wetlands. Green frogs are an exception among North American amphibian species in their ability to persist in urbanized contexts. In part, this hardiness stems from their largely aquatic habit; green frogs typically stay close to the shoreline, meaning that their dependence on upland environments is limited. Observational studies such as this one cannot elucidate the role that infectious disease may play in restricting the majority of amphibian species from urbanized contexts.

11.5 Conclusions

Most prior studies of macroparasite infection in wildlife have detected emergence or no response to urbanization (Table 11.1). This pattern, based on several independent studies, was echoed in our study of two parasite taxa and two host species. It is likely that distinctions in parasite biology and its interaction with host differences and environmental context are each critical to observed patterns. Such context dependence highlights the need for mechanistic studies to determine the conditions under which emergence is likely. Further, it would be fruitful to investigate the abundance and distribution of a greater number of species in these communities for signs of why emergence is likely in particular contexts. Given that disease emergence is a frequent side-effect of human development, there is even greater need to understand the consequences of infection to host individuals and populations.

For amphibians, this problem is acute. Infectious disease has been implicated in recent declines, extinctions, and deformity outbreaks (Stuart *et al.* 2004). In some cases, conversion of landscapes to human use may contribute to disease emergence

(Johnson and Chase 2004) and in fact could be a cryptic cause for population loss in disturbed landscapes, even when apparently suitable habitats remain.

Acknowledgments

Sincere thanks to S. Collinge and C. Ray for inviting our participation in this volume and for their helpful comments on a prior draft of this chapter. V. Tkach and M. Kinsella offered expert advice on the identification of parasites. J. Joseph provided field assistance. This research was supported by the NIH/NSF Ecology of Infectious Diseases Program.

References

Aizen, M. A., L. Ashworth, and L. Galetto. (2002). Reproductive success in fragmented habitats: do compatibility systems and pollination specialization matter? *Journal of Vegetation Science* **13**:885–892.

Amorim, M. N., A. Rabello, R. L. Contreras, and N. Katz. (1997). Epidemiological characteristics of *Schistosoma mansoni* infection in rural and urban endemic areas of Minas Gerais, Brazil. *Memorias do Instituto Oswaldo Cruz* **92**:577–580.

Anderson, J. W. and B. Fried. (1987). Experimental infection of *Physa heterostropha, Helisoma trivolvis*, and *Biomphalaria glabrata* (Gastropoda) with *Echinostoma revolutum* (Trematoda) cercariae. *Journal of Parasitology* **73**:49–54.

Appleton, C. C. (1978). Review of literature on biotic and abiotic factors influencing the distribution and life cycles of bilharziasis intermediate snail hosts. *Malacological Review* **11**:1–25.

Azazy, A. A. and A. S. Al-Tiar. (1999). A survey study on intestinal and blood parasites among school children in Sana'a province, Yemen. *Saudi Medical Journal* **20**:422–424.

Beasley, V. R., S. A. Faeh, B. Wikoff, J. Eisold, D. Nichols, R. Cole *et al.* (2004). Risk factors and the decline of the northern cricket frog, *Acris crepitans*: evidence for involvement of herbicides, parasitism, and habitat modifications. In M. Lannoo, ed. *The Status and Conservation of United States Amphibians*. University of California Press, Berkeley, CA.

Beaver, P. C. (1937). Experimental studies on *Echinostoma revolutum* (Froelich), a fluke from birds and mammals. *Illinois Biological Monographs* **15**:1–96.

Berger, L., R. Speare, P. Daszak, D. E. Green, A. A. Cunningham, C. L. Goggin *et al.* (1998). Chytridiomycosis causes amphibian mortality associated with population declines in the rain forests of Australia and Central America. *Proceedings of the National Academy of Sciences* **95**:9031–9036.

Brown, D. (1994). *Freshwater Snails of Africa and their Medical Importance*. 2nd Edition. Taylor and Francis, London.

Bush, A. O. and C. R. Kennedy. (1994). Host fragmentation and helminth parasites: hedging your bets against extinction. *International Journal for Parasitology* **24**:1333–1343.

Bustnes, J. O. and K. Galaktionov. (1999). Anthropogenic influences on the infestation of intertidal gastropods by seabird trematode larvae on the southern Barents Sea coast. *Marine Biology* **133**:449–453.

de Carneri, I., L. Di Matteo, and S. Tedla. (1992). A comparison of helminth infections in urban and rural areas of Addis Ababa. *Transactions of the Royal Society of Tropical Medicine and Hygiene* **86**:540–541.

Christensen, N. O., F. Frandsen, and M. Z. Roushdy. (1980). The influence of environmental conditions and parasite intermediate host-related factors on the transmission of *Echinostoma liei*. *Zeitschrift fur Parasitenkunde-Parasitology Research* **64**:47–63.

Dagoye, D., Z. Bekele, K. Woldemichael, H. Nida, M. Yimam, A. Hall *et al.* (2003). Wheezing, allergy, and parasite infection in children in urban and rural Ethiopia. *American Journal of Respiratory and Critical Care Medicine* **167**:1369–1373.

Daszak, P., A. A. Cunningham, and A. D. Hyatt. (2001). Anthropogenic environmental change and the emergence of infectious disease in wildlife. *Acta Tropica* **78**:103–116.

Daszak P., A. A. Cunningham, and A. D. Hyatt. (2003). Infectious disease and amphibian population declines. *Diversity and Distributions* **9**:141–150.

Dillon, R. T. (2000). *The Ecology of Freshwater Molluscs*. Cambridge University Press, Cambridge.

Ebenman, B., R. Law, and C. Borrval. (2004). Community viability analysis: the response of ecological communities to species loss. *Ecology* **85**:2591–2600.

Epstein, P. R., E. Chivian, and K. Frith. (2003). Emerging diseases threaten conservation. *Environmental Health Perspectives* **111**:A506–A507.

Fried, B. (2001). Biology of echinostomes except *Echinostoma*. *Advances in Parasitology* **49**:163–210.

Fried, B., S. Scheuermann, and J. Moore. (1987). Infectivity of *Echinostoma revolutum* miracidia for laboratory raised pulmonate snails. *Journal of Parasitology* **73**:1047–1048.

Gendron, A. D., D. J. Marcogliese, S. Barbeau, M.-S. Christin, P. Brousseau, S. Ruby *et al.* (2003). Exposure of leopard frogs to a pesticide mixture affects life history characteristics of the lungworm *Rhabdias ranae*. *Oecologia* **135**:469–476.

Gering J.C. and R. B. Blair. (1999). Predation on artificial bird nests along an urban gradient: predatory risk or relaxation in urban environments? *Ecography* **22**:532–541.

Gibbs, J. P. (1998). Distribution of woodland amphibians along a forest fragmentation gradient. *Landscape Ecology* **13**:263–268.

Gosner, K. (1960). A simplified table for staging anuran embryos and larvae with notes on identification. *Herpetologica* **16**:183–190.

Graczyk, T. K. and B. Fried. (1998). Echinostomiasis: a common but forgotten food-borne disease. *Journal of Tropical Medicine and Hygiene* **58**:501–504.

Gratz, N. G. (1999). Emerging and resurging vector-borne diseases. *Annual Review of Entomology* **44**:51–75.

Haas, W., M. Korner, E. Hutterer, M. Wegner, and B. Haberl. (1995). Finding and recognition of the snail intermediate hosts by three species of Echinostome cercariae. *Parasitology* **110**:133–142.

Habluetzel, A., G. Traldi, S. Ruggieri, A. R. Attili, P. Scuppa, R. Marchetti *et al.* (2003). An estimation of *Toxocara canis* prevalence in dogs, environmental egg contamination and risk of human infection in the Marche region of Italy. *Veterinary Parasitology* **113**:243–252.

Hanelt, B., L. E. Grother, and J. Janovy, Jr. (2001). Physid snails as sentinels of freshwater Nematomorphs. *Journal of Parasitology* **87**:1049–1053.

Hofer, S., S. Gloor, U. Müller, A. Mathis, D. Hegglin, and P. Deplazes. (2000). High prevalence of *Echinococcus multilocularis* in urban red foxes (*Vulpes vulpes*) and voles (*Arvicola terrestris*) in the city of Zürich, Switzerland. *Parasitology* **120**:135–142.

Huffman, J. E. and B. Fried. (1990). Echinostoma and echinostomiasis. *Advances in Parasitology* **29**:215–269.

Johnson, P.T.J. and J. M. Chase. (2004). Parasites in the food web: linking amphibian malformations and aquatic eutrophication. *Ecology Letters* **7**:521–526.

Johnson, P. T. J., K. B. Lunde, E. G. Ritchie, and A. E. Launer. (1999). The effect of trematode infection on amphibian limb development and survivorship. *Science* **284**:802–804.

Johnson P. T. J., K. B. Lunde, E. M. Thurman, E. G. Ritchie, S. N. Wray, D. R. Sutherland *et al.* (2002). Parasite (*Ribeiroia ondatrae*) infection linked to amphibian malformations in the western United States. *Ecological Monographs* **72**:151–168.

Johnson, P. T. J., K. B. Lunde, D. A. Zelmer, and J. K. Werner. (2003). Limb deformities as an emerging parasitic disease in amphibians: Evidence from museum specimens and resurvey data. *Conservation Biology* **17**:1724–1737.

Johnson, W. C. and S. K. Collinge. (2004). Landscape effects on black-tailed prairie dog colonies. *Biological Conservation* **115**:487–497.

Jokinen, E. H. (1983). *The Freshwater Snails of Connecticut* (Bulletin). State Geological and Natural History Survey of Connecticut.

Kanev, I., B. Fried, V. Dimitrov, and V. Radev. (1995). Redescription of *Echinostoma trivolvis* (Cort, 1914) (Trematoda, Echinostomatidae) with a discussion on its identity. *Systematic Parasitology* 32:61–70.

Martin, T. R. and D. B. Conn. (1990). The pathogenicity, localization, and cyst structure of echinostomatid metacercariae (Trematoda) infecting the kidneys of the frogs *Rana clamitans* and *Rana pipiens*. *Journal of Parasitology* 76:414–419.

Marzluff, J. M. (2001). Worldwide urbanization and its effects on birds. In J. M. Marzluff, R. Bowman, and R. Donnelly, eds. *Avian Ecology and Conservation in a Changing World*, pp. 19–47. Kluwer, Boston, MH.

Mason, P. R. and B. A. Patterson. (1994). Epidemiology of *Hymenolepis nana* infections in primary school children in urban and rural communities in Zimbabwe. *Journal of Parasitology* 80:245–250.

McAlpine, D. F. and M. D. B. Burt. (1998). Helminths of Bullfrogs, *Rana catesbeiana*, Green Frogs, *R. clamitans*, and Leopard Frogs, *R. pipiens* in New Brunswick. *Canadian Field Naturalist* 112:50–68.

McKinney, M. L. (2002). Urbanization, biodiversity, and conservation. *Bioscience* 52:883–890.

Mngomezulu, N., J. M. Govere, D. N. Durrheim, R. Speare, L. Viljoen, C. Appleton *et al.* (2002). Burden of schistosomiasis and soil-transmitted helminth infections in primary school children in Mpumalanga, South Africa, and implications for control. *South African Journal of Science* 98:607–610.

Morse, S. S., ed. (1993). *Emerging Viruses*. Oxford University Press, New York.

Morse, S. S. (1995). Factors in the emergence of infectious diseases. *Emerging Infectious Diseases* 1:7–15.

Mott, K. E., P. Desjeux, A. Moncayo, P. Ranqui, and P. de Raadt. (1990). Parasitic diseases and urban development. *Bulletin of the World Health Organization* 58:691–698.

Najarian, H. H. (1954). Developmental stages in the life cycle of *Echinoparyphium flexum* (Linton, 1892) Dietz, 1910 (Trematoda, Echinostomatidae). *Journal of Morphology* 94:165–197.

Nyan, O. A., G. E. L. Walraven, A. S. Banya, P. Milligan, M. Van der Sande, S. M. Ceesay *et al.* (2001). Atopy, intestinal helminth infection and total serum IgE in rural and urban adult Gambian communities. *Clinical and Experimental Allergy* 31:1672–1678.

Patz, J. A., T. K. Graczyk, N. Gellar, and A. Y. Vittor. (2000). Effects of environmental change on emerging parasitic diseases. *International Journal for Parasitology* 30:1395–1405.

Paul, M. J. and J. L. Meyer. (2001). Streams in the urban landscape. *Annual Review of Ecology and Systematics* 32:333–365.

Phiri, K., C. J. M. Whitty, S. M. Graham, and G. Ssembatya-Lule. (2000). Urban/rural differences in prevalence and risk factors for intestinal helminth infection in southern Malawi. *Annals of Tropical Medicine and Parasitology* 94:381–387.

Picquet, M., J. C. Ernould, J. Vercruysse, V. R. Southgate, A. Mbaye, B. Sambou *et al.* (1996). The epidemiology of human schistosomiasis in the Senegal river basin. *Transactions of the Royal Society of Tropical Medicine and Hygiene* 90:340–346.

Pietrock, M. and D. J. Marcogliese. (2003). Free-living endohelminth stages: at the mercy of environmental conditions. *Trends in Ecology and Evolution* 19:293–299.

Prudhoe, S. and R. A. Bray. (1982). *Platyhelminth Parasites of the Amphibia*. Oxford University Press, Oxford, England.

Richards, D. T., S. Harris, and J. W. Lewis. (1995). Epidemiological studies on intestinal helminth parasites of rural and urban red foxes (*Vulpes vulpes*) in the United Kingdom. *Veterinary Parasitology* 59:39–51.

Richter, K. O. and A. L. Azous. (1995). Amphibian occurrence and wetland characteristics in the Puget Sound basin. *Wetlands* 15:305–312.

Roche, J. and A. Benito. (1999). Prevalence of intestinal parasite infections with special reference to *Entamoeba histolytica* on the island of Bioko (Equatorial Guinea). *American Journal of Tropical Medicine and Hygiene* 60:257–262.

Schell, S. C. 1985. *Trematodes of North America*. University of Idaho Press, Moscow.

Schotthoefer, A. M., R. A. Cole, and V. R. Beasley. (2003). Relationship of tadpole stage to location of echinostome cercariae encystment and the consequences for tadpole survival. *Journal of Parasitology* 89:475–482.

Schrag, S. J. and P. Wiener. (1995). Emerging infectious disease: what are the relative roles of ecology and evolution? *Trends in Ecology and Evolution* 10:319–324.

Skelly, D. K. (1996). Pond drying, predators, and the distribution of *Pseudacris* tadpoles. *Copeia* 1996:599–605.

Smyth, J.D. and M.M. Smyth. (1980). *Frogs as Host–Parasite Systems I. An Introduction to Parasitology through the Parasites of Rana temporaria, R. esculenta and R. pipiens*. Macmillan Press, London.

Sprent, J. F. A. (1992). Parasites lost. *International Journal for Parasitology* 22:139–151.

Stuart, S. N., J. S. Chanson, N. A. Cox, B. E. Young, A. S. L. Rodriguez, D. L. Fischman *et al.* (2004). Status and trends of amphibian declines and extinctions worldwide. *Science* 306:1783–1786.

Thiemann, G. W. and R. J. Wassersug. (2000). Biased distribution of trematode metacercariae in the nephric system of *Rana* tadpoles. *Journal of Zoology* 252: 534–538.

Thompson, K. and A. Jones. (1999). Human population density and prediction of local plant extinction. *Conservation Biology* 13:185–189.

Tinsley, R. C. (1995). Parasitic disease in amphibians: control by the regulation of worm burdens. *Parasitology* 111:S153–S178.

Tkach, V., J. Pawlowski, and J. Mariaux. (2000). Phylogenetic analysis of the suborder Plagiorchiata (Platyhelminthes, Digenea) based on partial lsrDNA sequences. *International Journal for Parasitology* 30: 83–93.

Tkach, V. and J. Pawlowski. (1999). A new method of DNA extraction from the ethanol-fixed parasitic worms. *Acta Parasitologica* 44:147–148.

Turner, W. R., T. Nakamura, and M. Dinetti. (2004). Global urbanization and the separation of humans from nature. *Bioscience* 54:585–590.

United Nations. (2001). *The State of the World's Cities*. United Nations Centre for Human Settlements, UNHCS Habitat, Nairobi, Kenya.

Wellborn, G. A., D. K. Skelly, and E. E. Werner. (1996). Mechanisms creating community structure across a freshwater habitat gradient. *Annual Review of Ecology and Systematics* 27:337–363.

Williams, E. S., T. Yuill, M. Artois, J. Fischer, and S. A. Haigh. (2003). Emerging infectious diseases in wildlife. *Revue Scientifique et Technique de l'Office International des Epizooties* 21:139–157.

World Health Organization. (1993). The control of schistosomiasis: second report of the WHO expert committee. *WHO Technical Report Series 830*. World Health Organization, Geneva.

CHAPTER 12

Spatial-temporal dynamics of rabies in ecological communities

Leslie A. Real and James E. Childs

12.1 Background

The earliest historical records of human suffering due to infectious disease include two ancient Egyptian hieroglyphs; one depicting a man with a withered leg probably suffering from polio and another frieze depicting a man bitten by a dog and displaying symptoms of rabies (Bacon 1985). Culturally, rabies has assumed symbolic proportions representing destiny, madness, and racism. Many people are familiar with the iconic fate of *Old Yeller* and the end of mad-dog racism in *To Kill a Mockingbird*. Pasteur's development of a successful vaccine treatment for patients exposed to rabies was among the first grand successes of the Germ Theory of Disease and this success has been celebrated widely in literature and film. The 1936 Hollywood biography of Pasteur (with an Oscar winning performance by Paul Muni) has a striking scene from the period shortly after Pasteur invented his vaccine. A crowd of immigrants, all of whom have been bitten by rabid wolves on the Russian Steppe, emerge out of a fog bank and approach Pasteur's house begging for treatment. The symbolism is wonderful—out of the shrouded fog they emerge into the light of our new understanding that will bring relief and well-being! Yet despite the development of even safer and more successful treatments, better and more effective vaccines, rabies remains the most important and devastating viral zoonotic disease worldwide.

Our current understanding of the ecology and evolution of rabies virus (RABV) involves crucial inquiry into the structure and function of the virus (including aspects of its molecular organization and pathogenesis), the potential evolution of host specialization associated with distinct virus variants, the temporal dynamics of specific host variants within specific geographic areas, and the global geographic distribution of RABV host variants coupled to patterns of spatial dynamics associated with local and regional movement of virus in infected hosts. We now turn to each of these areas of current research interest.

12.2 The virus

Rabies and rabies-related viruses are members of the *Lyssavirus* genus (Family: Rhabdoviridae) of neurotropic, single-stranded, negative-sense RNA viruses (Fig. 12.1(a)), capable of producing fatal encephalitis in a wide variety of mammalian species (Nadin-Davis 2000). Lyssaviruses are characteristically bullet-shaped enveloped viral particles consisting of a tightly associated RNA-nucleoprotein (RNP) core surrounded by trimeric glycoproteins (G) embedded within the lipid by-layer membrane of the viral envelope (Wagner and Rose 1996). The viral genome, ~12 kB in size, consists of five protein coding regions: the nucleoprotein (N), matrix (M), phosphoprotein (P), glycoprotein (G), and replicase (L) genes. The functional significance of each of the five genes has been well characterized during the replication cycle of RABV over the course of infection (Nadin-Davis 2000).

Rabies virus, the type species, serotype 1/genotype 1, for the *Lyssavirus* genus, is distributed worldwide and is endemic throughout the tropical, subtropical, and temperate regions of Africa,

North and South America, Asia, Europe, and Australia. Within regions, RABV variants exhibit different degrees of host specialization and geographic compartmentalization. North American RABV variants in terrestrial carnivores show

significant species-specific geographic distributions (Fig. 12.1(b)). The classification of distinct variants of RABV to single or a few related species of mammalian hosts has been only recently appreciated and made possible through the use of monoclonal antibodies and genetic sequencing (Rupprecht *et al.* 1987, Smith *et al.* 1990, 1992; Smith and Seidel 1993). Molecular analysis of RABV suggests that geographic variants of major terrestrial carnivore hosts cluster phylogenetically within specific host lineages (Fig. 12.2(a)). Patterns of phylogenetic relatedness among viral variants are not directly related to the phylogenetic relatedness of terrestrial carnivore host species (Fig. 12.2(b)). RABV variants associated with bats, however, may show some degree of phylogenetic concordance between host and virus (Messenger *et al.* 2003).

Rabies Virus is also undergoing geographic expansion associated with three ongoing epidemics: one in Europe, one within the eastern United States, and one in Canada. The European rabies epidemic is largely associated with virus

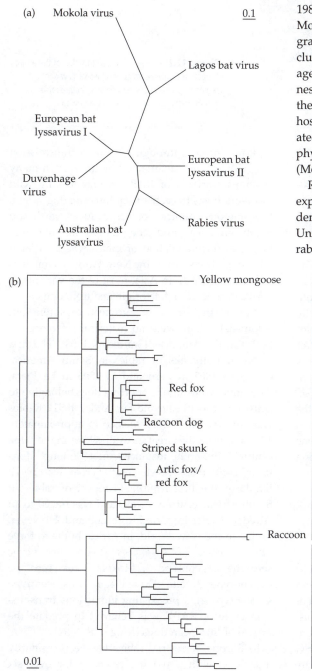

Figure 12.1 Phylogenetic relationships among rabies and other lyssaviruses. (a) Unrooted maximum likelihood tree of known lyssaviruses. Tree is based on the nucleoprotein gene (N, 1350 bp) using sequences available from GenBank and was constructed using a heuristic search under an HKY + I + G model in PAUP*4.0b10 (Swofford 2002). (b) Neighbor-joining tree of representative rabies virus N sequences assembled from GenBank by Holmes *et al.* (2002). Carnivora sequences were obtained from domestic dogs (worldwide) unless indicated otherwise. Chiroptera sequences were collected from various North and South American bat species. Tree was again constructed in Paup* based on maximum likelihood distances calculated under a HKY + I + G model and rooted using an Australian bat lyssavirus sequence as an outgroup (not shown).

(a)

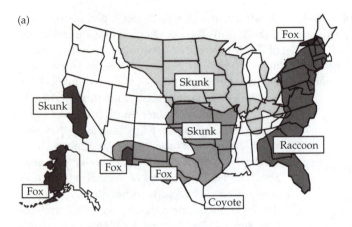

Figure 12.2(a) Geographic distribution of the major terrestrial carnivore hosts of rabies virus variants. Each region is largely characterized by a unique rabies variant specific to a single carnivore host.

spread in the red fox (*Vulpes vulpes*). The US rabies epidemic is associated with expansion of the raccoon (*Procyon lotor*) rabies variant following a presumed translocation of rabid animals from Florida to the West Virginia/Virginia border (Jenkins and Winkler 1987; Jenkins *et al.* 1988). Rabies has been endemic among raccoons in the southeastern United States for decades (Prather *et al.* 1975). The Canadian epidemic is associated with the expansion of rabies in the arctic fox (*Alopex lagopus*) into the southern provinces of Canada, especially Ontario. The southern expansion of arctic fox rabies through Canada has shifted to a red fox host after reaching Ontario. The Canadian epidemic meets the northern wave of raccoon-specific rabies expansion from the United States along the Canada/US border (Gordon *et al.* 2004). The expansion of the three epidemic waves has largely been controlled through a coordinated program of oral rabies vaccine (ORV) delivery along the front of the advancing wave (Wandeler 2000).

12.3 Global distribution of rabies virus among and affecting terrestrial mammals

No account of global rabies distribution can proceed without an introductory discussion of humans and the domestic dog. Domestic dogs serve as the major reservoir and principal source of RABV transmission to humans and other animals in many countries of Asia, Africa, and South America (WHO 1999). Other domestic and wild animals are typically infected through secondary transmission of RABV variants maintained by dogs, or in many locations, variants of RABV maintained by wild carnivore hosts traceable to a domestic dog origin. In numerous countries of Africa, Asia, North and South America, and the Caribbean, the first historical documentation of rabies was associated with dogs transported by New World colonialists (Smith *et al.* 1992). In Asia, most of the variants of RABV described to date originated from dogs.

Prior to the arrival of European explorers and colonialists, there were no historical references to rabies in the Americas (Smithcors 1958). The first recorded outbreaks of rabies in South America, dating to 1803 in Peru and in 1806 in La Plata, Argentina, were among sporting dogs belonging to British officers (Steele and Fernandez 1991). Rabies was first recorded from Mexico in approximately 1709 and from the Greater Antilles later in the same century, in both instances first among dogs (Smithcors 1958; Steele and Fernandez 1991). Similarly, the first irrefutable report of rabies in South Africa occurred in 1893 and was traced to an Airedale terrier imported from England. However, unlike in the New World, in Africa, home to three other species of *Lyssavirus* (Lagos bat virus, serotype 2/genotype 2, Mokola virus, serotype 3/genotype 3, and Duvenhage virus, serotype 4/genotype 4), a preexisting indigenous transmission cycle of RABV was believed to predate the arrival of European dogs (King *et al.* 1994).

In Europe, terrestrial rabies has been primarily associated with a red fox reservoir for over six

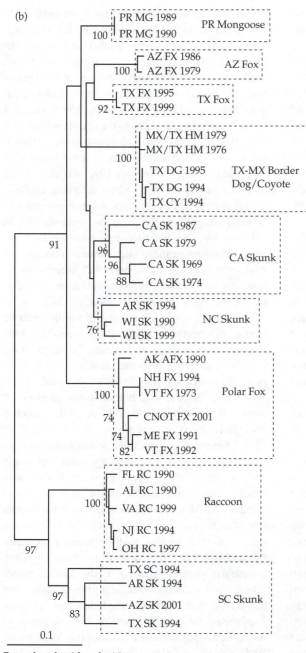

(b)

0.1

Rate of nucleotide substition

Figure 12.2(b) Neighbor-joining tree for nucleotide sequence of a 320-bp region of the nucleoprotein gene of selected RABV isolates from the Unites States, Mexico, and Canada. Each group of virus isolates that was sequenced to illustrate the unique RABV variants associated with terrestrial carnivores is boxed. The Polar Fox variant (artic and red fox) is no longer considered enzootic in the United States. Bootstrap values are shown at the branching points for clades recovered in > 700/1000 iterations of the data. Australian bat lyssavirus (ABLV) was used as the outgroup to root the tree. Samples from a rabid fox in Ontario, Canada (CN OT FX 2001?/4) and from two human rabies cases with exposures to rabid dogs in Mexico (MX/TX HM 1976 and 1979) are included to show variants of RABV shared across international boundaries. Unites States samples are identified by a two-letter abbreviation for the state and animal from which the sample originated followed by the year the case occurred. With the exception of the Canadian sample (GenBank accession U11735), all RABV sequences were derived from samples in a virus repository at the US Centers for Disease Control.

decades (Wandeler *et al.* 1974a, b). However, even in Europe, evidence suggests the RABV variant circulating among red foxes had a domestic dog origin (Bourhy *et al.* 1999), as does a related, second variant of European RABV established among raccoon dogs (*Nyctereutes procyonoides*). Geographic clustering of strains in both genetic lineages is evident in Europe, associated with physical barriers offered by rivers and mountains (Sacramento *et al.* 1992; Bourhy *et al.* 1999). The two species of European bat lyssaviruses (ELB-1 and ELB-2) have independent maintenance cycles among insectivorous bats in Europe, western Asia, and the United Kingdom (Fooks *et al.* 2004; Picard-Meyer *et al.* 2004), and bat-associated lyssaviruses have spilled-over to cause rabies among humans and wildlife (Fooks *et al.* 2003; Johnson *et al.* 2003b; Nathwani *et al.* 2003; Muller *et al.* 2004; Tjornehoj *et al.* 2004). New species of *Lyssavirus* continue to be discovered among central European and Asian insectivorous bats (Arai *et al.* 2003; Kuzmin *et al.* 2003).

In Asia, variants of domestic dog associated RABV are the causes of human and animal rabies. Evidence exists of genetic structuring of RABV variants maintained among dog populations according to geographic location in India (Jayakumar *et al.* 2004), Sri Lanka (Arai *et al.* 2001; Nanayakkara *et al.* 2003), Thailand (Susetya *et al.* 2003), and the Philippines (Nishizono *et al.* 2002). Although RABV circulates among mongooses (*Herpestes auropunctatus*) in some Asian countries (Patabendige and Wimalaratne 2003), the origin of the virus is presumably domestic dogs, as is also the case among mongooses introduced into the Caribbean in the 1800s to control rats (Everard and Everard 1992).

In South Africa (Nel *et al.* 1997), Zimbabwe (Bingham *et al.* 1999a, b), and Botswana (Johnson *et al.* 2004), two distinct RABV variants have been identified from specimens of over 30 different carnivore species belonging to four families of Carnivora: Viverridae, Canidea, Mustelidae, and Felidae. The two virus variants are maintained by independent cycles; one primarily associated with canids, originating with, and primarily involving domestic dogs, but also affecting several species of jackal (genus *Canis*), and bat-eared foxes (*Otocyon megalotis*); and the second cycle associated with viverrids and genets (genera *Cynictis, Herpestes, Suricata, Genetta, Civettictus*) (Nel *et al.* 1997; von Teichman *et al.* 1995). The viverrid subtype of RABV probably arose recently from spillover of the canid subtype and each of these RABV "biotypes" have crossed species barriers to infect other mammals, with no evidence of genetic modification in the virus recovered from non-reservoir host species (Nel *et al.* 1997).

In northern Africa and the Middle East, dog rabies remains the predominant threat, but wild carnivores, notably red foxes have been involved in rabies outbreaks in Oman (Novelli and Malankar 1991), Turkey (Johnson *et al.* 2003a), and, along with golden jackals (*Canis aureus*), in Israel (David *et al.* 2000). In East Africa, spillover from RABV maintained by domestic dogs occurs among many carnivore species, including lions (*Panthera leo*) and spotted hyenas (*Crocuta crocuta*) (Cleaveland and Dye 1995; East *et al.* 2001), and poses a conservation threat for existing populations of the African wild dog (*Lycaon pictus*) (Burrows 1992; Kat *et al.* 1996) and the Ethiopian wolf (*Canis simensis*) (Sillero-Zubiri *et al.* 1996). In the West African countries of Liberia, Ghana, and Nigeria the domestic dog is still regarded as the primary reservoir host for rabies affecting humans and animals (Alonge and Abu 1984; Ezeokoli and Umoh 1987; Monson 1985); however, few wildlife studies of rabies are available from these West African countries.

In Central America and most of South America north of northern Argentina, vampire bats (*Desmodus rotundus*) and domestic dogs have long been recognized as the most important independent reservoirs for RABV (Loza-Rubio *et al.* 1999), with animal and human cases ascribed to both variants in Brazil (Sato *et al.* 2004), Trinidad (Wright *et al.* 2002), and Mexico (De Mattos *et al.* 1999). However, as wildlife studies increase in countries originally struggling with epidemic canine rabies, new associations of RABV and wildlife are being found. In Mexico, a unique variant of RABV has been described from skunks (De Mattos *et al.* 1999). Bobcats (*Lynx rufus*) were found infected with a RABV variant previously thought restricted to gray foxes (*Urocyon cinereoargenteus*) in central Arizona in the United States (Steelman *et al.* 2000). Wildlife studies in Chile have implicated the Brazilian free-tailed bat (*Tadarida brasiliensis*) as a major source of infections in domestic animals in recent decades (De Mattos *et al.* 2000). Clearly, additional chiropteran and terrestrial mammal reservoirs will be discovered for RABV and other Lyssaviruses as wildlife studies continue in countries around the world. As recently as 1999, a new rabies-like virus was recovered from a sick pteropid bat in Australia, within months of the discovery of Australian bat lyssavirus (ABLV) (Gould *et al.* 1998).

12.4 Rabies and mammalian communities: big biases and little bodies

There are no published field data on the incidence and impact of rabies within any population of wildlife, with the exception of studies of endangered species where the appearance of rabies has threatened species already on the brink of extinction. The influence of rabies on the structure and dynamics of entire mammalian communities is nonexistent. No integrated ecological studies, with the exception of a few natural experiments, have assessed the magnitude of rabies impact on species other than medium-sized carnivores. Virtually all of the data on rabid wildlife in a geographic region are collected by national animal rabies surveillance systems. In the United States, this activity is co-ordinated by the Center for Disease Control and Prevention (CDC) and is designed to collect information to aid the prevention of disease in humans and domestic animals. As such, animal-based surveillance data provide only a crude and biased relative measure of monthly rates of rabies reported among different species, most of which are medium-sized carnivores that serve as the principal reservoir hosts for rabies virus variants to which humans and domestic animals are exposed. Unfortunately, these data are inadequate to measure or quantify rabies' impact upon any wildlife population or community process.

Nonetheless, the public health importance of rabies worldwide has generated the continuous and systematic collection of data on animal rabies, spanning more than five decades in the United States, which provides considerable information on the temporal–spatial patterns of rabies occurrence within selected wildlife hosts. The continuous, standardized collection of laboratory confirmed cases of rabies provides a dataset, irrespective of some inherent weaknesses, that can be used to explore, reveal and, through parameterization of models, predict some essential aspects of the spatiotemporal dynamics of RABV within wildlife serving as reservoir hosts.

An animal must not only survive the bite-wound inflicted during RABV transmission, but must also survive the incubation period, typically on the order of a month if rabies is to be diagnosed by methods

identifying antigen in fresh brain tissue. Therefore, surveillance counts of rabid animals should increase with the average body size of the species.

The inequality in rabies diagnoses among different sized mammals can be readily illustrated by sorting the 7970 cases of animal rabies reported in the United States in 2002 into three body-size bins. The bins chosen reflect typical average adult body-weight standards used to characterize mammalian communities (Bourliere 1975; Chew 1978); ≤ 2 kg = small, 2 to ≤ 45 kg = medium, and > 45 large = large.

Rodents represented <1% of all species tested for rabies in the United States (Childs *et al.* 1997), and virtually all of those tested and found rabid were large species such as woodchucks (*Marmota monax*) and beavers (*Castor canadensis*). An extreme under-representation of small terrestrial mammals was obvious in this dataset. However, the factors contributing to this size-bias are confounded by reliance on human observations of suspicious animal behavior, the problems inherent to mixing small body-size with RABV transmission by bite, the financial constraints that limit diagnostic laboratories to testing only specimens from animals directly involved in a human or domestic animal exposure to RABV (Wilson *et al.* 1997), and the public health community's general assumption that rodents, with the exception of large-bodied species, carry little risk of transmitting RABV. However, rodent species examined are fully susceptible to rabies infection, can transmit RABV by bite, and have been implicated in human rabies infection (Winkler 1991). In some countries rodents have been implicated in the maintenance of RABV, but critical data to support these contentions are elusive (Okoh 1986; Summa *et al.* 1987).

Small terrestrial mammals usually account for the greatest number of individuals and biomass in any mammalian community, and potentially these populations could benefit from rabies epizootics reducing predation pressure. However, virtually nothing is known of the direct effect of rabies on small mammal populations within a community. Therefore, any discussion of the community ecology of rabies is severely limited by the profound, possibly insurmountable, deficit of any representative information on wildlife rabies; most notably rabies among smaller mammals.

12.5 Rabies epizootic expansion

Given the public health importance of rabies, there has been a concerted effort to develop mathematical models to predict the trajectory and velocity of epizootic expansion of rabies in both Europe and North America, and often these models have been used to guide management and control strategies.

12.5.1 European red fox rabies epizootic

For reasons that are not at all clear, western Europe remained relatively rabies-free in the eigteenth and early-nineteenth centuries. The current European epizootic, primarily associated with rabies emergence in the red fox, appears to have begun in Poland sometime during 1939 and has spread westward at a relatively uniform rate of ~30–60 km per year. Red fox reach extraordinarily high densities in urban and suburban locations in Europe and these environments may have contributed to the current epizootic emergence. The current wave front stretches across Germany and most of eastern France where it has been stabilized through an ongoing wildlife control strategy employing oral vaccines whose efficacy has been optimized for the red fox host.

In a series of elegant and influential papers, Murray (Murray *et al.* 1986; Murray 1989; Murray and Seward 1992) modeled the wave front dynamics of red fox rabies as a diffusion process. In the simplest model, the fox population was divided into two groups: infectives (I) and susceptibles (S). Infectives consist of all rabid foxes and those in the incubation phase. More complex models further divide the fox population into an incubating sub-population as well as a recovered or immunized sub-population. For this simple model, however, all foxes once infected die at a rate a. The virus is transmitted to susceptible individuals at a rate r determined by the contact rate between infectives and susceptibles (rSI). Foxes are known to maintain rather fixed home ranges unless they are either rabid or young kits looking to establish a home range (Murray, 1989), so for a non-age-structured population model, the major spatial component will be due to the dispersal of infected animals across the landscape governed by the diffusion coefficient D km^2 per year. The dynamical equations for this simple system are:

$$\frac{\partial S}{\partial t} = -rIS$$

$$\frac{\partial I}{\partial t} = rIS - aI + D\frac{\partial^2 I}{\partial x^2} \qquad (12.1)$$

Although highly simplified, this system reveals many of the important properties of the spatial dynamics of fox rabies (Murray 1989). First, there is a critical threshold for rabies persistence and rabies will die out if the fox population declines below $S_c = a/r$. Second, in regions characterized by fox population densities above the critical threshold, rabies will advance with a wave front velocity:

$$c = 2[D(rS_0 - a)]^{\frac{1}{2}} \qquad (12.2)$$

where S_0 is the density of susceptible foxes prior to the introduction of rabies by infected foxes among neighboring populations.

Diffusion models for red fox rabies have been extended to include intrinsic population dynamics of the foxes, a sub-population of incubating infectives, and an immunized (and therefore non-susceptible) subpopulation. Addition of these biological features suggests a schematic for combined spatial–temporal dynamics of rabies, the overall features of which will be quite general (Box 12.1).

One substantial difficulty in using the diffusion model approach is incorporating habitat and environmental heterogeneity into predicting spatial dynamics. Most often we are interested in where the wave front will emerge from, rather than simply determining the average velocity of an advancing epizootic. The details of the wave front's location are often determined by small-scale environmental features that can cause the wave to bend and curl. One approach to incorporating environmental heterogeneity into a diffusion system is to assign different diffusion coefficients for sub-populations occurring within different habitats. Shigesada and Kawasaki (1997) used this approach in modeling fox-rabies spread across a

Box 12.1 General scheme for endemic and epizootic expansion of rabies

Modeling of rabies population dynamics in raccoons using Equation (12.1) reveals many of the most salient and predictable features of epidemic expansion. These features can be generalized to almost all epidemics. Following incursion of rabies into the "uninfected zone" (Fig. 12.3), the susceptible population declines but then is followed by recurrent epizootics with declining frequency and amplitude (the enzootic phase). The first period of raccoon rabies epizootic is about 48 months and declines at a rate of

approximately 5 months per cycle thereafter. Geographic expansion of rabies occurs at a rate of about 5 km per month. The schematic is a modified form of Murray's (1989) representation of fox rabies expansion in Europe. S_0 is the density of susceptible raccoons prior to the introduction of rabies by infected raccoons among neighboring populations, and S_c is a critical threshold for rabies persistence; rabies will die out if the raccoon population declines below $S_c = a/r$ (see text).

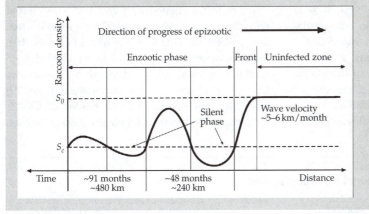

Figure 12.3 Depiction of raccoon rabies temporal dynamics, based on Murray's (1989) representation of fox rabies expansion in Europe. The diagram shows time increasing to the left of the epizootic front, and distance increasing to the right of the front.

heterogeneous landscape where there were two habitat types. Extension of this approach to multiple habitat types, however, can be very difficult.

The dynamics of spread over heterogeneous landscapes is most often influenced by local forces that are generally masked within the diffusion model structure. Alternative approaches (e.g. cellular automata, interactive networks, percolation models) construct the global spatial dynamics from explicit local (often heterogeneous) interactions. Using the North American raccoon rabies epizootic as a test system, we have used an interactive network approach to predict the spatial dynamics of rabies in raccoons.

12.5.2 North American raccoon rabies epizootic

The epizootic associated with raccoons in the eastern Unites States was most likely initiated in the mid-Atlantic region by the translocation of raccoons incubating rabies from an established focus of raccoon rabies in the southeastern Unites States for the

purpose of restocking dwindling local populations (Nettles *et al.* 1979; Smith *et al.* 1984). Since the mid-1970s, this raccoon-adapted variant of RABV has spread north to Maine and Ontario, Canada, and west to Ohio (Krebs *et al.* 2003b), causing one of the most intensive outbreaks of animal rabies ever recorded. The magnitude of this epizootic was enhanced by the spread of virus through naive raccoon populations of very high density, often in states that had not experienced terrestrial rabies for decades (Rupprecht *et al.* 1995). Coincident with epizootic spread has been an increased requirement for postexposure treatment (PET) in humans. For example, in New York (NY) state the number of individuals receiving PET increased from 84 in 1989, prior to the introduction of raccoon rabies, to 1125 in 1992 and 2905 in 1993 (Anonymous 1994).

Our first strategy in developing a predictive model for rabies spread relied on surveillance data from the epizootic that swept across the state of Connecticut (CT) from 1991 through 1996 (Wilson *et al.* 1997). Using an interactive network approach

(Box 12.2), we modeled the stochastic spread of raccoon rabies across the 169 CT townships, incorporating environmental heterogeneity, local transmission and long-distance translocation (LDT) (Smith *et al*. 2002). In our simulations, transport and movement of infected animals was at a smaller spatial scale than the translocation that initiated the east coast epidemic. The movement of individual animals across very great distances (such as the translocation across regions from Florida to the Virginia/West Virginia border) is very rare. However, shorter jumps well in advance of the wave-front (such as those crossing several state townships) may be quite common. In our simulations we included parameters that dictated the probability of these shorter LDT events.

We compared the predictive power of five alternative models where each model represented different weighted combinations of effects due to rivers, human population density, and global transport of infection. Our stochastic spatial simulator was able to mimic the spread of rabies only when environmental heterogeneity was incorporated into the model. The best fit model suggested that slower local spread of rabies was strongly associated with river crossings, that the global spread by translocation was relatively frequent, and that human population density had very little effect on the local spread of rabies. In a separate study, we demonstrated how human population density influenced the magnitude of raccoon rabies epizootics but not the time to first detection (Childs *et al*. 2001).

Townships separated by rivers had a seven-fold reduction in local transmission. All of the models that incorporated slowing at rivers had a better fit than the alternative models without rivers. Even though local transmission accounted for most transmission, LDT of rabid animals was important. Of the 159 townships not on the western border of CT, 21 townships (13%) recorded their first case of raccoon

---

Box 12.2 Interactive network model for rabies spread

An infected township, *i*, infects its adjacent neighbor, *j*, at a rate λ_{ij}. In addition, a township *j* may become infected because of translocation of rabid raccoons at a rate μ_j. Heterogeneity can be incorporated into the model by allowing the local rates from the neighbors $[\lambda_{ij}]$ and the rate of translocation $[\mu_j]$ to be functions of local habitat characteristics.

The probability that a township remained uninfected over time was modeled as a simple stochastic decay process, schematically represented in Fig. 12.4.

The simulation algorithm used to execute this process involves six steps. (1) First, compute the total rate of infection in the *j*th township, δ_j, where, $\delta_j = \mu_j X_j + \sum_i \lambda_{ij} X_j (1 - X_i)$, $X_j = 1$ if the *j*th township is uninfected and $X_j = 0$ otherwise. (2) Add the township rates to compute a total rate, $\Lambda = \sum_j \delta_j$.

(3) Third, compute the waiting time before a township becomes infected assuming that waiting times are exponentially distributed. (4) Fourth, check to see if any of the edges have become infected in the elapsed interval. (5) If no edges have become infected, select a random township to infect. (6) Infect the forced edge or the infected township, update the local rates, and repeat until each township becomes infected. Forced edges correspond to those

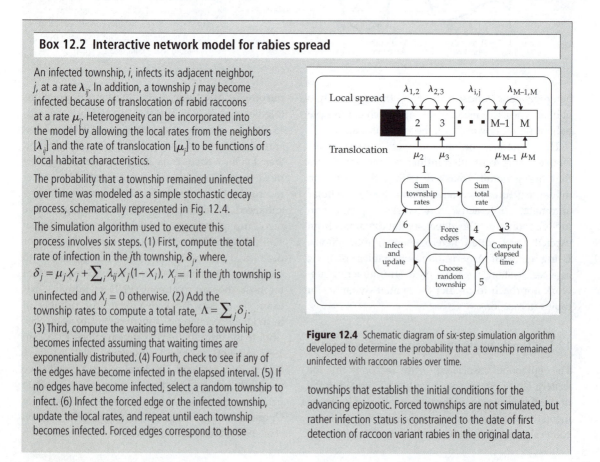

Figure 12.4 Schematic diagram of six-step simulation algorithm developed to determine the probability that a township remained uninfected with raccoon rabies over time.

townships that establish the initial conditions for the advancing epizootic. Forced townships are not simulated, but rather infection status is constrained to the date of first detection of raccoon variant rabies in the original data.

rabies when none of the adjacent townships were infected. All of the outlying townships identified by our model experienced rabies earlier than predicted probably caused in most circumstances by LDT.

The combined effects of spatial heterogeneity and LDT generate a complicated history of geographic spread. Our initial assessment, for example, does not adequately differentiate between LDT events that result in secondary foci for spread versus those LDT events that fade-out. Smith *et al.* (2005) have reformulated the interactive network model into a Network-Distance Model with different classes of LDT events and additional types of environmental heterogeneity. In our reanalysis, we found that most of the LDT events in the CT data failed to form secondary foci and that the river effect interacted with the degree of forest cover. Specifically, the effect of rivers on rates of spread was even greater when coupled with dense forest cover.

The interaction between forest cover and local transmission can lead to some direct recommendations for strategic management. In riparian areas with greater than 12% forest cover there was effectively no local transmission. Extensive riparian habitat may effectively contain the spread of rabies without vaccine intervention because these habitats are highly favored by raccoons. Once individuals have established home ranges in these habitats, they may show little propensity for dispersal and young animals may find it easier to establish new home ranges in these resource rich areas. Consequently, vaccine bait delivery might be most effective when targeted for areas of riparian habitat with less than 12% forest cover.

To assess the consequences of a seven-fold delay crossing rivers on the overall dynamics of rabies, we further simulated the epizootic with and without rivers and with and without LDT. Rivers delayed the appearance of rabies in southeastern CT by approximately 16 months without translocation and by 11 months with translocation (Lucey *et al.* 2002). We conclude that environmental heterogeneities have played a significant role in determining the rate and direction of epizootic expansion of this important disease.

We tested the predictive power of the spatial simulator against an independent spatiotemporal dataset for time-to-first-detection of raccoon rabies across the 754 townships of NY (Russell *et al.* 2004).

We simulated the spread of rabies across NY using the previously derived best-fit parameters for CT. Using these simulation parameters, we tested the predictive capabilities of the model for the first 106 months corresponding to the available surveillance data indicating the northernmost extent of the raccoon rabies epizootic. The model captured the dynamics of the first 48 months but we witnessed a significant deviation away from the predicted rate of spread after month 48 (Fig. 12.5).

After month 48 the predicted trajectory for rabies spread in the northeastern townships (Fig. 12.5, gray triangles, $y = 0.9521x$) was similar to that of the first 48 months. However, the rate of rabies spread in townships in the northwestern portion of the state was approximately 30% lower than our model predicted ($y = 0.667x$, $R^2 = 0.27$, $P < 0.001$, Fig. 12.5, black triangles). Month 49 corresponded with the epizootic wave front colliding with two very different spatial obstacles; townships distributing vaccine for raccoon rabies control and the Adirondack Mountains.

By 1995, the NY Department of Health and Cornell University had begun distributing oral

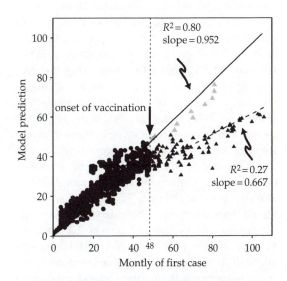

Figure 12.5 Relationship between model predictions and observed time to first appearance for the first 106 months of the New York epidemic. The best-fit line for the first 48 months (black circles) is shown by the solid black line ($y = 0.9521x$, $R^2 = 0.7974$, $P < 0.0001$). The best-fit line after the onset of vaccination (black triangles) is shown by the dashed line ($y = 0.667x$, $R^2 = 0.27$, $P < .001$). The gray triangles correspond to townships in the northern portion of New York State along the Hudson River – Lake Champlain corridor. Post vaccination townships experience a 30% reduction in rate of spread relative to that predicted by the general model. From Russell *et al.* (2004).

vaccine for immunizing raccoons against rabies (Hanlon and Rupprecht 1998) at two primary sites at the northeastern and northwestern edges of the Adirondack Mountain range in front of the advancing epizootic (C. Trimarchi, *personal communication*). Our observation that the average rate of rabies spread declined markedly from the predicted rate at a time and location coincident with vaccination is consistent with an interpretation of vaccine-mediated reduction in the rate of epizootic spread. However, this attractive conclusion is confounded. The coniferous forests of the Adirondack Mountains are not a preferred habitat for raccoons (Merriam 1886) and raccoon population density in this region is extremely low (Godin 1977). The abrupt change in habitat and forest composition (coniferous forest from deciduous forest) would have a substantial effect on raccoon population densities and contact rates, which influence transmission dynamics.

Simulation of raccoon rabies spread into novel geographic areas can be used for more than model validation. It can be an essential tool for strategic planning and control. In late July, 2004, raccoon rabies was detected in Lake County, Ohio (OH), 11 km west of the ORV vaccine barrier along the OH and Pennsylvania (PA) border. In collaboration with the US Department of Agriculture (USDA), the State of OH, and CDC, and using the geographic locations of rabid raccoons, we simulated the likely trajectory of rabies spread across OH using the CT–NY model (Russell *et al.* 2005). The picture that emerged from several different scenarios suggests that rabies, if unchecked, will spread across the middle of the state where there are few environmental impediments or barriers. With no effective physical barriers in this region, rabies would reach the western boundary of OH in only 36 months and could travel at over 2.5 times the velocity of any previously recorded rabies epizootic. If the disease is not confined within OH the limits to raccoon variant rabies spread are defined only by the geographic distribution of its host and rabies would rapidly establish itself in raccoons throughout the mid-western Unites States.

Once the epizootic wave front passes through a geographic region rabies will establish itself endemically and be governed by local density-dependent dynamics (Box 12.1). The long-term behavior of time-series of case occurrence at a given geographic location should then reveal the underlying density dependent host–pathogen population dynamics, which we address below.

12.6 Temporal dynamics within geographic locations

The temporal dynamics of epizootic rabies in red foxes in Europe was first modeled by Anderson *et al.* (1981). They constructed a simple dynamical systems model for the interaction between fox populations (partitioned into subclasses representing susceptible, infectious, and recovered/immune hosts) and rabies in a nonspatial framework. Their model accounted for many of the salient features of the temporal dynamics of red fox rabies, which includes predicting the observed 3–5 year population cycle of foxes infected with rabies, the existence of a critical threshold for local rabies epidemics, and predictions on average prevalence. They also extended the models to incorporate control strategies, that is, a mixture of culling or vaccinating foxes.

Coyne *et al.* (1989) used an analogous form of the Anderson *et al.* (1981) model to explore raccoon rabies temporal population dynamics, including an inquiry into the relative efficacy of culling versus vaccination of raccoons. They partitioned the total raccoon population into categories of susceptible raccoon hosts (X), exposed hosts (i.e. H_1, infected but not infectious), hosts exposed that develop immunity (H_2), rabid hosts (Y), and hosts that are immune (I).

The population dynamics were governed by the following differential equations:

$$\frac{dX}{dt} = a(X + I) - (b + \beta Y + \gamma N)X$$

$$\frac{dH_1}{dt} = \rho\beta XY - (b + \sigma + \gamma N)H_1$$

$$\frac{dH_2}{dt} = (1 - \rho)\beta XY - (b + \sigma + \gamma N)H_2 \qquad (12.3)$$

$$\frac{dY}{dt} = \sigma H_1 - (b + \alpha + \gamma N)Y$$

$$\frac{dI}{dt} = \sigma H_2 - (b + \gamma N)I$$

where N is the total raccoon population size $(X+H_1+H_2+Y+I)$. The dynamic changes in the five compartments of this model are governed by the parameter values for birth rate = a, death rate = b, density-dependent mortality = γ, incubation period = $1/\sigma$, rabies-induced mortality = α, transmission rate = β, and proportion of raccoons that develop natural immunity = $(1-\rho)$.

The *qualitative* predictions of this model are: (1) the first epizootic period should be approximately 48 months, (2) subsequent epizootics should occur with diminishing period (i.e. increasing frequency), and (3) epizootics should occur with decreasing amplitude. The *quantitative* predictions of this model, particularly the rate of diminishing period and amplitude, i.e., the rate of damping in oscillation, depends most strongly on $(1-\rho)$, the proportion of infected raccoons developing viral immunity (see Box 12.1).

To match predictions from the SEIR model to observed data, we constructed a phenomenological algorithm for defining when epizootics occurred based on the time series of reports on rabid raccoon numbers by US counties along the eastern seaboard (Childs *et al.* 2000). First, for each county the median number of reported rabid raccoons per month was determined from CDC data. Second, an epizootic was defined as beginning when the monthly number of rabid raccoons reported was greater than the county median for two consecutive months and ended when this number was less than the county median for two consecutive months. We also required that an epizootic have a minimum duration of five months to reduce the short-term variation in reporting. We applied this algorithm to empirical data gathered through national surveillance to measure the duration of successive epizootic and inter-epizootic intervals which together define the epizootic period.

Marked periodicity in rabid raccoons was apparent in many of the time series of county surveillance data. The median value for the first epizootic period was 48 months and there was a dominant mode between 41 and 60 months. The epizootic period declined by approximately 5 months between each successive epizootic.

We then applied the same epizootic algorithm to numerical solutions to the SEIR model for different parameter sets of the SEIR. Our observed median values of 14 months for the duration of the first epizootic and 48 months for the first epizootic period fit the predicted time series from the SEIR at the parameter set corresponding to low levels of immunity, $\rho = 1\text{--}5\%$. Variation in the transmission rate β by ± 25% had little effect on the quantitative structure of the model predictions. Epizootic periods subsequent to the first also were predicted to decline to about 65–80% of the first epizootic period by the fourth epizootic.

The combined use of data- and model-analysis suggests that raccoon rabies, once established in a specific spatial location, undergoes predictable damped oscillatory dynamics with a first epidemic period of approximately 48 months; the period of subsequent epizootic cycles declined by approximately 5 months per cycle. Our analysis illustrates how models when judged against data can be used to establish the most likely values of important population parameters; in our case, establishing bounds on the probability of acquiring natural immunity. Previous studies had suggested the likelihood of acquiring immunity may be as high as 20% in raccoons, but our analysis suggests that the maximum immunity expected would be < 5%. We are sure that sensitivity analyses of population parameters coupling models and data will become a standard feature of future research in disease ecology.

12.7 Host population dynamics and rabies virus spillover

Our results show distinctive *and predictable* temporal patterning to epizootic rabies occurring among raccoons at the level of counties. Although models of rabies–host population dynamics were developed for a single RABV variant circulating within the specific reservoir host population, public and veterinary health officials and, increasingly, conservation biologists are most concerned about spillover of RABV to domestic animals, livestock, wildlife, and to humans. The dynamic pattern of sequential epizootic and inter-epizootic intervals predicted from the time series data from individual counties provides a qualitative measure of each county's unique history with raccoon rabies (Box 12.1). This qualitative pattern can then be combined with quantitative values captured by national surveillance for animal rabies (Krebs *et al.* 2003a) to model the risk of rabies occurring among secondarily, and incidentally infected species (Gordon *et al.* 2004).

We developed logistic regression models to assess the risk of rabies among domestic cats as a function of the temporal stage of an epizootic within a county, the magnitude of monthly reports of rabid raccoons and total raccoons tested, and the human population size within the reporting county (Gordon *et al.* 2004). Domestic cats were chosen because they have been the domestic animal most frequently reported rabid in the Unites States since 1992 (Krebs *et al.* 2003a), and are responsible for many of the human PET for rabies in the United States (Moore *et al.* 2000; Moran *et al.* 2000). We included surveillance data on rabid skunks and all skunks tested for rabies as an independent covariate with raccoons. Several northeastern states, most notably Massachusetts (MA) and Rhode Island (RI), have recently reported greater numbers of rabid

skunks than rabid raccoons in their regions suggesting that skunks may serve to maintain raccoon-variant RABV transmission for a time when raccoon numbers are low (Guerra *et al.* 2003).

Our analysis included 129 counties from CT, MA, New Hampshire (NH), NY, RI, and Vermont (VT) (Fig. 12.6). After excluding cases of rabid animals infected with a red fox variant of RABV in counties along the Canadian border, we found that the risk for rabies among cats, measured as the odds ratio (OR), was strongly linked to the temporal dynamics of raccoon rabies, based on increases relative to the pre-raccoon epizootic era (defined as the time period including all months from the pre-raccoon variant interval and the pre-epizootic interval). Because the risk for rabies among cats was identical among epizootic cycles subsequent to the first, we only distinguished the components of the first epizootic cycle, epizootic and inter-epizootic intervals (Fig. 12.6). Rabies risk for cats was greatest during the first raccoon epizootic stage (greater than 12-fold the pre-epizootic level) declined to

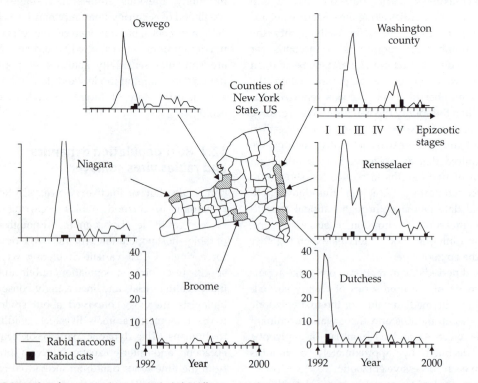

Figure 12.6 Number of raccoons and cats reported rabid at different epizootic temporal stages in Oswego, Washington, Rensselaer, Dutchess, Broome, and Niagara counties, New York (NY), from 1992 to 2000.

approximately 6-fold baseline risk into the first inter-epizootic interval, and then remained elevated at 7.5-fold baseline risk into intervals subsequent to the end of the first epizootic cycle. Independent of the temporal stage of raccoon rabies, risk for rabies in cats increased with the increasing number of rabid skunks (OR = 2.5 per 10 positive skunks). The risk for rabies among cats was significantly lowest among counties with the highest quartile of human population density and increased significantly with decreasing quartiles of human population density to 1.7-, 1.9-, and 2.5-fold the highest density quartile, indicating a pronounced urban–rural gradient. Rural cat owners are more prone to allowing their cats to roam freely in the outdoors, and large populations of stray and feral cats exist in rural areas. Unvaccinated cats from rural locations have disproportionately contributed to annual counts of rabid cats (Jenkins and Winkler 1987; Eng and Fishbein 1990).

These analyses demonstrated a strong association between risks of rabies spillover to an important secondary species and the temporal dynamics of rabies in a wildlife reservoir. The greatest risk for rabies among cats was associated with epizootics among the raccoon host, but notably, the monthly counts of rabid skunks also contributed to the logistic model outcome. There was a persistent, elevated risk for rabies among cats subsequent to the termination of the first epizootic cycle, as had been noted by descriptive studies. For example, in Maryland, the number of rabid cats did not decline over a 9-year period, even as rabid raccoon counts dwindled, but remained at relatively stable levels far higher than existed before the raccoon variant entered the state (Fogelman *et al.* 1993). The mechanism(s) for rabies spillover remains unclear, although transient transmission by skunks may play a role; there are no molecular data or epidemiologic data to suggest that host shifts have established an independent cycle of maintenance among skunks (Guerra *et al.* 2003).

12.8 Research priorities

In closing, we highlight what we believe to be the major research questions in rabies evolutionary and community ecology. The research questions are directed at each of the major subheadings above,

that is, issues relating to the virus, issues relating to spatial dynamics, temporal dynamics, and spillover and host-shift within a community context:

1. What determines the conditions under which an epidemic will originate? Are there community changes that give rise to conditions for epidemic emergence? For example, are the population densities of meso-predators, such as raccoons and foxes, influenced by the removal of top-level carnivores, such as wolves, in such a way as to increase the likelihood of rabies emergence?
2. What are the community effects of rabies? How does the rabies mediated decline in meso-predators influence the population densities and species interactions among the prey (e.g. small mammals, birds) of these meso-predators?
3. What are the major phylogeographic distributions of RABV variants and how are these distributions affected by patterns of epidemic expansion and host range distribution?
4. What is the role of long distance translocation/ dispersal on patterns of epidemic expansion and phylogeographic variation at a variety of spatial scales?
5. How, and under what circumstances, do new reservoir hosts arise? For example, as dog rabies decreases in Asia and Africa, will new wildlife reservoirs emerge?
6. What are the molecular adaptations in RABV variants that promote or maintain species-specific distributions and geographic differentiation? Are there molecular correlates with novel host emergence?
7. What are the mechanisms that maintain persistence in endemic rabies? Given the high lethality of RABV, why does it not just burn out? Are communities with higher richness of potential host species more or less likely to maintain the virus?

By addressing at least this minimal set of questions, we hope to illustrate how rabies can remain a major model for understanding the ecology and evolution of host–pathogen systems in general.

Acknowledgments

We would like to thank Caroline Henderson, David Smith, Colin Russell, Lance Waller, Tracy Lambert

Jack, Susan Nadin-Davis, Roly Tinline, Chuck Rupprecht, Cathy Hanlon, and Roman Biek for their many helpful suggestions on research issues and collaboration on rabies projects. Roman Biek kindly constructed the phylogenetic trees in Fig. 12.1. This research was supported by NIH RO1 AI047498 and USDA 03 7100 4129 CA (to LAR).

References

Alonge, D. O. and S. A. Abu. (1984). Rabie is Ghana, West Africa. *Journal of Zoonoses* **11**:53–58.

Anderson, R. M., H. C. Jackson, R. M. May, and A. M. Smith. (1981). Population dynamics of fox rabies in Europe. *Nature* **289**:765–771.

Anonymous. (1994). Raccoon rabies epizootic—United States 1993. *Morbidity and Mortality Weekly Report* **43**:269–273.

Arai, Y. T., H. Takahashi, Y. Kameoka, T. Shiimo, O. Wimalaratne, and D. L. Lodmell. (2001). Characterization of Sri Lanka rabies virus isolates using nucleotide sequence analysis of nucleoprotein gene. *Acta Virologica* **45**:327–333.

Arai, Y. T., I. V. Kuzmin, Y. Kameoka, and A. D. Botvinkin. (2003). New lyssavirus genotype from the Lesser Mouse-eared Bat (*Myotis blythi*) Kyrghystan. *Emerging Infectious Diseases* **9**:333–337.

Bacon, P. J. (1985). Population dynamics of rabies in wildlife, Pages 358pp. Academic Press, London, Orlando.

Bingham, J., C. M. Foggin, A. I. Wandeler, and F. W. Hill. (1999a). The epidemiology of rabies in Zimbabwe. 1. Rabies in dogs (*Canis familiaris*). *Onderstepoort Journal of Veterinary Research* **66**:1–10.

Bingham, J., C. M. Foggin, A. I. Wandeler, and F. W. Hill. (1999b). The epidemiology of rabies in Zimbabwe. 2. Rabies in jackals (*Canis adustus* and *Canis mesomelas*). *Onderstepoort Journal of Veterinary Research* **66**:11–23.

Bourliere F. (1975). Mammals, small and large: the ecological implications of size. In *Small Mammals: Their Productivity and Population Dynamics*, ed. F.B. Golley, K. Petrusewicz, L. Ryszkowski, 1.1:1–8. Cambridge University Press, Cambridge.

Bourhy, H., B. Kissi, L. Audry, M. Smreczak, M. Sadkowska-Todys, K. Kulonen *et al.* (1999). Ecology and evolution of rabies virus in Europe. *Journal of General Virology* **80**:2545–2557.

Burrows, R. (1992). Rabies in wild dogs. *Nature* **359**:277.

Chew R. M. (1978). Impact on the ecosystem. In D. P. Snyder, ed. *Populations of Small Mammals Under Natural Conditions*, pp. 167–180. University of Pittsburgh Press, Pittsburgh, PA.

Childs J. E., L. Colby, J. W. Krebs, T. Strine, M. Feller *et al.* (1997). Surveillance and spatiotemporal associations of rabies in rodents and lagomorphs in the United States 1985–1994. *Journal of Wildlife Diseases* **33**(1):20–27.

Childs, J. E., A. T. Curns, M. E. Dey, L. A. Real, L. Feinstein, O. N. Bjornstad, *et al.* (2000). Predicting the local dynamics of epizootic rabies among raccoons in the United States [comment]. *Proceedings of the National Academy of Sciences of the United States of America* **97**:13666–13671.

Childs, J. E., A. T. Curns, M. E. Dey, A. L. Real, C. E. Rupprecht, and J. W. Krebs. (2001). Rabies epizootics among raccoons vary along a North–South gradient in the Eastern United States. *Vector Borne & Zoonotic Diseases* **1**:253–267.

Cleaveland, S. and C. Dye. (1995). Maintenance of a microparasite infecting several host species: rabies in the Serengeti. *Parasitology* **111**:S33–S47.

Coyne, M. J., G. Smith, and F. E. McAllister. (1989). Mathematic model for the population biology of rabies in raccoons in the mid-Atlantic states. *American Journal of Veterinary Research* **50**:2148–2154.

David, D., B. Yakobson, J. S. Smith, and Y. Stram. (2000). Molecular epidemiology of rabies virus isolates from Isreal and other middle- and Near-Eastern countries. *Journal of Clinical Microbiology* **38**:755–762.

De Mattos, C. A., M. Favi, V. Yung, C. Pavletic, and C. C. De Mattos. (2000). Bat rabies in urban centers in Chile. *Journal of Wildlife Diseases* **36**:231–240.

De Mattos, C. C., C. A. De Mattos, E. Loza-Rubio, A. Aguilar-Setien, L. A. Orciari, and J. S. Smith. (1999). Molecular characterization of rabies virus isolates from Mexico: implications for transmission dynamics and human risk. *American Journal of Tropical Medicine and Hygiene* **61**:587–597.

East, M. L., H. Hofer, J. H. Cox, U. Wulle, H. Wiik, and C. Pitra. (2001). Regular exposure to rabies virus and lack of symptomatic disease in Serengeti spotted hyenas. *Proceedings of the National Academy of Sciences of the United States of America* **98**:15026–15031.

Eng, T. R. and D. B. Fishbein. (1990). Epidemiologic factors, clinical findings, and vaccination status of rabies in cats and dogs in the United States in 1988. National Study Group on Rabies. *Journal of the American Veterinary Medical Association* **197**:201–209.

Everard, C. O. and J. D. Everard. (1992). Mongoose rabies in the Caribbean. *Annals of the New York Academy of Sciences* **653**:356–366.

Ezeokoli, C. D. and J. U. Umoh. (1987). Epidemiology of rabies in northern Nigeria. *Transactions of the Royal Society of Tropical Medicine and Hygiene* **81**:268–272.

Fogelman, V., H. R. Fischman, J. T. Horman, and J. K. Grigor. (1993). Epidemiologic and clinical characteristics of rabies in cats. *Journal of the American Veterinary Medical Association* **202**:1829–1833.

Fooks, A. R., L. M. McElhinney, D. J. Pounder, C. J. Finnegan, K. Mansfield, N. Johnson *et al.* (2003). Case report: isolation of a European bat lyssavirus type 2a from a fatal human case of rabies encephalitis. *Journal of Medical Virology* **71**:281–289.

Fooks, A. R., D. Selden, S. M. Brookes, N. Johnson, D. A. Marston, T. A. Jolliffe, *et al.* (2004). Identification of a European bat lyssavirus type 2 in a Daubenton's bat found in Lancashire. *The Veterinary Record* **155**:606–607.

Godin, A. J. (1977). *Wild Mammals of New England.* Johns Hopkins University Press, Baltimore.

Gordon, E. R., A. T. Curns, J. W. Krebs, C. E. Rupprecht, L. A. Real, and J. E. Childs. (2004). Temporal dynamics of rabies in a wildlife host and the risk of cross-species transmission. *Epidemiology and Infection* **132**:515–524.

Gould, A.R., A. D. Hyatt, R. Lunt, J. A. Kattenbelt, S. Hengstberger, and S. D. Balcksell. (1998). Characterization of a novel lyssavirus isolated from Pteropid bats in Australia. *Virus Research* **54**: 165–187.

Guerra, M. A., A. T. Curns, C. E. Rupprecht, C. A. Hanlon, J. W. Krebs, and J. E. Childs. (2003). Skunk and raccoon rabies in the eastern United States: temporal and spatial analysis. *Emerging Infectious Diseases* **9**:1143–1150.

Hanlon, C. A. and C. E. Rupprecht. (1998). The reemergence of rabies. In W. M. Scheld, D. Armstrong, and J. M. Hughes, eds. *Emerging infections*, pp. 59–80. Washington, DC, ASM Press.

Holmes, E. C., C. H. Woelk, R. Kassis, and H. Bourhy. (2002). Genetic constraints and the adaptive evolution of rabies virus in nature. *Virology* **292**:247–257.

Jayakumar, R., K. G. Tirumurugaan, G. Ganga, K. Kumanan, and N. A. Mahalinga. (2004). Characterization of nucleoprotein gene sequence of an Indian isolate of rabies virus. *Acta Virologica* **48**:47–50.

Jenkins, S. R. and W. G. Winkler. (1987). Descriptive epidemiology from an epizootic of raccoon rabies in the Middle Atlantic States, 1982–1983. *American Journal of Epidemiology* **126**:429–437.

Jenkins, S. R., B. Perry, and W. Winkler. (1988). Ecology and epidemiology of raccoon rabies. *Reviews of Infectious Diseases* **10**(suppl.):S620–S625.

Johnson, N., C. Black, J. Smith, H. Un, L. M. McElhinney, O. Aylan *et al.* (2003a). Rabies emergence among foxes in Turkey. *Journal of Wildlife Diseases* **39**:262–270.

Johnson, N., D. Selden, G. Parsons, D. Healy, S. M. Brookes, L. M. McElhinney, *et al.* (2003b). Isolation of a European bat lyssavirus type 2 from a Daubenton's bat in the United Kingdom. *The Veterinary Record* **152**:383–387.

Johnson, N., M. Letshwenyo, E. K. Baipoledi, G. Thobokwe, and A. R. Fooks. (2004). Molecular epidemiology of rabies in Botswana: a comparison between antibody typing and nucleotide sequence phylogeny. *Veterinary Microbiology* **101**:31–38.

Kat, P. W., K. A. Alexander, J. S. Smith, J. D. Richardson, and L. Munson. (1996). Rabies among African wild dogs (*Lycaon pictus*) in the Masai Mara, Kenya. *Journal of Veterinary Diagnostic Investigation* **8**:420–426.

King, A. A., C. D. Meredith, and G. R. Thomson. (1994). The biology of southern African lyssavirus variants. *Current Topics in Microbiology and Immunology* **187**: 267–295.

Krebs, J. W., J. T. Wheeling, and J. E. Childs. (2003a). Rabies surveillance in the United States during 2002. *Journal of the American Veterinary Medical Association* **223**:1736–1748.

Krebs, J. W., S. M. Williams, J. S. Smith, C. E. Rupprecht, and J. E. Childs. (2003b). Rabies among infrequently reported mammalian carnivores in the United States, 1960–2000. *Journal of Wildlife Diseases* **39**:253–261.

Kuzmin, I. V., L. A. Orciari, Y. T. Arai, J. S. Smith, C. A. Hanlon, Y. Kameoka, *et al.* (2003). Bat lyssaviruses (*Aravan and Khugand*) from Central Asia: phylogenetic relationships according to N, P and G gene sequences. *Virus Research* **97**:65–79.

Loza-Rubio, E., A. Aguilar-Setien, C. Bahloul, B. Brochier, P. P. Pastoret, and N. Tordo. (1999). Discrimination between epidemiological cycles of rabies in Mexico. *Archives of Medical Research* **30**:144–149.

Lucey, B. T., C. A. Russell, D. Smith, M. L. Wilson, A. Long, L. A. Waller, *et al.* (2002). Spatiotemporal analysis of epizootic raccoon rabies propagation in Connecticut, 1991–1995. *Vector Borne and Zoonotic Diseases* **2**:77–86.

Merriam, C. H. (1886). *The Mammals of the Adirondack Region: Northeastern New York.* Clinton Holt and Company, New York.

Messenger, S. L., C. E. Rupprecht, and J. S. Smith. (2003). Bats, emerging virus infections, and the rabies paradigm. In T. H. Kunz and M. B. Fenton, eds. *Bat Ecology*, pp. 622–679. University of Chicago Press, Chicago.

Monson, M. H. (1985). Practical management of rabies and the 1982 outbreak in Zorzor District, Liberia. *Tropical Doctor* **15**:50–54.

Moore, D. A., W. M. Sischo, A. Hunter, and T. Miles. (2000). Animal bite epidemiology and surveillance for rabies postexposure prophylaxis. *Journal of the American Veterinary Medical Association* **217**:190–194.

Moran, G. J., D. A. Talan, W. Mower, M. Newdow, S. Ong, J. Y. Nakase, *et al.* (2000). Appropriateness of rabies postexposure prophylaxis treatment for animal exposures. Emergency ID Net Study Group. *Journal of the American Medical Association* **284**:1001–1007.

Muller, T., J. Cox, W. Peter, R. Schafer, N. Johnson, L. M. McElhinney, *et al.* (2004). Spill-over of European bat lyssavirus type 1 into stone marten (*Martes foina*) in Germany. *Journal of Veterinary Medicine Series B: Infectious Diseases and Public Health* **51**:49–54.

Murray, J. D. (1989). *Mathematical Biology*, Springer-Verlag, New York.

Murray, J. D. and W. L. Seward. (1992). On the spatial spread of rabies among foxes with immunity. *Journal of Theoretical Biology* **156**:327–348.

Murray, J. D., E. A. Stanley, and D. L. Brown. (1986). On the spatial spread of rabies among foxes. *Proceedings of the Royal Society of London, Biology* **229**:111–150.

Nadin-Davis, S. A. (2000). Rabies and rabies-related viruses. In R. C. A. Thompson, ed. *Molecular Epidemiology of Infectious Diseases*, pp. 245–257. Arnold, London.

Nanayakkara, S., J. S. Smith, and C. E. Rupprecht. (2003). Rabies in Sri Lanka: splendid isolation. *Emerging Infectious Diseases* **9**:368–371.

Nathwani, D., P. G. McIntyre, K. White, A. J. Shearer, N. Reynolds, D. Walker, *et al.* (2003). Fatal human rabies caused by European bat Lyssavirus type 2a infection in Scotland. *Clinical Infectious Diseases* **37**:598–601.

Nel, L., J. Jacobs, J. Jaftha, and C. Meredith. (1997). Natural spillover of a distinctly Canidae-associated biotype of rabies virus into an expanded wildlife host range in southern Africa. *Virus Genes* **15**:79–82.

Nettles, V. F., J. H. Shaddock, R. K. Sikes, and C. R. Reyes. (1979). Rabies in translocated raccoons. *American Journal of Public Health* **69**:601–602.

Nishizono, A., K. Mannen, L. P. Elio-Villa, S. Tanaka, K. S. Li, K. Mifune, *et al.* (2002). Genetic analysis of rabies virus isolates in the Philippines. *Microbiology and Immunology* **46**:413–417.

Novelli, V. M. and P. Malankar. (1991). Epizootic of fox rabies in the Sultanate of Oman. *Transactions of the Royal Society of Tropical Medicine and Hygiene* **85**:543.

Okoh, A. E. (1986). Investigation of possible rabies reservoirs in rodents in Nigeria. *International Journal of Zoonoses.* **13**:1–5.

Patabendige, C. G. and O. Wimalaratne. (2003). Rabies in mongooses and domestic rats in the southern province of Sri Lanka. *Ceylon Medical Journal* **48**:48–50.

Picard-Meyer, E., J. Barrat, E. Tissot, M. J. Barrat, V. Bruyere, and F. Cliquet. (2004). Genetic analysis of European bat lyssavirus type 1 isolates from France. *The Veterinary Record* **154**:589–595.

Prather, E. C., W. J. Bigler, G. L. Hoff, and J. A. Tomas. (1975). *Rabies in Florida: History, Status, and Trends.* Jacksonville, FL, Division of Health, Department of Health and Rehabilitative Services, State of Florida.

Rupprecht, C. E., L. T. Glickman, P. A. Spencer, and T. J. Wiktor. (1987). Epidemiology of rabies virus variants: differentiation using monoclonal antibodies and discriminant analysis. *American Journal of Epidemiology* **126**:298–309.

Rupprecht, C. E., J. S. Smith, M. Fekadu, and J. E. Childs. (1995). The ascension of wildlife rabies: a cause for public health concern or intervention? *Emerging Infectious Diseases* **1**:107–114.

Russell, C. A., D. L. Smith, L. A. Waller, J. E. Childs, and A. L. Real. (2004). *A priori* prediction of disease invasion dynamics in a novel environment. *Proceedings of the Royal Society of London, Biology* **271**:21–25.

Russell, C. A., D. L. Smith, J. E. Childs, and L. A. Real. (2005). Predictive spatial dynamics and strategic planning for raccoon rabies emergence in Ohio. *PloS Biology* **3**(3):e88.

Sacramento, D., H. Badrane, H. Bourhy, and N. Tordo. (1992). Molecular epidemiology of rabies virus in France: comparison with vaccine strains. *Journal of General Virology* **73**:1149–1158.

Sato, G., T. Itou, Y. Shoji, Y. Miura, T. Mikami, M. Ito, *et al.* (2004). Genetic and phylogenetic analysis of glycoprotein of rabies virus isolated from several species in Brazil. *Journal of Veterinary Medical Science* **66**:747–753.

Shigesada, N. and K. Kawasaki. (1997). *Biological Invasions.* Oxford University Press, Oxford.

Sillero-Zubiri, C., A. A. King, and D. W. Macdonald. (1996). Rabies and mortality in Ethiopian wolves (*Canis simensis*). *Journal of Wildlife Diseases* **32**:80–86.

Smith, D. L., B. Lucey, L. A. Waller, J. E. Childs, and L. A. Real. (2002). Predicting the spatial dynamics of rabies epidemics on heterogeneous landscapes. [comment]. *Proceedings of the National Academy of Sciences of the United States of America* **99**:3668–3672.

Smith, D. L., L. A. Waller, C. A. Russell, J. E. Childs, and L. A. Real. (2005). Assessing the role of long-distance translocation and spatial heterogeneity in the raccoon rabies epizootic in Connecticut. *Preventive Veterinary Medicine* (*in press*).

Smith, J. S. and H. D. Seidel. (1993). Rabies: a new look at an old disease. *Progress in Medical Virology* **40**:82–106.

Smith, J. S., J. W. Sumner, L. F. Roumillat, G. M. Baer, and W. G. Winkler. (1984). Antigenic characteristics of isolates associated with a new epizootic of raccoon rabies in the United States. *Journal of Infectious Disease* **149**:769–774.

Smith, J. S., P. A. Yager, W. J. Bigler, and E. C. J. Hartwig. (1990). Surveillance and epidemiologic mapping of monoclonal antibody-defined rabies variants in Florida. *Journal of Wildlife Diseases* **26**:473–485.

Smith, J. S., L. A. Orciari, P. A. Yager, H. D. Seidel, and C. K. Warner. (1992). Epidemiologic and historical relationships among 87 rabies virus isolates as determined by limited sequence analysis. *Journal of Infectious Diseases* **166**:296–307.

Smithcors, J. F. (1958). The history of some current problems in animal diseases VII. Rabies. *Veterinary Medicine* **53**:149–154.

Steele, J. H. and P. J. Fernandez. (1991). History of rabies and global aspects. In G. M. Baer, ed. *The natural history of rabies*, pp. 1–24. CRC Press, Boca Raton, FL.

Steelman, H. G., S. E. Henke, and G. M. Moore. (2000). Bait delivery for oral rabies vaccine to gray foxes. *Journal of Wildlife Diseases* **36**:744–751.

Summa M. E., M. L. Carrieri, S. R. Favoretto, and E. L. Chamelet. (1987). Rabies in the state of Sao Paulo: the rodents question. *Revista do Instituto de Medicina Tropical de Sao Paulo* **29**:53–58.

Susetya, H., M. Sugiyama, A. Inagaki, N. Ito, K. Oraveerakul, N. Traiwanatham, *et al.* (2003). Genetic characterization of rabies field isolates from Thailand. *Microbiology and Immunology* **47**:653–659.

Swofford, D. (2002). *PAUP*. Phylogenetic Analysis Using Parsimony (*and Other Methods), Version 4.0b10*. Sinauer Associates, Sunderland, MA.

Tjornehoj, K., L. Ronsholt, and A. R. Fooks. (2004). Antibodies to EBLV-1 in a domestic cat in Denmark. *The Veterinary Record* **155**:571–572.

von Teichman, B. F., G. R. Thomson, C. D. Meredith, and L. H. Nel. (1995). Molecular epidemiology of rabies virus in South Africa: evidence for two distinct virus groups. *Journal of General Virology* **76**:73–82.

Wagner, R. R. and J. K. Rose. (1996). Rhabdoviridae. In B. N. Fields, D. M. Knipe, and P. M. Howley, eds. *Fields Virology*, pp. 1121–1136. Lippincott-Raven Publishers, Philadelphia, PA.

Wandeler, A., J. Muller, G. Wachendorfer, W. Schale, U. Forster, and F. Steck. (1974a). Rabies in wild carnivores in central Europe. III. Ecology and biology of the fox in relation to control operations. *Zentralblatt Fur Veterinarmedizin- Reihe B* **21**:765–773.

Wandeler, A., G. Wachendorfer, U. Forster, H. Krekel, W. Schale, J. Muller, *et al.* (1974b). Rabies in wild carnivores in central Europe. I. Epidemiological studies. *Zentralblatt Fur Veterinarmedizin- Reihe B* **21**:735–756.

Wandeler, A. I. (2000). Oral immunization against rabies: afterthoughts and foresight. *Schweizer Archiv fur Tierheilkunde* **142**:455–462.

WHO. (1999). World Survey of Rabies No 33. *WHO/CDS/ CSR/APH/* 99 4:1–29.

Wilson, M. L., P. M. Bretsky, J. G. H. Cooper, S. H. Egbertson, H. J. V. Kruiningen, and M. L. Carter. (1997). Emergence of raccoon rabies in Connecticut, 1991–1994: spatial and temporal characteristics of animal infection and human contact. *American Journal of Tropical Medicine & Hygiene* **57**:457–463.

Winkler W. G. (1991). Rodent rabies. In G. M. Baer, ed. *The Natural History of Rabies*, pp. 405–410. CRC Press, Boca Raton, FL.

Wright, A., J. Rampersad, J. Ryan, and D. Ammons. (2002). Molecular characterization of rabies virus isolates from Trinidad. *Veterinary Microbiology* **87**:95–102.

CHAPTER 13

The emergence of Nipah and Hendra virus: pathogen dynamics across a wildlife-livestock-human continuum

Peter Daszak, R. K. Plowright, J. H. Epstein, J. Pulliam, S. Abdul Rahman, H. E. Field, A. Jamaluddin, S. H. Sharifah, C. S. Smith, K. J. Olival, S. Luby, K. Halpin, A. D. Hyatt, A. A. Cunningham, and the Henipavirus Ecology Research Group (HERG)

13.1 Background

Emerging zoonotic pathogens represent a key threat to global public health and constitute around 75% of all known emerging pathogens (Taylor *et al.* 2001, Smolinski *et al.* 2003). Of particular concern are a number of viruses that emerged recently from wildlife, are lethal to humans (e.g. Ebola virus), capable of spreading rapidly (e.g. SARS coronavirus), and have caused recent pandemics (e.g. HIV-1 and Influenza virus) (Morse 1993; Burke 1998). For many of the emerging infectious diseases (EIDs) caused by these viruses, there are few effective therapies, vaccines, or other preventative strategies. Consequently, surveillance and control programs and the development of drug and vaccine candidates are a high priority for public health programs (Smolinski *et al.* 2003). However, control programs require an understanding of the causes of emergence and of host and pathogen population dynamics. This is a challenge because many emerging zoonotic viruses have multiple wildlife reservoir hosts (e.g. hantavirus, West Nile virus) or emerge via complex transmission pathways (e.g. Ebola virus, Nipah virus). To understand this process therefore requires study of viral dynamics within each important wildlife reservoir species (e.g. among age classes and sexes), among reservoir species as well as between reservoir, domestic animal, and human populations. Because viral transmission often requires direct contact between animals, understanding the population dynamics and contact rates at different spatial and temporal scales is also important to understanding disease emergence. The process of disease emergence is usually driven by environmental, ecological, and socio-economic factors that influence wildlife reservoir, vector, and human population dynamics (Daszak *et al.* 2001; Weiss and McMichael 2004). These add new layers of complexity to the process and require an understanding of how these changes affect contact rates and viral dynamics within and among populations, species, and communities.

In this chapter, we review recent research on the emergence of Nipah and Hendra viruses, two lethal zoonotic paramyxoviruses that first emerged from fruit bat reservoirs in Malaysia in 1999 and Australia in 1994, respectively (Murray *et al.* 1995; Chua *et al.* 2000). This research suggests that despite the complexity of Nipah and Hendra virus ecology, their emergence can be understood using a combination of field, laboratory, and simple modeling approaches. These ultimately provide a new predictive strategy for control of future outbreaks.

13.2 Nipah virus

13.2.1 Outbreak in Malaysia, 1998–9

Nipah virus is one of four recently discovered paramyxoviruses: Nipah virus, Hendra virus, Menangle virus, and Tioman virus (Mackenzie 1999; Chua *et al.* 2000). These viruses are all members of the family *Paramyxoviridae*, which includes a number of viruses that have emerged following transmission to a new host species: for example, measles virus, which is thought to have emerged in humans around 10,000 years ago from a host jump by a common ancestor of the cattle viruses rinderpest and peste des petits ruminants (Dobson and Carper 1996); and canine distemper virus, which has emerged in lion, various marine mammals, and ferrets from its domestic dog host (Cleaveland *et al.* 2001). Nipah and Hendra viruses belong to the order *Mononegavirales*, family *Paramyxoviridae*, subfamily *Paramyxovirinae* and genus *Henipavirus* and are thus distinct from all other members of the family. Menangle virus and Tioman virus belong to the same subfamily but genus *Rubulavirus*. Measles, canine distemper and other paramyxoviruses are more distant in evolutionary terms. Serological and viral isolation suggest all four viruses have *Pteropus* spp. fruit bats (flying foxes) as their natural reservoir hosts (Hyatt *et al.* 2004). Three of these viruses have spilled over into human populations following outbreaks in livestock "amplifier" hosts (pigs for Nipah and Menangle viruses; horses for Hendra virus) (Philbey *et al.* 1998; Johara *et al.* 1999; Halpin *et al.* 2000; Chua *et al.* 2002b). Hendra virus emerged in 1994, 1995, 1999, and in 2004 in Australia, causing the death of 19 horses and two of four people who became ill (Field *et al.* 2000, 2001, Field *et al.*, unpublished data). Menangle virus was responsible for extensive mortality of pigs in a 1997 outbreak, and caused severe febrile illness in two pig farmers (Philbey *et al.* 1998).

Nipah virus emerged with dramatic consequences in Malaysia and Singapore in 1999, infecting 265 people and causing the death of 105 people—a case fatality rate of over 39% (Chua *et al.* 2000). The virus was isolated from pigs which exhibited respiratory and often neurological syndromes. The respiratory syndrome was characterized by a loud barking cough, and it was assumed that transmission of Nipah virus among pigs and from pigs to humans occurred via aerosolized droplets containing infectious virus from sloughing of infected epithelial cells of the respiratory tract (Hyatt *et al.* 2001; Middleton *et al.* 2002). Epidemiological investigations revealed that although the majority of human cases were in the Negri Sembilan and Selangor regions of central peninsular Malaysia, the index case (the first human to be infected by the virus) occurred at a large pig farm over six months earlier in the town of Ipoh, Perak State (Fig. 13.1). It appears that movement of infected pigs from the index farm spread the disease into the two southern states, leading to the outbreak (Chua *et al.* 1999, 2000; Field *et al.* 2001; Chua 2003). Approximately one million pigs were slaughtered to control the outbreak, and it is estimated that this virus caused the loss of 36,000 jobs and US$120 million in exports (Nor and Ong 2000). Despite extensive epidemiological investigations, there is little evidence that human-to-human transmission of Nipah virus occurred during this outbreak.

13.2.2 Causes of Nipah virus emergence in Malaysia

To understand the emergence of Nipah virus in Malaysia, we examined two broad environmental changes: deforestation and livestock production. Both have the potential to affect the population dynamics, behavior, or movement of Nipah virus hosts, with deforestation affecting fruit bats (reservoir hosts) and livestock production affecting the abundance of pigs (amplifier hosts). We used data from the Food and Agricultural Organization (www.fao.org) to assess the rate of change in these factors over the past four decades in Malaysia (Fig. 13.2). Pig production has increased in Malaysia over the past 45 years, but not in a dramatic manner. Oil palm production has increased exponentially, but most palm production occurs on lands previously cleared for the rubber industry, which declined rapidly during this period. Forest cover in Malaysia decreased from 49% in 1979 to 45.3% in 1992, and agricultural land use has expanded from 4.2 to 7.9 million hectares from 1961 to 2001. This does not appear to represent a significant increase in the rate of deforestation relative to Sumatra and

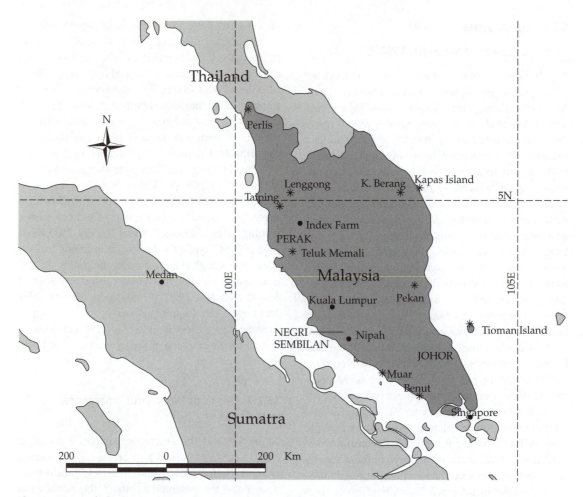

Figure 13.1 A map of peninsular Malaysia, showing sites of Nipah virus disease outbreak (Nipah) and sites where serological surveys of fruit bats have shown Nipah virus-positive bats (asterisks). The human and pig index cases for Nipah virus occurred in Ipoh (Index Farm), whereas most of the human cases occurred in the Negri Sembilan region.

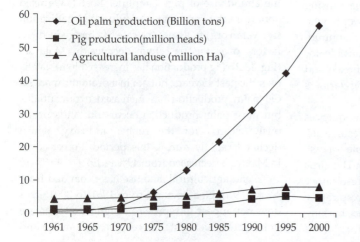

Figure 13.2 Pig production, oil palm production and agricultural land use (a proxy for deforestation) in Malaysia over the past four decades. Note the slight dip in pig production following the 1999 Nipah virus outbreak.

Borneo, or other tropical regions (Achard *et al.* 2002).

A recent paper proposed that ENSO-related (El Niño Southern Oscillation) drought in the mid-1990s in Sumatra and related anthropogenic forest fires may have driven fruit bats, infected with Nipah virus, to migrate into Malaysia in search of fruiting or flowering trees (Chua *et al.* 2002a). This paper provided circumstantial evidence for a link between ENSO drought, forest fires, and a large spike in airborne particulates in mid-1997 caused by these fires. The authors proposed that fruit bats in Sumatra would migrate away from this haze to seek food in peninsular Malaysia, and that the common practice of planting fruit tree crops (rambutan, mango, durian, and others) around pig farms would have drawn bats to the index farm (Chua *et al.* 2002a). More than 100 ha of durian (*Durio zibethinus*) and rambutan (*Nephelium lappaceum*) orchards surround the pig-farming area where the index case of human encephalitis and index cases of pig diseases due to Nipah virus were reported. At the piggeries associated with the index human case of Nipah virus disease, pig-sties were purposely constructed such that the low concrete walls that confined the pigs extended beyond the edge of the roof to allow rainwater run-off from the roof to collect inside the enclosure for bathing the pigs. Partially eaten fruits were also found within pigsties, suggesting a direct mechanism for Nipah virus transmission from fruitbats to pigs (Chua *et al.* 2002a).

The hypothesis that NiV emergence was driven by ENSO-related changes in flying fox movement patterns relies on two key assumptions: first, that flying fox movement from Sumatra to peninsular Malaysia is a relatively rare event prompted by unfavorable conditions (drought and haze) in Sumatra and, second, that under normal conditions flying foxes are not found in the area surrounding the index farm or, if they are, that the virus does not normally circulate among them. To test this hypothesis, we examined the distribution of the two fruit bats found in Malaysia, *P. vampyrus* and *P. hypomelanus*, tested individuals of these species from colonies across Malaysia for antibodies to Nipah virus, and used satellite telemetry to follow fruit bat migration in a non-drought period (2003–4) (Box 13.1).

We found that, contrary to the assumptions of this hypothesis, fruit bats were found to migrate between peninsular Malaysia and Sumatra during non-ENSO years. Home range analysis suggests that some bats forage equally in Sumatra and Malaysia during non-drought years (Epstein *et al.*, *unpublished data*). We found that Nipah virus seropositive fruit bats were present in Malaysia throughout the year and across a multiyear period (Abdul Rahman *et al.*, *unpublished data*). We discovered two large, seasonal colonies of *P. vampyrus* within 50 km of the index farm, and a smaller temporary colony (camp) present each year for around 4–6 months within 5 km of the farm (Epstein *et al.*, *unpublished data*) (Figs 13.1, 13.3). The larger colonies contained Nipah virus seropositive bats throughout the year and over the multiyear period (Table 13.1). Together, these data suggest that Nipah virus is present continually in fruit bats in peninsular Malaysia, and therefore was probably available for introduction into pigs at the index farm prior to the large ENSO drought in the mid-1990s. The index human case for Nipah virus in January 1997 and a rise in the rate of pig abortions at the index farm in late 1996 also precede the ENSO drought and further refute the hypothesis. It is still possible, however, that ENSO-related fluctuations in fruit bat migration from Sumatra to Malaysia play a role in increasing the number of Nipah virus positive bats present at the index site over time.

The Nipah virus index farm in Ipoh, Perak had a standing pig population of over 31,000 head at the time it was culled in 1999 (Nor *et al.* 2000) (Hume Field, *personal communication*). This farm was representative of a small number of intensively managed farms in the area that produced pork for export to Singapore. The pig herd was managed to optimize production by maximizing birth rates and maintaining a high rate of turnover in the young pig population. In order to understand how farm management may have affected NiV emergence in pig populations, we developed a simple SEIR model for NiV dynamics on a pig farm (J. Pulliam, *unpublished data*). The model describes population and disease

Box 13.1 Identifying hosts in extended communities

Studying viral spillover in a system that includes a reservoir host, an amplifier host, and humans requires a multidisciplinary approach. The work described in this chapter involved virologists, ecologists, veterinarians, and modelers, working to understand contact rates within and between hosts, viral transmission dynamics and risk of viral spillover between species within the reservoir hosts. For the different aspects of viral transmission, the following three approaches were taken:

1. *Viral dynamics within the reservoir host, Pteropus* spp. *fruit bats.* To understand this, we need to measure population size and dynamics and viral prevalence across the host population. Measuring population size in fruit bats is difficult due to migration between discrete colonies. Our approach is to use satellite telemetry to assess routes of migration, and seasonal changes in colony size to gain some insights into rates of migration between colonies. Viral dynamics are also not easily measured. Both Nipah and Hendra virus have short infectious periods in fruit bats, and viral prevalence is extremely low. Instead, we measure prevalence of antibodies to Nipah and Hendra viruses, using an ELISA test and confirmation by serum neutralization. This gives us an indication of *changes* in antibody prevalence, suggesting recent transmission. Finally, to understand routes of viral excretion, infectious period, pathogenesis, and other aspects of transmission between individual fruit bats, we use experimental infection of captive animals. This has its own difficulties because of the lethal nature of the viruses to people and the lack of effective therapies. All experimental infections have to take place under the highest level of biosecurity (BSL-4) and therefore involve a series of logistical issues.

2. *Viral dynamics within the amplifier host, domestic pigs.* Currently no pig farms in Malaysia are known to be infected by Nipah virus, therefore measuring viral dynamics directly is not possible. Similarly for Hendra virus, spillover to and transmission between horses seems to be a rare, transient event and has therefore not been directly observed. We are able to understand viral dynamics for Nipah virus in pigs due to the nature of the pig farms in Malaysia. The index farm is part of a series of farms designated to export live pigs for slaughter in Singapore, a large pork market. These designated farms have historically been required to keep detailed logs of population dynamics,

such as birth rates, death rates in each age class, and other data. These data are entered into a standard pig management program called "PigChamp". At the time of the Nipah virus outbreak, detailed information on test results from the index and other infected farms was collected by the Malaysian government scientists, and those involved in outbreak investigation from the Centers for Disease Control and Prevention, USA and CSIRO, Australia. We have also worked closely with another export farm that is still running in Malaysia and has similar management to the index farm. Access to these data has allowed us to parameterize our model of the dynamics of Nipah virus in the index farm prior to spillover to humans.

3. *Dynamics of the spillover event (reservoir host-amplifier host-human transmission).* Spillover for both viruses appears to be a rare occurrence. Therefore our approach has been to examine transmission pathways and to understand factors that increase the risk of spillover. For Nipah virus, we are currently conducting experimental infections in bats, to examine routes of virus excretion. We have also conducted Nipah and Hendra virus culture experiments on fruit, under a range of temperature, humidity, and pH conditions. This will provide us with relative capacity for viral transmission from bats to pigs or horses via fomites. For amplifier host spillover to people, we assume simply that contact between humans and amplifier hosts is a measure of the intensity of pig and horse production and human population density.

We are currently examining changes in pig and horse distribution and production management over the past five decades in Malaysia and Australia, respectively. The risk of spillover is related to factors that can affect the transmission of virus across this host continuum. Here, complex relationships need to be measured between bat population or migration and climate, changes in forest cover, fruiting and flowering tree phenology, season etc. For amplifier hosts, temporal and spatial changes in populations and changes to the management of livestock need to be assessed. Accurately assessing risk of future spillover is clearly a challenge, but the combination of bench virology, epidemiology, veterinary pathology and ecology allows us to begin to understand what promotes these rare, but devastating events.

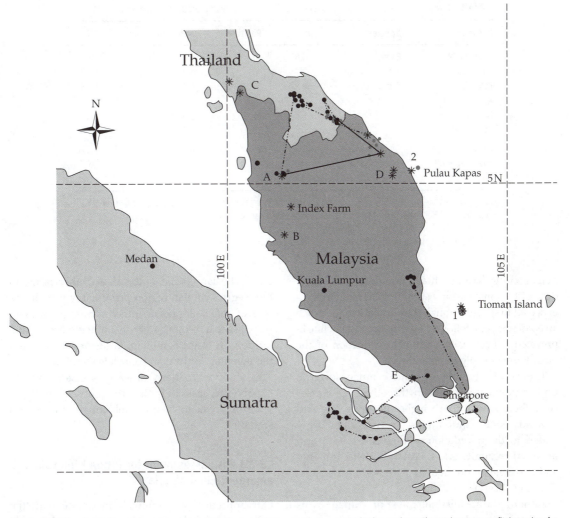

Figure 13.3 The distribution and seroprevalence of Nipah virus in Malaysian *P. vampyrus* and *P. hypomelanus*. The tracks represent flight paths of satellite-collared fruit bats. The time between points is 10 days. Colony locations with seropositive bats are identified by an asterisk and labeled for reference with Table 13.1.

dynamics of four distinct age classes of pigs: sows (adult females kept for breeding purposes), piglets (young pigs—up to about one month of age—housed in pens adjacent to their mother's for the purpose of suckling), and weaners and porkers (young pigs that have been weaned from their mother's milk and are housed separately until ready to be sent off to market at about 6 months of age). Weaners differ from porkers in that they are young enough to retain maternal antibodies to NiV infection. We derived population-dynamic parameters using pig management data from an

intensively managed active pig farm similar in size and operation to the index farm' and disease-dynamic parameters using data from experimental infections and observations made during the NiV outbreak (Mohd Nor *et al.* 2000; Middleton *et al.* 2002).

Since the rate of transmission of the virus within a farm is unknown, we manipulated the transmission coefficient to examine the progression of an epidemic under various transmission scenarios. Figure 13.4 shows the results of numerical integration of the ODE (ordinary differential equation) model, showing NiV dynamics on an intensively

Table 13.1 Nipah virus seroprevalence in *Pteropus* spp. bats summarized by location and species

Location[a]	Species	n	Positive[b]	Seroprevalence	SE
Leggong (A)	*P. vampyrus*	28	15	0.54	0.09
T. Memali (B)	*P. vampyrus*	7	2	0.29	0.17
Perlis (C)	*P. vampyrus*	7	1	0.14	0.13
K. Berang (D)	*P. vampyrus*	12	4	0.33	0.14
Benut (E)	*P. vampyrus*	24	13	0.54	0.10
Total (A–E)		78	35	0.45	0.06
Pulau Tioman (1)	*P. hypomelanus*	251	59	0.24	0.026
Pulau Kapas (2)	*P. hypomelanus*	30	3	0.10	0.05
Total (1–2)		281	62	0.22	

Bats from colonies "A" and "B", which are 50 km from the index farm, have a seroprevalence of 54% (+ 9%) and 29% (−17%), respectively. Means ± SE of seroprevalence are presented.

[a] Location labels correspond to colonies in Figs 13.3 and 13.4.

[b] Positive samples tested by C-ELISA.

managed pig farm, such as the index farm, under different transmission scenarios. The virus is expected to spread through the population and reach an epidemic peak followed by a monotonic decline in prevalence, eventually leading to extinction of the virus within the pig population.

The decline of viral prevalence is much slower in porker populations than in the other age classes since these have a much higher turnover rate and new susceptible individuals are constantly being added to the population as piglets are born and maternal immunity is lost. Peak prevalence is higher and is reached more quickly with higher transmission (Fig. 13.4(a)).

Although transmission rates of Nipah virus among pigs is unknown, transmission of the virus via aerosol suggests that R_0 is likely to be relatively high. The closely related measles virus, for example, which also spreads via aerosol has an R_0 value that varies between 12.5 and 18.0, depending on properties of the community where it is introduced (Anderson and May 1982). If Nipah virus is highly transmissible between pigs within a farm setting, intensive management results in a rapid initial epidemic phase. An additional spillover event following this initial epidemic is likely to result in maintenance of the virus within porker populations. Our results suggest that the pig populations at the index farm were able to maintain Nipah virus infection within their population for an extensive

time. The large-scale outbreak on other farms in the Negri Sembilan region presumably was due to sale of infected pigs to other farms, perhaps in response to a recognized problem in pig production in Ipoh. In Negri Sembilan, farms are smaller and the potential for human contact is therefore greater. The observed pattern of early sporadic human Nipah virus cases in Ipoh, with a subsequent large-scale outbreak in Negri Sembilan fits this model scenario.

13.2.3 Risk assessment for future Nipah virus emergence in Malaysia

Our approach of combining modeling with the collection of field and laboratory data has provided unique insight into this recently emerged pathogen. We envisage that Nipah virus emergence in 1998–9 was primarily a product of the development of intensive pig farms in Malaysia. Our fruit bat distribution and serosurveillance data suggest that Nipah virus-infected bats are historically present in Malaysia, and that the virus may have been repeatedly introduced into pig farms prior to the outbreak. However, the high turnover of weaners at the export farm allowed Nipah virus to become endemic and ultimately cause an outbreak in humans as infected pigs were sold to other farms in the more densely populated region of Negri Sembilan and Selangor. We can

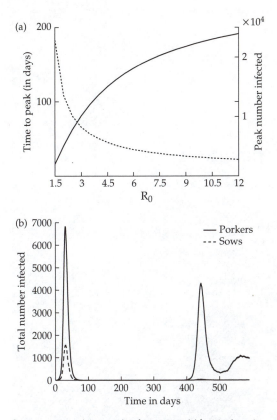

Figure 13.4 Simulation results of an SEIR model for NiV dynamics on the index farm. (a) Simulations predict that peak prevalence is higher (solid line) and is reached more quickly (dashed line) with higher values of R_0 (shown here for a standing pig population of 30,000 individuals). (b) Stochastic simulation ($R_0 = 6$) with rare spillover events (here, exponentially distributed with a mean of 1/90 days) demonstrate that high birthrates and rapid turnover of porkers for exports create a sustained input of susceptibles, which allows NiV maintenance. The figure represents a single realization of the stochastic simulation for a farm with a standing pig population of approximately 30,000 pigs. The total numbers of infected porkers (solid line) and sows (dashed line) are shown.

make some broad assessments of the risk for future emergence of Nipah virus based on our analyses:

1. Nipah virus is more likely to re-emerge with increasing intensity of management of pig farms in Malaysia.

2. The process of growing fruiting trees adjacent to pigsties at these intensively managed farms is a high-risk strategy for spillover from bats to pigs.

Simple measures such as mandatory buffer zones where fruit trees are excluded, or increased biocontainment of pig farms would help prevent future outbreaks.

3. The wide temporal and spatial distribution of NiV in peninsular Malaysian fruit bats suggest that fruit bats are likely to harbor Nipah virus across their geographical distribution in South and Southeast Asia. Many of these areas support extensive pig production, and are therefore at risk of spillover into these amplifier hosts.

Nipah virus is listed as a select agent of potential bioterrorism use (www.bt.cdc.gov/agent/agentlist-category.asp) due to its high case fatality rate in humans and the lack of adequate therapies or vaccines (Lam 2003). The ability to identify risk factors for emergence should also prove useful in preventing bioterrorism scenarios such as collection of Nipah virus-infected pig tissues or samples from an active outbreak farm. By identifying high risk livestock practices in areas at high risk for Nipah virus emergence, it will be possible to set up rapid response teams which would vaccinate/cull pigs at the first signs of outbreak and reduce the availability of infected animal tissues for uncontrolled use.

13.2.4 Nipah virus emergence in India and Bangladesh

Since the 1999 Malaysia outbreak, Nipah virus (or at least a virus extremely closely related to Nipah virus) has been identified in *Pteropus* spp. fruit bats in Cambodia (Olson *et al.* 2002), Sumatra, Indonesia (Field *et al.* unpublished data), and Haryana State, India (Epstein *et al.*, unpublished data). It has also been implicated in an outbreak of human encephalitis in Siliguri, West Bengal, India (Kumar 2003). Most significantly, it has been confirmed as the cause of human illness and mortality in a series of outbreaks in Bangladesh between 2001 and 2005. Five outbreaks of human Nipah virus infection have been recognized in Bangladesh during this period, and all occurred between the months of January and May (WHO 2004) (Fig. 13.5, S. Luby, *unpublished data*). A total of 90 human cases of Nipah infection

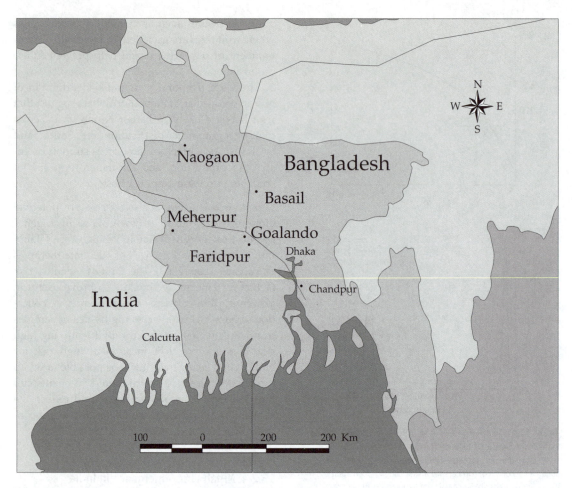

Figure 13.5 Map of Bangladesh showing locations of Nipah virus outbreaks 2001–5.

have been documented; 66 (73%) died. As occurred in human cases of Nipah virus infection in Malaysia, the disease caused fever and central nervous system symptoms, with a high case fatality rate (Parashar *et al.* 2000). Pteropid bats (*P. giganteus*) were the only wild animal sampled that had serologic evidence of infection (Hsu *et al.* 2004). In Meherpur and Naogaon in 2003, serum samples were collected from 10 birds, 6 pigs, 2 shrews, 5 rodents, and 56 bats including 44 *P. giganteus*. Antibodies against Nipah virus antigen were detected in two *P. giganteus* adult females. Serum specimens from all of the other animals were negative (Hsu *et al.* 2004). In Goalando district in 2004, of 92 *P. giganteus* captured, 14 (15%) had antibodies to Nipah virus in contrast to no detectable antibodies

among 5 rodents, 40 shrews, 36 other small fruit bats, and 4 insectivorous bats (D. Carrol, *personal communication*).

There were important differences between the multiple outbreaks in Bangladesh and the single outbreak in Malaysia and Singapore. First, in Bangladesh there was consistent evidence of person-to-person transmission of Nipah virus (Hsu *et al.* 2004). In the first outbreak, in the Meherpur district, the index patient died six days after first developing symptoms. Five other persons in the household developed Nipah virus disease 10–18 days after the index case. Nine of the 13 Nipah virus-infected people in this outbreak were relatives of the index case. Living with a person who had Nipah was a risk factor for illness (Hsu *et al.* 2004). In the

Naogon outbreak in January 2003, the head of one household became ill, followed two weeks later by his wife and three eldest daughters. All died of Nipah virus infection. In Goalando in January 2004, contact with a person who had symptoms of Nipah encephalitis was strongly associated with developing Nipah infection (J. Montgomery, *personal communication*). In the Faridpur outbreak between February and April 2004, the virus appears to have undergone four transmission cycles in people (E. Gurley and S. Luby, *unpublished data*).

Second, there is no evidence for livestock amplifier hosts between pteropid bats and humans in the Bangladesh outbreaks. Pigs are uncommon in Bangladesh, though a pig herd was present in Meherpur two weeks before the outbreak (Jahangir Hossain, *unpublished data*). Contact with a sick cow was significantly associated with illness in the Meherpur outbreak but the cow was not tested for Nipah virus, and so it is still unclear what role domestic animals play in Nipah virus transmission in Bangladesh (Hsu *et al*. 2004).

Therefore, it seems that the epidemiology of Nipah virus in Bangladesh differs substantially from that in Malaysia in that: (1) It has spilled over repeatedly and independently; (2) Spillover appears to be seasonal; (3) Spillover occurred seemingly without livestock amplifier hosts; and (4) there appears to have been human-to-human transmission. These factors significantly heighten the threat of Nipah virus as a potentially pandemic pathogen that is likely to continue to emerge in humans.

13.3 Hendra virus

13.3.1 Outbreaks in Queensland, Australia, 1994–2004

In 1994, the racehorse "Drama Series" developed symptoms of respiratory disease while pregnant and at pasture. She was moved to a racing stable in the suburb of Hendra, Brisbane. Within two weeks, 21 horses and two humans became ill. Of these, 14 horses died or were killed following an illness characterized by high fevers and severe respiratory difficulties (sometimes characterized by frothy nasal discharge). Of the infected humans, one was admitted to intensive care with severe influenza-like

symptoms but died shortly after. Racing was temporarily halted in northern Australia. This was the first identified case of Hendra virus, a new paramyxovirus endemic in Australian flying fox (fruit bat) populations (Murray *et al*. 1995; Field *et al*. 2001). To date, this virus is known to have emerged into horses and humans five times, with all four human cases (two fatal) attributed to contact with infected horses (Hooper *et al*. 1996; Field *et al*. 2000, 2001). The most recent spillover event was in 2004 near Cairns, northern Queensland, where one person was infected but not fatally (Field *et al*., *unpublished data*).

Hendra virus has not emerged in Australia with the explosive impact of Nipah virus for a number of reasons. First, unlike pigs, horses are housed at low density and hence there is limited opportunity for secondary transmission among these amplifier hosts. Second, although Hendra virus causes respiratory infection in horses, it does not seem to lead to a coughing syndrome; limiting the probability of transmission (Hooper *et al*. 1997). Third, whereas Nipah virus (in pigs) exhibits a tropism for epithelial cells, Hendra virus (in horses) exhibits a tropism for endothelial cells. This is an important point, because it is likely that this tropism is in part related to the infected host species. It is unknown if Hendra virus is able to infect pigs with the same respiratory pathogenesis as Nipah virus. If this is the case, and should a future spillover occur into a pig farm in Australia, the consequences for livestock production and human health will be significant. Hendra virus is the closest fully characterized relative of Nipah virus, and there are no effective vaccines or therapies (Chong *et al*. 2001; Wang *et al*. 2001). It has a high case fatality rate: two of the four known human infections have resulted in death (one by encephalitis after a prolonged remission). Serological studies suggest that Hendra virus is widespread in Australian flying fox populations and therefore has the potential to re-emerge (Halpin *et al*. 2000; Field *et al*. 2001). Finally, like Nipah virus, it is considered a select agent of potential bioterrorism use (www.bt.cdc.gov/agent/agentlist-category.asp).

Understanding the causes of Hendra virus emergence is likely to be more difficult than for Nipah virus because of the small number of cases and the sporadic nature of horse ranching compared with pig farming in Malaysia (Field *et al*. 2001). Our approach has been to first use Hendra virus in flying foxes as a model for the ecology of Henipaviruses in their wildlife reservoir hosts. We aim to then identify peaks of virus transmission in bats and related environmental risk factors for spillover.

13.3.2 Hendra virus dynamics in flying fox reservoirs

Australian flying foxes (fruit bats of the genus *Pteropus*) have three ecological traits that are likely to play key roles in Hendra virus emergence. First, they occur in very large, dense colonies, which number from 10,000 for a small nursery colony of black flying foxes (*P. alecto*) to millions of individuals for little red flying foxes in Far North Queensland, Australia (Nowak 1994). They migrate in response to flowering and fruiting phenology, and although discrete populations move independently, there is thought to be some mixing (Eby 1991; Vardon *et al.* 2001). This suggests that something similar to a metapopulation model may describe their population dynamics most accurately. Finally, they respond to anthropogenic land use by changing their colony location, size, and structure and by altering their migration patterns (Markus and Hall 2004), thus providing a potential link between land use change in Australia and the emergence of Hendra virus.

Experimental data suggest that Hendra virus has a short infectious phase and immunity is lifelong (Williamson *et al.* 1998, 2000; Hooper *et al.* 2001). Therefore, like the human paramyxovirus, measles virus, Hendra virus may require large host populations to provide enough susceptibles to ensure viral persistence (Bolker and Grenfell 1995). For measles virus, the threshold host population size (below which the virus cannot be maintained) is around 350,000–500,000 people. A human population of this size produces enough newborn susceptibles to maintain endemicity of the virus (Black 1996). However, flying foxes undergo synchronous birthing, which equates to a rapid pulse of susceptibles, a likely increased transmission of Hendra virus, followed by a period outside the birthing season when susceptibles drop below the density required for maintenance. This seasonal reproduction is likely to raise the threshold density for Hendra virus.

We tested this hypothesis by modeling Hendra virus dynamics using an SEIR model in a closed population of flying foxes. Hendra virus was unable to persist when the model was parameterized using field and experimental data. Thus, if this hypothesis is correct, either one or more of our assumptions (of direct horizontal transmission, or of a short infectious phase followed by lifelong immunity) is wrong, or there is an alternative mechanism by which the virus maintains itself in flying foxes. We have proposed three strategies for Hendra virus persistence in Australian flying foxes (Field 2003):

1. *Via the presence of discrete populations that sometimes mix.* As specialist nectarivores and frugivores, flying foxes are highly nomadic, traveling large distances to track resources, occasionally gathering in mass congregations during resource concentration, and separating into smaller groups when resources are scarce or widely distributed (Hall and Richards 2000; Vardon *et al.* 2001). These complex spatial dynamics may facilitate viral persistence in a similar manner to the metapopulation dynamics that maintain some animal populations via asynchronous dynamics and the "rescue effect" (Lloyd and May 1996; McCallum and Dobson 2002; Park *et al.* 2002). Hendra virus antibodies are consistently found in all four species of flying foxes in mainland Australia (Field *et al.* 2001). RNA sequences of isolates cultured from three of these species are identical, strongly suggesting that Hendra virus may circulate between species (Halpin 2000). However, the percentage of individuals with antibodies differs markedly between species, indicating either different viral population dynamics within species or different species-specific host–viral interactions. Further study is required to understand the spatial dynamics of Hendra virus in flying fox populations and to demonstrate that metapopulation dynamics enable viral persistence.

2. *Via latent or chronic infections.* The threshold host density required for persistence tends to be lower for pathogens that employ strategies involving sexual, vertical or vector-mediated transmission, latent or chronic infections, immune evasion, reservoir hosts, or long-lived and resistant external stages (Dobson and Carper 1996). For Hendra virus, there is some evidence that the virus can be transmitted

vertically (Halpin *et al.* 2000; Williamson *et al.* 2000). High viral loads in fetal membranes, and the concurrence of Hendra virus outbreaks within bat birthing seasons have led to the hypothesis that transmission to horses may occur via contamination of pasture with fetal membranes during parturition or abortion (Halpin *et al.* 2000). Testing hypotheses involving various pathogen persistence strategies is an area of active research involving transmission experiments and field research.

3. *Via loss of immunity.* Waning immunity causes previously resistant individuals to reenter the susceptible class. If Hendra virus immunity is highly transient in flying foxes, it is possible that this could lead to a significant increase in the number of available susceptibles and provide a mechanism for the virus to persist. Although this has not been shown for other paramyxoviruses, there appears to be considerable heterogeneity in short-term antibody response to infection with Hendra virus in *Pteropus* spp. and the duration of immunity has not yet been measured.

13.3.3 Potential causes of Hendra virus emergence

Flying foxes require large tracts of forested area to find food, making them highly sensitive to landscape change (Eby *et al.* 1999). Across their range in the Old World Tropics and into southeastern Australia, fruit bat habitat has been degraded on a large scale. This has resulted in population declines, population concentration during resource scarcity, distributional changes, and increasing dependency on native and introduced flowering or fruiting trees planted in suburban or urban gardens (a recent trend in Australia) (Mickleburg *et al.* 1992; Eby *et al.* 1999; Tidemann 1999; Hall 2000; Parry-Jones and Augee 2001). All of these processes may lead to increased contact with domestic animals and humans and opportunities for viral spillover. In Australia it has been estimated that at current rates of land clearing, all remnant stands of little red flying fox habitat (lowland eucalypt woodland greater than 100 m in diameter and outside protected areas in the northeastern rangelands) will be cleared between 2016 and 2040 (Catterall *et al.* 1997). While this threatens flying foxes in their native habitat, it

may also result in increasing numbers of flying foxes seeking food in suburban and urban settings and increasing livestock or human contact with these reservoirs of Hendra virus.

13.4 Conclusions

For Nipah and Hendra viruses, the emergence of a pathogen from a wildlife reservoir seems to signify a change in the system. These changes appear to be due to alterations in structure and composition of wildlife communities, habitat loss or modification, or shifts in human population distribution and human activity patterns (Box 13.2). This can be extrapolated to most cases of emerging infectious diseases with wildlife reservoirs (Daszak *et al.* 2000; Morens *et al.* 2004; Weiss and McMichael 2004). For example, HIV/AIDS is caused by HIV-1 and -2, which evolved from simian immunodeficiency viruses that jumped host from chimpanzees and sooty mangabees to humans, respectively. Here, changes in the contact rate between bushmeat hunters and their prey, concurrent with demographic changes in Central Africa, appear to have resulted in large-scale emergence of a new zoonosis (Hahn *et al.* 2000). For SARS coronavirus, farming of wild mammals (civets), increasing demands for wildlife species as food, and the increasingly diverse array of live wildlife in "wet markets" seems to have led to another pandemic emerging disease (Guan *et al.* 2003; Webster 2004). For hantavirus pulmonary syndrome, which is caused by Sin Nombre virus carried by the deer mouse (*Peromyscus maniculatus*), changes in human demography and climatic patterns in the southwestern United States have led to repeated, though small-scale, outbreaks (Mills *et al.* 1999).

Despite our understanding of these broad patterns in emergence, studying and ultimately predicting the process of emergence is hindered by three major issues. First, the complexity of pathogen dynamics in wildlife, particularly when the pathogen is present in a range of wildlife reservoir species. This leads to complex dynamics in the risk of spillover throughout seasons, wildlife population cycles and as anthropogenic changes alter wildlife community composition and ecology. Second, in many cases, evolutionary constraints on emerging zoonotic

Box 13.2 Viral emergence and community ecology

Due to the involvement of three hosts in the chain of Nipah and Hendra virus emergence, different aspects of community ecology are important at different points in the process of emergence. The following are two key questions that we need to answer to understand emergence, and its community ecology context:

1. What factors determine the temporal and spatial dynamics of reservoir hosts? Fruit bats migrate large distances in response to food availability. Because they feed exclusively on the flowers and fruit of forest and orchard trees, understanding their population dynamics is essentially a study of fruiting and flowering tree phenology. Fruit bat colony size, species composition, and location alter with seasonal availability of food. Indentifying the niche of the key reservoir hosts is fundamental to understanding their dynamics. However, more important is an assessment of how phenology changes in response to abiotic factors

such as climate and season. Because of the large scale of fruit crop cultivation in Malaysia, studying the phenology of agricultural products is also important. Thus, we are dealing with another community ecology concept—that of disturbance. In this case, there are significant changes to the spatial structure of production that results in changes to population dynamics and distribution of the primary consumers—and ultimately to the risk of viral emergence.

2. How do livestock amplifier hosts contribute to viral emergence? This can be viewed in the context of species introductions. In Malaysia, pig populations are much larger and densities higher than the Australian horse populations within which Hendra virus emerged. These differences can be viewed as differences in "success" of an introduced species, which leads to differences in contact rates between fruit bats and the amplifier host and therefore differences in likelihood of spillover.

pathogens may be fundamental to the process of emergence. For example, the ability of influenza virus to reassort genes allows it to move whole genes between viral strains in animals coinfected with multiple strains. This has led to repeated rapid shifts in virulence historically and is a high risk factor for future emergence (Alexander and Brown 2000). New models that fuse viral phylogeny and emerging disease ecology are the first step in unifying theories on disease emergence (Boots *et al.* 2004; Grenfell *et al.* 2004). For Nipah and Hendra virus, the causes of emergence are almost certainly ecological rather than evolutionary, because all isolates so far sequenced are highly conserved (Halpin 2000). Third, the precise mechanics of the interaction between complex, often multifactorial drivers of disease emergence and the risk of spillover into humans is hard to analyze. These complexities require multidisciplinary approaches from diverse disciplines and take many years to come to fruition. For example, studies of Lyme disease in the northeastern United States have begun to show clear patterns of landscape change that promote spillover between rodent reservoirs and humans (LoGiudice *et al.* 2003). This work has involved intensive collection of field data on reservoir hosts, vectors, pathogens and landscape characteristics and many

years of work. Given the importance of zoonoses in emerging diseases (Taylor *et al.* 2001), understanding the ecology of zoonotic disease emergence is a key challenge to ecologists and public health researchers alike.

Acknowledgments

This work was supported in part by an NIH/NSF "Ecology of Infectious Diseases" (R01-TW05869) award from the John E. Fogarty International Center and by core funding to the Consortium for Conservation Medicine from the V. Kann Rasmussen Foundation. This work is published as part of a collaboration with the Australian Biosecurity Cooperative Research Center for Emerging Infectious Diseases. We acknowledge Mike Bunning (US Air Force, Office of Surgeon General, Bolling Air Force Base, Washington, DC, USA and Centers for Disease Control and Prevention, Fort Collins, Colorado, USA) for allowing access to PigChamp data from the Nipah virus index farm.

References

Achard, F., H. Eva, H.-J. Stibig, P. Mayaux, J. Gallego, T. Richards *et al.* (2002). Determination of deforestation rates of the World's humid tropical forests. *Science* **297**:999–1002.

Alexander, D. J. and I. H. Brown. (2000). Recent zoonoses caused by influenza A viruses. *Revue Scientifique et Technique de L'Office International des Epizooties* **19**:197–225.

Anderson, R. M. and R. M. May. (1982). Directly transmitted infectious diseases: control by vaccination. *Science* **215**:1053–1060.

Black, F. L. (1996). Measles endemicity in insular populations: critical community size and its evolutionary implication. *Journal of Theoretical Biology* **11**:207–211.

Bolker, B. and B. T. Grenfell. (1995). Space, persistence and dynamics of measles epidemics. *Philosophical Transactions of the Royal Society of London Series B, Biological Sciences*:309–320.

Boots, M., P. J. Hudson, and A. Sasaki. (2004). Large shifts in pathogen virulence relate to host population structure. *Science* **303**:842–844.

Burke, D. S. 1998. The evolvability of emerging viruses. In A. M. Nelson and C. R. Horsburgh, eds. *Pathology of emerging infections*, pp. 1–12. American Society for Microbiology, Washington D.C.

Catterall, C., R. Storey, and M. B. Kingston. (1997). Reality versus rhetoric: a case study monitoring regional deforestation. In P. Hale and D. Lamb, eds. *Conservation Outside Nature Reserves*, pp. 367–377. Centre for Conservation Biology, Queensland, Brisbane.

Chong, H. T., A. Kamarulzaman, C. T. Tan, K. J. Goh, T. Thayaparan, R. Kunjapan *et al.* (2001). Treatment of acute Nipah encephalitis with ribavirin. *Annals of Neurology* **49**:810–813.

Chua, K. B. (2003). Nipah virus outbreak in Malaysia. *Journal of Clinical Virology* **26**:265–275.

Chua, K. B., W. J. Bellini, P. A. Rota, B. H. Harcourt, A. Tamin, S. K. Lam *et al.* (2000). Nipah virus: A recently emergent deadly paramyxovirus. *Science* **288**:1432–1435.

Chua, K. B., K. J. Goh, K. T. Wong, A. Kamarulzaman, P. S. K. Tan, T. G. Ksiazek, *et al.* (1999). Fatal encephalitis due to Nipah virus among pig-farmers in Malaysia. *Lancet* **354**:1257–1259.

Chua, K. B., B. H. Chua, and C. W. Wang. (2002a). Anthropogenic deforestation, El Nino and the emergence of Nipah virus in Malaysia. *Malaysian Journal of Pathology* **24**:15–21.

Chua, K. B., C. L. Koh, P. S. Hooi, K. F. Wee, J. H. Khong, B. H. Chua *et al.* (2002b). Isolation of Nipah virus from Malaysian Island flying-foxes. *Microbes and Infection* **4**:145–151.

Cleaveland, S., M. K. Laurenson, and L. H. Taylor. (2001). Diseases of humans and their domestic mammals: pathogen characteristics, host range and the risk of emergence. *Philosophical Transactions of the Royal Society of London Series B-Biological Sciences* **356**:991–999.

Daszak, P., A. A. Cunningham, and A. D. Hyatt. (2000). Emerging infectious diseases of wildlife—threats to biodiversity and human health. *Science* **287**:443–449.

Daszak, P., A. A. Cunningham, and A. D. Hyatt. (2001). Anthropogenic environmental change and the emergence of infectious diseases in wildlife. *Acta Tropica* **78**: 103–116.

Dobson, A. P. and E. R. Carper. (1996). Infectious diseases and human population history. *Bioscience* **46**:115–126.

Eby, P. (1991). Seasonal movements of gray-headed flying-foxes, *Pteropus-Poliocephalus* (Chiroptera, Pteropodidae), from 2 maternity camps in northern New-South-Wales. *Wildlife Research* **18**:547–559.

Eby, P., G. Richards, L. Collins, and K. Parry-Jones. (1999). The distribution, abundance and vulnerability to population reduction of a nomadic nectarivore, the grey-headed flying-fox *Pteropus poliocephalus* in New South Wales, during a period of resource concentration. *Australian Zoologist* **31**:240–253.

Field, H. E. (2003). Hendra virus in Australian flying foxes: possible maintenance strategies. *Journal of Clinical Virology* **28S**:S87–S108.

Field, H. E., P. Young, J. M. Yob, J. Mills, L. Hall, and J. Mackenzie. (2001). The natural history of Hendra and Nipah viruses. *Microbes and Infection* **3**:307–314.

Field, H. E., P. C. Barratt, R. J. Hughes, J. Shield, and N. D. Sullivan. (2000). A fatal case of Hendra virus infection in a horse in north Queensland: clinical and epidemiological features. *Australian Veterinary Journal* **78**:279–280.

Grenfell, B. T., O. G. Pybus, J. R. Gog, J. L. N. Wood, J. M. Daly, J. A. Mumford *et al.* (2004). Unifying the epidemiological and evolutionary dynamics of pathogens. *Science* **303**:327–332.

Guan, Y., B. J. Zheng, Y. Q. He, X. L. Liu, Z. X. Zhuang, C. L. Cheung *et al.* (2003). Isolation and characterization of viruses related to the SARS coronavirus from animals in Southern China. *Science* **302**:276–278.

Hahn, B. H., G. M. Shaw, K. M. de Cock, and P. M. Sharp. (2000). AIDS as a zoonosis: scientific and public health implications. *Science* **287**: 607–614.

Hall, L. and G. Richards. (2000). *Flying Foxes: Fruit and Blossom Bats of Australia*, 1st edition. Krieger Publishing Company.

Halpin, K. (2000). Genetic studies of Hendra virus and other novel Paramyxoviruses. University of Queensland.

Halpin, K., P. L. Young, H. E. Field, and J. S. Mackenzie. (2000). Isolation of Hendra virus from pteropid bats: a natural reservoir of Hendra virus. *Journal of General Virology* **81**:1927–1932.

Hooper, P., S. Zaki, P. Daniels, and D. Middleton. (2001). Comparative pathology of the diseases caused by Hendra and Nipah viruses. *Microbes and Infection* **3**: 315–322.

Hooper, P. T., A. R. Gould, G. M. Russell, J. A. Kattenbelt, and G. Mitchell. (1996). The retrospective diagnosis of a second outbreak of equine morbillivirus infection. *Australian Veterinary Journal* **74**:244–245.

Hooper, P. T., P. J. Ketterer, A. D. Hyatt, and G. M. Russell. (1997). Lesions of experimental equine morbillivirus pneumonia in horses. *Veterinary Pathology* **34**:312–322.

Hsu, V. P., M. J. Hossain, U. D. Parashar, M. A. Mohammed, T. G. Ksiazek, I. Kuzmin *et al*. (2004). Nipah virus encephalitis reemergence, Bangladesh. *Emerging Infectious Diseases* **10**:2082–2087.

Hyatt, A. D., S. R. Zaki, C. S. Goldsmith, T. G. Wise, and S. G. Hengstberger. (2001). Ultrastructure of Hendra virus and Nipah virus within cultured cells and host animals. *Microbes and Infection* **3**:297–306.

Hyatt, A. D., P. Daszak, A. A. Cunningham, H. Field, and A. R. Gould. (2004). Henipaviruses: gaps in the knowledge of emergence. *Ecohealth* **1**:25–38.

Johara, M. Y., H. Field, A. R. Sohayati, J. Maria, M. R. Azmin, and C. Morrissy. (1999). Preliminary investigation of probable reservoir host of Nipah virus. In *Proceedings of the National Congress on Animal Health Production* Alor Gajah, Malaysia.

Kumar, S. (2003). Inadequate research facilities fail to tackle mystery disease. *British Medical Journal* **326**:12d.

Lam, S. K. (2003). Nipah virus—a potential agent of bioterrorism? *Antiviral Research* **57**:113–119.

Lloyd, A. L. and R. M. May. (1996). Spatial heterogeneity in epidemic models. *Journal of Theoretical Biology* **179**: 1–11.

LoGiudice, K., R. S. Ostfeld, K. A. Schmidt, and F. Keesing. (2003). The ecology of infectious disease: effects of host diversity and community composition on Lyme disease risk. *Proceedings of the National Academy of Sciences of the United States of America* **100**:567–571.

Mackenzie, J. S. (1999). Emerging viral diseases: An Australian perspective. *Emerging Infectious Diseases* **5**:1–8.

Markus, N. and L. Hall. (2004). Foraging behaviour of the black flying-fox (*Pteropus alecto*) in the urban landscape of Brisbane, Queensland. *Wildlife Research* **31**:345–355.

McCallum, H. and A. Dobson. (2002). Disease, habitat fragmentation and conservation. *Proceedings of the Royal Society of London, B* **269**:2041–2049.

Mickleburg, S., A. Hutson, and P. Racey. (1992). *Old World Fruit Bats: An Action Plan for Their Conservation*. IUCN, Gland, Switzerland.

Middleton, D. J., H. A. Westbury, C. J. Morrissy, B. M. van der Heide, G. M. Russell, M. A. Braun *et al*. (2002).

Experimental Nipah virus infection in pigs and cats. *Journal of Comparative Pathology* **126**:124–136.

Mills, J. N., T. G. Ksiazek, C. J. Peters, and J. E. Childs. (1999). Long-term studies of Hantavirus reservoir populations in the Southwestern United States: a synthesis. *Emerging Infectious Diseases* **5**:135–142.

Mohd Nor, M. N., C. H. Gan, and B. L. Ong. (2000). Nipah virus infection of pigs in peninsular Malaysia. *Revue Scientifique et Technique de l'Office International des Epizooties* **19**:160–165.

Morens, D. M., G. K. Folkers, and A. S. Fauci. (2004). The challenge of emerging and re-emerging infectious diseases. *Nature* **430**:242–249.

Morse, S. S. (1993). *Emerging Viruses*. Oxford University Press, New York.

Murray, K., P. Selleck, P. Hooper, A. Hyatt, A. Gould, L. Gleeson *et al*. (1995). A morbillivirus that caused fatal disease in horses and humans. *Science* **268**:94–97.

Nor, M. and B. Ong. (2000). The Nipah virus outbreak and the effect on the pig industry in Malaysia. In *Proceedings of the 16th International Pig Veterinary Congress*, pp. 548–550. Ocean Grove, USA.

Nor, M. N. M., C. H. Gan, and B. L. Ong. (2000). Nipah virus infection of pigs in peninsular Malaysia. *Revue Scientifique Et Technique De L'Office International Des Epizooties* **19**:160–165.

Nowak, R. M. (1994). *Walker's Bats of the World*. Johns Hopkins University Press, Baltimore, MD.

Olson, J. G., C. Rupprecht, P. E. Rollin, U. S. An, M. Niezgoda, T. Clemins *et al*. (2002). Antibodies to Nipah-like virus in bats (*Pteropus lylei*), Cambodia. *Emerging Infectious Diseases* **8**:987–988.

Parashar, U. D., L. M. Sunn, F. Ong, A. W. Mounts, M. T. Arif, T. G. Ksiazek *et al*. (2000). Case-control study of risk factors for human infection with a new zoonotic paramyxovirus, Nipah virus, during a 1998–1999 outbreak of severe encephalitis in Malaysia. *Journal of Infectious Diseases* **181**:1755–1759.

Park, A. W., S. Gubbins, and C. A. Gilligan. (2002). Extinction times for closed epidemics: the effects of host spatial structure. *Ecology Letters* **5**:747–755.

Parry-Jones, K. and M. Augee. (2001). Factors affecting the occupation of a colony site in Sydney, New South Wales by the grey-headed flying-fox *Pteropus poliocephalus* (Pteropodidae). *Australian Ecology*, **26**:47–55.

Philbey, A. W., P. D. Kirkland, A. D. Ross, R. J. Davis, A. B. Gleeson, R. J. Love *et al*. (1998). An apparently new virus (family Paramyxoviridae) infectious for pigs, humans, and fruit bats. *Emerging Infectious Diseases* **4**:269–271.

Smolinski, M. S., M. A. Hamburg, and J. Lederberg. (2003). *Microbial Threats to Health: Emergence, Detection, and Response*. The National Academies Press, Washington D.C.

Taylor, L. H., S. M. Latham, and M. E. J. Woolhouse. (2001). Risk factors for human disease emergence. *Philosophical Transactions of the Royal Society of London, B* **356**:983–989.

Tidemann, C. (1999). Biology and management of the grey-headed flying-fox, *Pteropus poliocephalus*. *Acta Chiropterologica* **1**:151–164.

Vardon, M. J., P. S. Brocklehurst, J. C. Z. Woinarski, R. B. Cunningham, C. F. Donnelly, and C. R. Tidemann. (2001). Seasonal habitat use by flying-foxes, *Pteropus alecto* and *P. scapulatus* (Megachiroptera), in monsoonal Australia. *Journal of Zoology* **253**:523–535.

Wang, L. F., B. H. Harcourt, M. Yu, A. Tamin, P. A. Rota, W. J. Bellini *et al.* (2001). Molecular biology of Hendra and Nipah viruses. *Microbes and Infection* **3**:279–287.

Webster, R. G. (2004). Wet markets—a continuing source of severe acute respiratory syndrome and influenza? *Lancet* **363**:234–236.

Weiss, R. A. and A. J. McMichael. (2004). Social and environmental risk factors in the emergence of infectious diseases. *Nature Medicine* **10**:S70–S76.

WHO. (2004). Nipah virus outbreak(s) in Bangladesh, January–April 2004. *Weekly Epidemiological Record* **79**:168–172.

Williamson, M. M., P. T. Hooper, P. W. Selleck, L. J. Gleeson, P. W. Daniels, H. A. Westbury. (1998). Transmission studies of Hendra virus (equine morbillivirus) in fruit bats, horses and cats. *Australian Veterinary Journal* **76**:813–818.

Williamson, M. M., P. T. Hooper, P. W. Selleck, H. A. Westbury, and R. F. Slocombe. (2000). Experimental Hendra virus infection in pregnant guinea-pigs and fruit bats (*Pteropus poliocephalus*). *Journal of Comparative Pathology* **122**:201–207.

CHAPTER 14

Potential effects of a keystone species on the dynamics of sylvatic plague

Chris Ray and Sharon K. Collinge

14.1 Background

Of all zoonoses, plague has the most notorious record of emergence, being responsible for three human pandemics since the fifth century AD. The third pandemic, which began in the nineteenth century, currently involves at least several hundred (confirmed and reported) human cases each year worldwide (World Health Organization, www.who.int). This modern pandemic began with increased trade and introduction of diseased rodents from ancient foci in Eurasia and Africa to ports around the world (Pollitzer 1954; Barnes 1982). Introduced to the west coast of North America just over a century ago, plague is now recognized as an emerging threat to humans and naive wildlife throughout western North America (Daszak *et al.* 2000; Biggins and Kosoy 2001). In this chapter, we focus on relationships between plague and the structure of prairie communities in grasslands of the United States. We report new data on the structure of these communities, and use simple models to explore how community interactions may affect plague prevalence.

14.1.1 The host–pathogen system

Sylvatic plague is maintained within an extensive and variable network of mammalian species and their fleas (Pollitzer and Meyer 1961; Poland and Barnes 1979). "In this complex and shifting milieu, it is often difficult to separate the principals from the bit players, especially since their roles may change with time and in space" (Barnes 1982, p. 253). This is particularly true in North America,

where the relationships between hosts and pathogen are still settling out (Biggins and Kosoy 2001). Although there is some evidence for host–pathogen coevolution within the enzootic foci of plague in Asia, there is less evidence in North America for stable plague foci, resistant host populations, or host-related variants of the pathogen (Biggins and Kosoy 2001; Gage and Kosoy 2005).

The plague bacterium, *Yersinia pestis*, appears to have evolved recently (< 20,000 years ago) from a relatively benign gastrointestinal parasite, *Y. pseudotuberculata* (Achtman *et al.* 1999; Parkhill *et al.* 2001). Key features in the evolution of *Y. pestis* include the acquisition of virulence factors essential for effective use of fleas as vectors (Hinnebush *et al.* 2002) and for transmission via subcutaneous routes (Parkhill *et al.* 2001). These options for transmission (Box 14.1) contribute to the spectacular generalism of *Y. pestis*, which has been found to occur naturally in more than 200 species of mammal worldwide (Pollitzer and Meyer 1961; Poland and Barnes 1979). Of these species, rodents that construct flea-friendly burrows or middens are the most important hosts (Gage and Kosoy 2005). Rodents in general tend to support high levels of bacteremia, and their burrows and nests tend to support the vector populations necessary to perpetuate the vector-mediated circulation of *Y. pestis*. Natural infections of *Y. pestis* have been reported from over 260 species of fleas worldwide (Gage and Kosoy 2005). Of these species, 85% specialize on rodent hosts and 55% specialize further on cricetid rodents. Less than 23% occur in North America.

Box 14.1 Modes of plague transmission

Plague may be transmitted by infectious fleas, by direct contact with infectious host tissues or, more rarely, by inhalation of respiratory droplets from an infectious host. The mode of transmission affects the pathology of the disease. Bubonic plague, which infects the lymphatic system causing painfully swollen lymph nodes or "buboes", generally arises from flea bites or contact with infectious tissues. Septicemic plague, which infects the blood system, develops from bubonic plague or as a primary infection resulting from any mode of transmission. Pneumonic plague, which infects the respiratory system, develops from septicemic plague or as a primary infection resulting from inhalation of infectious agents (Gage *et al.* 1995; Perry and Fetherston 1997).

Sylvatic plague is most likely maintained through transmission involving fleas (Pollitzer and Meyer 1961; Perry and Fetherston 1997). Fleas can transmit plague in two ways. Fleas that have recently fed on an infectious host may transmit *Y. pestis* mechanically via contaminated mouth parts. Although often considered rare and inefficient (Perry and Fetherston 1997), mechanical transmission requires no bacterial incubation within the flea gut, and may result in quick spread of infection when fleas are numerous (Pollitzer and Meyer 1961; Gage and Kosoy 2005). *Y. pestis* also employs a much more efficient mechanism for vector-mediated transmission, known as "blocking".

Blocking was first described by Bacot and Martin (1914), using the rat flea *Xenopsylla cheopis* as a model (Fig. 14.1(a)). Blocking begins with the production of a protein (*Yersinia* murine toxin) that allows *Y. pestis* to colonize, survive, and grow within the midgut of the flea (Hinnebusch *et al.* 2002). Under appropriate environmental conditions, *Y. pestis* can multiply quickly to fill the midgut. Aggregates of *Y. pestis* may then spill over to block the proventriculus, a valve connecting the esophagus to the midgut (Fig. 14.1(b)). A blocked flea can draw a blood meal into its esophagus, but not into its midgut. Instead, the aborted meal is regurgitated back into the host, along with any plague bacteria that are dislodged from the proventriculus (Bacot and Martin 1914; Perry and Fetherston 1997; Hinnebusch *et al.* 2002). Because they are starving, blocked fleas attempt to feed more often, and may regurgitate many thousands of bacilli into a host (Perry and Fetherston 1997).

Efficient transmission of *Y. pestis* has been demonstrated in at least 31 flea species, and may be common in most flea species under certain environmental conditions or levels of host bacteremia (Perry and Fetherston 1997). Temperature affects the speed and success of blocking, and optimal blocking temperatures vary among flea species (as reviewed in Gage and Kosoy 2005). Flea species also vary markedly in their tendency to become blocked. Because flea species tend to be host-specific, variation in blocking rates may contribute to variation in vectorial capacity (see Chapter 6, this volume) and the potential for enzootic and epizootic plague in different host–vector communities (Pollitzer and Meyer 1961; Poland and Barnes 1979; Gage and Kosoy 2005). Blocking may also lead to a breakdown in host–vector specificity, if starving fleas are more likely to bite any available host. So blocking may serve the dual purpose of increasing both intra- and interspecific transmission of *Y. pestis* (Cully and Williams 2001).

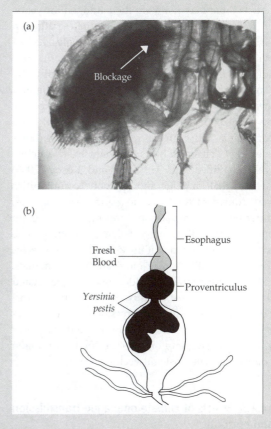

Figure 14.1 Under certain conditions, plague bacteria form a bolus between the esophagus and the midgut, preventing fleas from completing a blood meal. (a) Blocked *Xenopsylla cheopis* (photo from the Centers for Disease Control). (b) Detail showing engorged esophagus, bacterial bolus and midgut infection (redrawn from Bacot and Martin 1914).

14.1.2 The nature and maintenance of plague foci

Many authors suggest that *Y. pestis* cannot persist locally without tracking the more abundant hosts (and vectors) available within a region, through at least occasional interspecific transmission (as reviewed in Pollitzer and Meyer 1961; Poland and Barnes 1979; Gage and Kosoy 2005). This view is supported by the structure of host communities in the relatively ancient plague foci of Asia, which tend to include closely interacting assemblages of two or more species of gerbils, jirds, susliks, pikas, marmots, voles, jerboas, or rats (Biggins and Kosoy 2001). Other mechanisms for the long-term maintenance of *Y. pestis* include alternate vectors (such as ticks) that may maintain the pathogen for years, or reversible mutations that attenuate pathogen virulence. Perry and Fetherston (1997) note a lack of evidence for these mechanisms. Instead, they suggest that plague is maintained locally by "enzootic" hosts that exhibit high bacteremia and low mortality and that plague is spread regionally by "epizootic" hosts that exhibit both high bacteremia and high mortality. They admit, however, that "enzootic hosts have not been conclusively identified" (p. 55). Gage and Kosoy (2005) suggest that enzootic and epizootic communities may consist of the same host and vector species, differing only in rates of transmission. Keeling and Gilligan (2000) suggest that epizootic plague may be maintained within a single host species through extinction–recolonization dynamics. However, their model considers only plague-related fluctuations in host density. If host (and vector) populations are often depressed due to factors other than disease, the long-term maintenance of *Y. pestis* may depend on interspecific transmission among alternate host and vector species.

14.1.3 Effects of climate on plague transmission and epizootics

Plague has a nearly worldwide distribution, but current plague foci occur primarily in semiarid to arid grasslands and uplands of Asia, Africa, and western North America (Barnes 1982; Perry and Fetherston 1997; Biggins and Kosoy 2001; Boisier

et al. 2002; Hoar *et al.* 2003). Although these regions can be hot and dry, plague epizootics tend to occur during seasons that are "warm" but not "hot" (Pollitzer and Meyer 1961; Cavanaugh and Marshall 1972; Boisier *et al.* 2002). This effect of temperature is often attributed to a peak in the efficiency of flea-mediated transmission of *Y. pestis* at intermediate temperatures (Box 14.1). Effects of soil humidity on flea survival and growth may also affect the potential for epizootics (Pollitzer and Meyer 1961). Because the survival and growth of fleas may peak somewhere in the range of 50–95% soil humidity (Silverman and Rust 1981, 1983; Thomas 1996), it has been suggested that flea populations and disease transmission increase after periods of higher than average precipitation in dry climates, and conversely in wet climates (Parmenter *et al.* 1999).

Precipitation has also been linked more directly to epizootics of plague in North America. Parmenter *et al.* (1999) suggested a trophic-cascade hypothesis in which increased precipitation leads to increase in plant productivity followed by increase in rodent population density and disease transmission. In agreement with this hypothesis, they found that human plague cases in the southwestern United States occurred more frequently following periods of higher than average local precipitation. Enscore *et al.* (2002) used similar datasets to model human plague as a function of recent temperatures and time-lagged precipitation. For two separate datasets in the southwestern United States, their results suggested that the number of human plague cases tracked periods of spring and monsoon precipitation with a 1- to 2-year lag. The number of cases in a given year was also positively related to the number of "warm" (e.g. daily maximum >26°C) days in that year, and negatively related to the number of "hot" (>30°C) days. The models of Enscore *et al.* (2002) were suggested both by the trophic-cascade hypothesis of Parmenter *et al.* (1999) and by the effects of hot, dry weather on flea populations and flea-mediated transmission of *Y. pestis*. Collinge *et al.* (2005a) found additional support for this temperature-modulated, trophic-cascade model in one of two datasets on plague occurrence in prairie dogs, as described in Section 14.3.1. Stapp *et al.* (2004) also noted that epizootics in prairie dogs appear to follow periods of higher precipitation associated with the El Niño Southern Oscillation Index.

14.1.4 Effects of plague on humans and wildlife in North America

The transmission gap between sylvatic plague sources and human communities was traditionally bridged by commensal rodents and their fleas (Pollitzer 1954; Pollitzer and Meyer 1961; Poland and Barnes 1979), although commensal shrews have provided similar links in parts of Madagascar and Southeast Asia (Boisier *et al.* 2002). In more recent times, and especially in North America, human plague cases are more likely to derive directly from contact with sylvatic sources (Barnes 1982; Perry and Fetherston 1997). For example, many cases of plague in Native Americans have been traced to contact with wildlife occurring on tribal lands (Barnes 1982). Plague results in high bacteremia and high mortality in many wild rodents of North America, especially sciurids and woodrats, and die-offs in these species may result in questing fleas that pose a risk to humans or their pets (Pollitzer and Meyer 1961; Barnes 1982; Gage *et al.* 1995; Perry and Fetherston 1997). Consequently, efforts to estimate human plague risk in the United States have featured serological surveys for plague exposure in predators, such as the coyote, and surveillance for die-offs in conspicuous sciurids, such as the prairie dog (Barnes 1982).

Prairie dogs (*Cynomys* spp.) are particularly susceptible to plague, which causes nearly 100% mortality in some species (Hoogland 1995; Cully *et al.* 1997; Cully and Williams 2001). This high mortality has played a significant role in the recent decimation of the most widespread *Cynomys* species, the black-tailed prairie dog (*C. ludovicianus*) (US Fish and Wildlife Service 2000). Loss of the black-tailed prairie dog is likely to affect the ecological function of prairie communities, because many species appear to benefit from the ecological services provided by prairie dogs (Kotliar *et al.* 1999). Prairie dogs may also affect the epidemiological function of prairie communities. They may affect disease prevalence if the resources available on prairie-dog colonies (especially burrows) attract and concentrate host (and vector) species, increasing opportunities for interspecific transmission (Cully and Williams 2001).

Will plague eliminate a keystone of prairie ecology? Do prairie dogs play a key role in the maintenance of sylvatic plague? We address these possibilities in light of field data and the predictions of graphical models that include a generalist pathogen, two host species, and differential effects of a third (keystone) species on the strength of interspecific host competition and interspecific pathogen transmission. Our observations suggest alternative roles for prairie dogs in the maintenance of sylvatic plague.

14.2 Study sites and methods

We study plague in the midwestern United States. Our "Colorado" study area covers most of Boulder County, Colorado, an area of considerable and continuing urban development. We also collaborate with colleagues studying plague in undeveloped areas of Colorado, Kansas, Oklahoma, Wyoming, Montana and South Dakota. All of these study areas lie in short- and mixed-grassed prairies occupied by black-tailed prairie dogs. We focus here on observations drawn from our Colorado study with reference to our collaborative studies where appropriate.

Our Colorado study area consists of 20 "on-colony" trapping sites located on prairie-dog colonies, each of which is paired with a nearby "off-colony" trapping site. Paired trapping sites are generally separated by 0.5–2.0 km, and matched in gross habitat characteristics (topography, vegetation, and land use). At each trapping site, we trap small rodents annually during early and late summer. We also trap prairie dogs annually at on-colony sites, primarily in mid-summer. Similar designs and protocols for small-rodent trapping have been followed in all study areas listed above (J. Cully and B. Holmes, *personal communication*).

Each study area yields annual data on whether each prairie-dog colony is occupied. Historical data on occupancy are also available for two of these study areas: the "Colorado" study area described above and a "Montana" study area comprising most of southern Phillips County, Montana (Collinge *et al.* 2005a, b). In both study areas, whole colonies of prairie dogs often die-off between annual censuses. Local land managers are confident that past die-offs were caused by plague, and *Y. pestis* was often confirmed present in prairie dogs or their fleas during a die-off (Collinge *et al.* 2005a). We have used these observations to infer the spatial and temporal patterns of plague occurrence within both Colorado and Montana study areas.

14.3 Study results to date

Our long-term data on the locations of prairie-dog colony die-offs provide opportunities to relate plague epizootics to climate, colony characteristics (e.g. size or connectivity), and landscape context (e.g. urban or riparian cover around a colony). Our trapping efforts provide further data on the structure of host–vector communities in areas with and without prairie dogs. Here, we use these data to address several questions regarding the potential interactions between plague and community structure in North American prairies.

14.3.1 Is plague occurrence affected by climate, through a trophic cascade?

Although Brown and Ernest (2002) argue well that any link between "rain and rodents" is nonlinear at best, others have noted links between plague and precipitation that naturally suggest a trophic cascade leading from increased precipitation through increased rodent density and disease prevalence (Pollitzer and Meyer 1961; Barnes 1982; Parmenter *et al.* 1999; Enscore *et al.* 2002; Stapp *et al.* 2004). Brown and Ernest (2002) predicted that it would be difficult to detect a linear relationship between disease prevalence and time-lagged precipitation, due to the complexity of rodent responses to precipitation. In the case of plague, an additional complication is the potential for ambient temperatures to modulate an incipient epizootic (Box 14.1; Enscore *et al.* 2002). Nevertheless, Enscore *et al.* (2002) were able to explain human plague cases in the southwestern United States using the (temperature-modulated) trophic-cascade model as shown in Figure 14.2(a). If it can explain plague in humans, this model may do even

better given data from a species in closer contact with small rodents.

Collinge *et al.* (2005a) tested this model against long-term data on epizootics in prairie dogs. First, we developed a suite of predictors based on the temperature thresholds and time-lagged precipitation variables identified by Enscore *et al.* (2002). This suite of predictors differed slightly from those used by Enscore *et al.*, because the range of diurnal temperatures and the timing of annual precipitation in our study areas differ from those in the southwestern United States. Next, we developed a set of linear models, each based on a unique combination of our predictor variables. We ignored interaction effects, having no *a priori* reason to suspect them. Finally, we used model selection, based on an information criterion (Burnham and Anderson 2002), to determine the relative support for each model given data from each study area.

This approach, which involved pitting the data against a large number of models, might easily suggest a spurious relationship between epizootics and climate (Burnham and Anderson 2002; Collinge *et al.* 2005a). We would only claim support for the Enscore *et al.* (2002) hypothesis if two criteria were met: (1) all of the models with good support were in agreement with the hypothesis (i.e. none indicated negative effects of lagged precipitation or "warm" days, positive effects of "hot" days), and (2) models based on similar predictor variables shared similar support (suggesting that no model had spuriously high support).

We did not find support for the (temperature-modulated) trophic-cascade model for plague in Colorado (Fig. 14.2(b)), but the model was supported by data from Montana (Fig. 14.2(c)) (Collinge *et al.* 2005a). In Montana, the number of prairie-dog colony die-offs was predicted well by a suite of models including positive effects of time-lagged precipitation and 'warm' days, and negative effects of 'hot' days (Fig. 14.2(c)). In Colorado, only one model was supported by the data (similar models had no support) and that model did not agree with the Enscore *et al.* (2002) hypothesis. This apparent failure of the hypothesis in Colorado may be due to limited data. Only two regional epizootics were observed in Colorado (Fig. 14.2(b)). The timing of annual precipitation

(a)

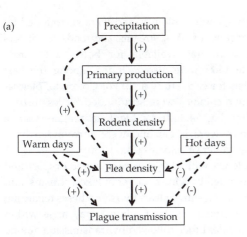

also varies markedly among years within our Colorado study area, which may decouple any relationship between rain and rodents (Collinge *et al.* 2005a).

14.3.2 Is plague occurrence related to prairie-dog colony structure and context?

If epizootics are spread among colonies through dispersal of infected prairie dogs or their infected fleas, then isolated colonies should be less likely to die off (Cully and Williams 2001). The probability that a colony will die off may also be related to

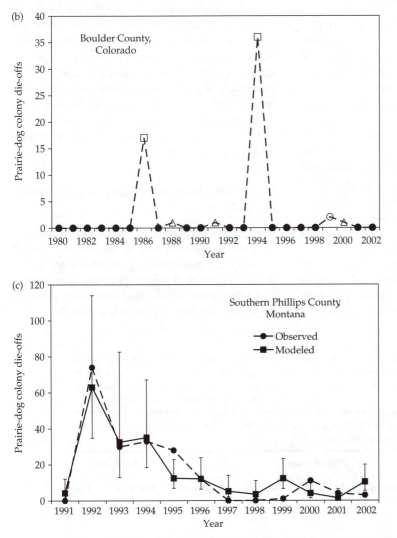

Figure 14.2 The Enscore *et al.* (2002) trophic-cascade model for plague (a), and data on plague in prairie dogs from study areas in Colorado (b) and Montana (c). Open symbols in (b) distinguish the quality of each plague year (square=many colony die-offs, circle=few, triangles=fewer still). Regardless of how the data were coded, neither the quantitative nor qualitative data from Colorado could be fit reliably by this trophic-cascade model. But it fit the Montana data quite well (R^2 rescaled for Poisson regression=0.91). The model in (c) is the Akaike-weighted average of all models with good support (ΔAIC < 4), representing the following predictors (and effects): April–July precipitation in the previous year (positive effect), and number of days in the current year above 26.7°C (positive effect) and 29.4°C (negative effect). Error bars indicate Akaike-weighted 95% confidence intervals. Adapted from Collinge *et al.* (2005a) with kind permission of Springer Science and Business Media.

features in the surrounding landscape that affect the movement or density of plague hosts and vectors. For example, riparian corridors may be used by dispersing prairie dogs (Roach *et al.* 2001), increasing opportunities for the entry of plague into colonies that lie along streams (T. Johnson and J. Cully, *personal communication*). Conversely, riparian habitats may be inhabited by communities with low potential for supporting or transmitting plague.

Collinge *et al.* (2005b) used data from Colorado and Montana to model plague in this spatial context. We identified each prairie-dog colony as either "plague-positive" or "plague-negative," depending on whether it had experienced an epizootic within the study period. Using GIS (Geographic Information System) techniques (e.g. see Chapter 7, this volume), we then characterized features of each colony and its context—features that may affect the transmission of *Y. pestis* through effects on community structure or on the movement of hosts and vectors (Table 14.1). We treated each feature as a predictor, developed a set of logistic regression models, and used model selection to determine the relative support for each model (as described above). Because we considered a large number of models, we hoped that the suite of models with best support would be consistent within and between study areas. Any other result would raise the suspicion of spurious relationships.

The results of this spatial analysis were consistent among models and between study areas (Collinge *et al.* 2005b). Plague-positive colonies in both Colorado and Montana were closer to previously

plague-positive colonies, and were surrounded by lower cover of lakes, streams, and roads. Predictors that were not available for both study areas (Table 14.1) were also included among the best models for each study area: For Colorado, plague-positive colonies were surrounded by less urbanization (Fig. 14.3(a)); for Montana, plague-positive colonies were larger and were surrounded by a higher cover of colonies (Fig. 14.3(b)).

Colonies with plague were clustered in space and surrounded by a lower cover of lakes, streams, and roads, suggesting at least two hypotheses regarding plague dynamics. First, plague may arise within independent foci, followed by transmission among closely spaced colonies through the movement of infected hosts or vectors. Lakes, streams, and roads may retard host or vector movement. Second, plague may arise at the scale of colony complexes, simultaneously affecting adjacent colonies. An abundance of prairie-dog colonies and a dearth of riparian habitats may encourage host–vector communities that can support enzootic or epizootic plague at scales larger than a single colony (Collinge *et al.* 2005b).

14.3.3 Is the black-tailed prairie dog a keystone species?

The general consensus among studies involving more than one trophic level is that plant and animal diversity, and animal density, are higher on prairie-dog colonies than in similar off-colony sites (Kotliar *et al.* 1999). Whether this trend indicates that prairie dogs have "keystone" effects is less clear. The classic

Table 14.1 Relative importance of variables used to predict epizootics of plague in black-tailed prairie dogs in study areas within Colorado and Montana. Higher values indicate higher support (Akaike weight) for models that include this variable as a predictor. Signs in parentheses indicate how this variable was related to plague occurrence in all models with good support (ΔAIC < 4). "Isolation" was the distance to the nearest plague-positive colony in the previous census. Urbanization was lacking in the Montana study area. Colony area and cover were not consistently recorded in the Colorado study area. There was no significant covariance among predictors. Adapted from Collinge *et al.* (2005b) with kind permission of Springer Science and Business Media.

	Percent cover					Focal colony	
	Lakes	Streams	Roads	Urbanization	Colonies	Isolation	Area
Colorado	1.00 (–)	0.99 (–)	0.34 (–)	0.28 (–)	N/A	0.56 (–)	N/A
Montana	1.00 (–)	0.46 (–)	0.33 (–)	N/A	0.28 (+)	1.00 (–)	1.00 (+)

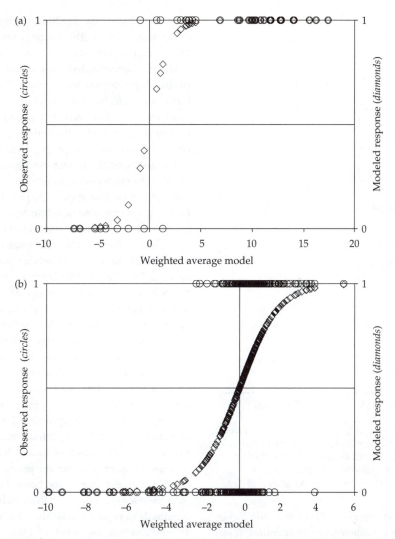

Figure 14.3 Fitted models of plague occurrence in prairie-dog colonies, based on colony structure and landscape context in two study areas. Models for both areas include negative relationships between plague occurrence (response = 1) and colony isolation plus surrounding cover of lakes, streams and roads. Additional predictors are described in Table 14.1. The model for each study area is the Akaike-weighted average of all models with good support (ΔAIC < 4, Burnham and Anderson 2002). (a) For the Colorado study area, percent concordant = 99% and |modeled–observed| < 0.5 for 95% of colonies (97% of plague-positives, 89% of plague-negatives). (b) For Montana, percent concordant = 79% and |modeled–observed| < 0.5 for 70% of colonies (81% of plague-positives, 56% of plague-negatives). Adapted from Collinge *et al.* (2005b) with kind permission of Springer Science and Business Media.

keystone effect is predator-mediated coexistence among a number of prey species that would otherwise dwindle through competition (see Chapter 2, this volume). Predator-mediated coexistence can be facilitated by frequency-dependent predation by a generalist. Density-dependent predation by a generalist can induce the opposite effect: predator-mediated exclusion of some prey species. Here, we

suggest that prairie dogs may have a similar effect, facilitating the exclusion of some small mammals that would otherwise occur in prairie landscapes.

In contrast to their effects on total species diversity, we have evidence from study areas throughout the range of the black-tailed prairie dog (Conlin 2005, Cully *et al.*, *in preparation*) that the richness of small-mammal species is lower within prairie-dog

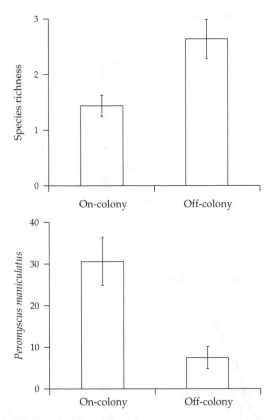

Figure 14.4 Differences in the communities of small rodents found on or near colonies of the black-tailed prairie dog. Species richness (a) and number of deer mice captured per 100 trap-nights (b) were averaged over four trapping periods during 2003–4 on each of 20 on-colony and 20 off-colony sites. Error bars indicate 95% confidence intervals.

colonies than at similar off-colony sites (Fig. 14.4(a)). Previous studies have also found fewer species of small mammals on prairie-dog colonies (as reviewed in Kotliar 1999; Lomolino and Smith 2003). Although the abundance of small rodents is often higher on colonies than off, this pattern is generally due to high abundance of a single species (Fig. 14.4(b)), such as the deer mouse (*Peromyscus maniculatus*) or the Northern grasshopper mouse (*Onychomys leucogaster*) (O'Meilia *et al.* 1982; Agnew *et al.* 1986; Mellink and Madrigal 1993; Cully *et al.*, *in preparation*). The apparent reduction in small-mammal diversity on prairie-dog colonies is compelling given the potential relationships between host diversity, pathogen "dilution," and disease emergence (see Chapter 3, this volume, for discussion of the dilution effect).

Prairie dogs may facilitate direct or apparent competition (or both) among small mammals. *Direct competition* may rise in response to the spatially concentrated resources available on prairie-dog colonies: for example, shelter and food (arthropods, forbs) may be enhanced through the burrowing and selective foraging behavior of prairie dogs. Species attempting to use these concentrated resources may find themselves in frequent interspecific contact. An increase in the ratio of inter- to intraspecific interactions tends to favor competitive exclusion (see Chapter 2, this volume). Prairie dogs may also facilitate *apparent competition*, by providing favorable conditions for generalist parasites. If the density of a parasite follows the total density of a suite of similar (competing) host species, then the more susceptible host species may be excluded through parasitism rather than directly through competition. If small-mammal parasites are easily maintained within prairie-dog burrows by the host–vector community using these burrows, then these parasites may preclude local persistence of the more susceptible host species. Each of these factors may also affect the potential for plague in the community (Box 14.2).

The potential for prairie dogs to facilitate parasite-mediated apparent competition may or may not extend to predator-mediated effects. Although coyotes commonly occur on prairie-dog colonies, these generalist predators have been shown to mediate coexistence (rather than exclusion) of small mammals in prairie landscapes (Henke and Bryant 1999). However, the work of Holt and colleagues (Chapter 2, this volume) suggests that such a keystone predator may also facilitate parasite-mediated apparent competition by affecting coexistence of alternate host species. The outcome of this predator-*and*-parasite-mediated apparent competition may be complex, depending on which species is the better competitor, which is more robust to predation, and which is more robust to disease. In any case, if prairie-dog activities attract keystone predators as well as generalist parasites, they may facilitate apparent competition in complex ways! We will not speculate on the relative importance of predation and parasitism in structuring these communities, but note that episodes of rinderpest virus in ungulates and canine distemper in lions

Box 14.2 An application of isocline methods to sylvatic plague

Plague may persist at very low frequency in a complex landscape if localized conditions favorable for its outbreak occur with sufficient frequency in time and space. Here we use the graphical methods discussed by Holt and colleagues (Holt *et al.* 2003, Chapter 2, this volume) to explore local community structures and dynamics that may be of disproportionate importance for plague maintenance.

Zero-growth isoclines and thresholds describe the bounds within which populations can grow. A specialist pathogen may require a threshold density of susceptible hosts in order for pathogen transmission to exceed pathogen loss through death or recovery of hosts. A generalist pathogen has more options, and may be maintained as long as host density within the *community* is sufficient. If we describe the host community on two axes, we may be able to divide this plane into regions of positive and negative pathogen growth, separated by the zero-growth isocline (as defined mathematically in Chapter 2, Box 2.2).

Figure 14.5 (a) shows three, hypothetical zero-growth isoclines for *Y. pestis* within a community of two host species. The axes describe the density of susceptible individuals of each species (S_i). Pathogen growth is negative between each isocline and the origin, and positive for higher densities of susceptible hosts. Isocline 1 describes a typical condition for pathogen invasion when transmission is density dependent (Holt *et al.* 2003, Chapter 2). Note that mosquitoes, ticks, and other generalist vectors may facilitate frequency-dependent transmission resulting in pathogen-growth isoclines with positive slope (Dobson 2004). But for host-specific flea species, we suggest that pathogen transmission between host species may be much lower than transmission within species, resulting in pathogen-growth isoclines that bow out from the origin. Such isoclines indicate that the pathogen requires nearly the full threshold density of each host species in order to invade, with little benefit gained by interspecific host interactions. Isocline 2 indicates that the pathogen can more easily invade a community when both host species are present, implying a significant effect of interspecific host interactions. This effect may be facilitated by resources that can be shared by several host and vector species; for example, prairie-dog burrows. Especially if each host species is territorial, interspecific use of prairie-dog burrows may increase interspecific relative to intraspecific interactions. This effect may be enhanced if the traffic through prairie-dog burrows, combined with a favorable microclimate for fleas, increases the potential for nonspecific host–vector contacts. Isocline 3 represents an

additional effect of bacterial "blocking" in the flea gut (see Box 14.1), which may starve the flea and further promote nonspecific host–vector contacts. Given the potential for prairie-dog burrows to enhance contacts between multiple species of hosts and vectors, the presence of prairie dogs within a community may enhance the potential for plague. But that is only part of the story.

Prairie dogs may also affect the potential for coexistence of multiple host species. Figure 14.5 (b) shows hypothetical carrying capacities for two consumer species (C_i) competing to some degree for similar resources (Tilman 1982; Grover 1997). Line 1 represents weak competition, with each competitor able to persist near its own carrying capacity even when both occur together. Such coexistence among small rodents could theoretically be facilitated by small-scale habitat heterogeneity and associated opportunities for niche partitioning (Kotler and Brown 1999; Chase and Leibold 2003). Line 1 may be precluded in habitat engineered by prairie dogs (see text). Line 2 indicates that inter- and intraspecific competition are equal in strength, such that the carrying capacity of the community follows the proportion of each species present. Line 3 indicates strong interspecific competition, with less likelihood of coexistence. In the text, we present evidence that the species richness of small rodents is lower on prairie-dog colonies, even though the on-colony abundance of rodents generally exceeds off-colony abundance. This evidence, combined with the obvious opportunities for interspecific interactions within prairie-dog burrows, suggests that line 3 may be the better model when prairie dogs are present.

The full potential for plague in prairie communities may be related to the interaction between patterns of pathogen transmission (Fig. 14.5(a)) and patterns of host competition (Fig. 14.5(b)). Here we consider models in which the presence of active prairie-dog burrows may alter the relative strength of interspecific interactions among two rodent host species and their specific fleas. We adopt the simplifying assumption of Holt and Dobson (Chapter 2) that host density is fixed by factors other than disease, which precludes apparent competition. (This assumption may be relaxed at larger scales, as discussed below.)

If the zero-growth isocline for *Y. pestis* lies completely outside the carrying capacity of the host community (cf. solid and upper dashed lines in Fig. 14.5(c)), there may never be enough susceptible hosts for *Y. pestis* to invade. In the presence of prairie dogs, however, burrow sharing among species may boost the relative strength of

continues

Box 14.2 *continued*

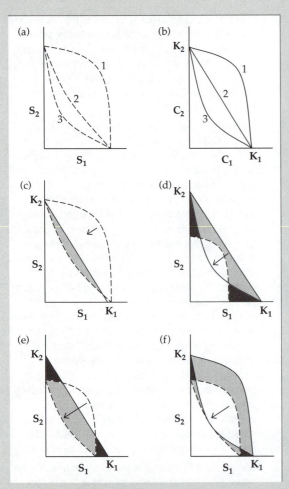

Figure 14.5 Zero-growth isoclines for a generalist pathogen (dashed lines) and carrying capacities for two hosts that are in direct competition for resources (solid lines). Isoclines in (a) describe the potential for a pathogen to invade a susceptible host community, which is *negative* between each isocline and the origin. Lines in (b) describe the potential for population growth within the host community, which is *positive* between each line and the origin. S_i or C_i = density of susceptible host or consumer species *i*. K_i = carrying capacity of species *i*. Isoclines in (a) indicate low (1), intermediate (2), and high (3) levels of interspecific pathogen transmission. Lines in (b) indicate low (1), intermediate (2), and high (3) levels of interspecific host competition. Shaded regions in (c)–(f) indicate host densities that should support disease outbreaks (but not necessarily persistence; see text). Arrows indicate possible shifts in isocline shape and disease potential accompanying an increase in interspecific interactions. These hypothetical scenarios represent possible keystone effects of prairie dogs on the community ecology and epidemiology of small rodents that share prairie-dog burrows.

interspecific transmission sufficiently to allow positive growth of this generalist pathogen when both host species are present (shaded region of Fig. 14.5(c)).

Alternatively, if the isocline for *Y. pestis* lies completely inside the carrying capacity for the community (cf. dashed and upper solid lines in Fig. 14.5(d)), there may often be a sufficient density of susceptible hosts to support plague (shaded regions of Fig. 14.5(d)). But an increase in interspecific competition could dramatically reduce the opportunities for plague persistence (darker regions of Fig. 14.5(d)).

Figure 14.5(d) suggests that the presence of prairie dogs may create conditions favorable for three alternative states of community structure: host 1 or 2 dominant with plague (dark regions under lower solid curve), or both hosts without plague (clear region near origin). These same

alternative states may also exist if the transmission isocline bulges through the carrying capacity (Fig. 14.5(e)). If interactions within prairie-dog burrows boost interspecific transmission but not competition, plague may persist even when neither host dominates, although any equilibrium community would likely lie on one host axis (Tompkins *et al.* 2000, Chapter 2).

Figure 14.5(f) represents effects of prairie-dog burrows on both pathogen transmission and host competition for resources. This example indicates that on-colony opportunities for plague may be much more restricted, but the direction and magnitude of this effect will depend on details of the relative effects of prairie-dog burrows on transmission and competition within and between alternate hosts for plague.

continues

Box 14.2 *continued*

These graphical models are based on assumptions that the community is at equilibrium and overall host densities are not affected by plague, contrary to observations. Communities of small rodents in this region are extremely variable (Brown and Ernest 2002), as are their fleas (Barnes 1982). Plague is known to effectively remove prairie dogs from entire communities (see text). It is also likely that plague causes significant morbidity or mortality among other rodent hosts. Adding asymmetric, plague-induced host morbidity or mortality to these models would foment apparent competition, affecting the carrying capacity of hosts and setting up a feedback between intensities of competition and transmission.

A full model delineating the potential for localized, enzootic plague must address at least this level of complexity. But such complex models may not be warranted, as observations of localized, enzootic plague are the rare exception in North America (K. Gage and M. Kosoy, *personal communication*).

Despite their simplicity, the models in Fig. 14.5 can be used to suggest conditions—perhaps local in time and space—that should enhance the probability of a plague epizootic. Given sufficient frequency of epizootics, plague may persist through extinction–colonization dynamics (Keeling and Gilligan 2000) across a network of communities. This scenario would require timely recovery of post-plague communities. It will be important to determine whether prairie dogs and their associates are resilient enough to withstand current (and future) frequencies of plague epizootics.

have awakened ecologists to the potentially dominant role played by parasites even in the Serengeti (McCallum and Dobson 1995).

14.3.4 Is plague enzootic in prairie communities?

There is some discord in the literature regarding the importance of resistant, enzootic hosts in the maintenance of plague. Some authors suggest that enzootic foci are spatially rare or nonexistent, with most plague taking the form of epizootics that sweep more or less rapidly across the landscape (Barnes 1982; Gage and Kosoy 2005). Others suggest that epizootics result from localized transmission from resistant enzootic hosts to susceptible ones (Perry and Fetherston 1997; Antolin *et al.* 2002).

Few North American rodents are considered to be potential enzootic hosts for plague, as few exhibit both high bacteremia and low mortality. Two possible exceptions are deer mice (*P. maniculatus*) and California voles (*Microtus californicus*): in limited clinical trials, both have responded to *Y. pestis* infection with high bacteremia and low mortality (Gage *et al.* 1995). Another candidate is the white-tailed prairie dog (*Cynomys leucurus*), the least social of the prairie-dog species (Cully and Williams 2001). Individual white-tailed prairie dogs are highly susceptible to plague, but the density of individuals within colonies and the frequency of their social interactions may be low enough to reduce transmission and sustain *Y. pestis* (Cully and Williams 1997; Anderson and Williams 1997). It has also been suggested that *Y. pestis* is sustained at the metapopulation level in black-tailed prairie dogs, through limited transmission among colonies (Cully and Williams 2001). Yet another hypothesis for the local maintenance of *Y. pestis* involves low-level infections sustained by fleas (Gage and Kosoy 2005).

Several observations suggest that plague commonly persists at least at low frequency within North American host–vector communities. In many regions, serological evidence of exposure to *Y. pestis* is common among mid-sized carnivores, such as coyotes, even in the absence of recent epizootics (Barnes 1982; Gese *et al.* 1997; Hoar *et al.* 2003). When even a single case of plague is identified in a human, a domestic pet, or a prairie-dog colony, local sampling commonly reveals *Y. pestis* within small mammals or their fleas (Barnes 1982; Madon *et al.* 1995). Relationships between climate and plague epizootics (Parmenter *et al.* 1999; Enscore *et al.* 2002), especially the relatively small-scale relationship found by Collinge *et al.* (2005a), also suggest that *Y. pestis* is available locally to respond to climate.

How does evidence from intensive trapping studies bear on this question? Evidence of *Y. pestis* is almost universally lacking from studies of small mammals undertaken before a plague case is detected (K. Gage, Centers for Disease Control, *personal communication*). Our study is no exception. Although we targeted host and vector species suspected to maintain *Y. pestis* during inter-epizootic periods, and despite the spatial, temporal, and numeric scale of our sampling, we found no evidence of *Y. pestis* among approximately 3900 rodent hosts and their many fleas sampled throughout our Colorado study area during 2003–4.

We recognize several potential reasons for this failure to detect *Y. pestis* among our samples. Because the last major epizootic occurred in 1994, and the last minor epizootic was detected in 2000, perhaps sufficient time had passed for *Y. pestis* to be cleared from these communities. Perhaps *Y. pestis* persists at such low frequencies in hosts or vectors that our sampling intensity was not sufficient to detect it. Perhaps it persists locally in species or locations not targeted by our sampling scheme. Today, just months after our last round of sampling in 2004, there is renewed evidence of plague activity throughout this study area. If the pathogen did not persist locally within the community of small rodents, prairie dogs and their fleas, this sudden and region-wide appearance of plague suggests very rapid spread through interspecific transmission.

14.4 Synthesis

Despite the long history of human struggle with plague, little is known regarding the dynamics of *Y. pestis* in its natural host–vector communities. Especially in the newly invaded communities of North American wildlife, it has proven difficult to identify classic reservoir hosts associated with reliable vectors. For this reason, the analyses we present here are exploratory in nature, and offer no confirmation of how plague works. But the results of our analyses suggest one primary direction for further research. Each of our analyses suggests that the dynamics of sylvatic plague may be determined largely by interspecific interactions, often across multiple trophic levels. We will need the tools of community ecology to identify the relative frequency, timing, and strength of these interactions to evaluate their importance in plague

dynamics. New molecular tools may aid in this work. Girard *et al.* (2004) have demonstrated patterns of genetic differentiation in *Y. pestis* at several geographic scales. Further knowledge of these patterns may help reveal the frequency, timing, and relative strength of intra- and interspecific transmission. With this knowledge, we may begin to evaluate the feedbacks between the structure of prairie communities and the potential for plague to structure those communities.

References

Achtman, M., K. Zurth, G. Morrelli, G. Torrea, A. Guiyoule, and E. Carniel. (1999). *Yersinia pestis*, the cause of plague, is a recently emerged clone of *Yersinia pseudotuberculosis*. *Proceedings of the National Academy of Sciences of the United States of America* **96**:14043–14048.

Agnew, W., D. W. Uresk, and R. M. Hansen. (1986). Flora and fauna associated with prairie dog colonies and adjacent ungrazed mixed-grass prairie in western South Dakota. *Journal of Range Management* **39**:135–139.

Anderson, S. H. and E. S.Williams. (1997). Plague in a complex of white-tailed prairie dogs and associated small mammals in Wyoming. *Journal of Wildlife Diseases* **33**:720–732.

Antolin, M. F., P. Gober, B. Luce, D. E. Biggins, W. E. Van Pelt, D. B. Seery *et al.* (2002). The influence of sylvatic plague on North American wildlife at the landscape level, with special emphasis on black-footed ferret and prairie dog conservation. In *Transactions of the 67th North American Wildlife and Natural Resources Conference*, pp. 104–127.

Bacot, A. W. and C. J. Martin. (1914). Observations on the mechanism of the transmission of plague by fleas. *Journal of Hygiene* **13**(Suppl. III):423–439.

Barnes, A. M. (1982). Surveillance and control of bubonic plague in the United States. *Symposium of the Zoological Society of London.* **50**:237–270.

Biggins, D. and M. Y. Kosoy. (2001). Influences of introduced plague on North American mammals: implications from ecology of plague in Asia. *Journal of Mammalogy* **82**:906–916.

Boisier, P., L. Rahalison, M. Rasolomaharo, M. Ratsitorahina, M. Mahafaly, M. Razafimahefa *et al.* (2002). Epidemiologic features of four successive annual outbreaks of bubonic plague in Mahajanga, Madagascar. *Emerging infectious diseases* **8**:311–316.

Brown, J. H. and S. K. M. Ernest. (2002). Rain and rodents: complex dynamics of desert consumers. *BioScience* **52**:979–987.

Burnham, K. P. and D. R. Anderson. (2002). *Model Selection and Inference: A Practical Information-Theoretic Approach.* New York, Springer-Verlag.

Cavanaugh, D. C. and J. D. Marshal, Jr. (1972). The influence of climate on the seasonal prevalence of plague in the Republic of Vietnam. *Journal of Wildlife Diseases* **8**:85–94.

Chase, J. M. and M. A. Leibold. (2003). *Ecological niches: linking classical and contemporary approaches.* University of Chicago Press, Chicago, IL.

Collinge, S. K., W. C. Johnson, C. Ray, R. Matchett, J. Grensten, J. F. Cully, Jr. *et al.* (2005a). Testing the generality of a trophic-cascade model for plague. *EcoHealth* **2**:1–11.

Collinge, S. K., W. C. Johnson, C. Ray, R. Matchett, J. Grensten, J. F. Cully, Jr. *et al.* (2005b). Landscape structure and plague occurrence in black-tailed prairie dogs on grasslands of the western USA. *Landscape Ecology, in press.*

Conlin, D. (2005). Abundance of rodents on grasslands characterized by a patchy distribution of prairie dogs, urban development, and plague epidemics. MS thesis, University of Colorado, Boulder, CO. 77 pp.

Cully, J. F., Jr. and E. S. Williams. (2001). Interspecific comparisons of sylvatic plague in prairie dogs. *Journal of Mammalogy* **82**:894–905.

Cully, J. F., Jr., A. M. Barnes, T. J. Quan, and G. Maupin. (1997). Dynamics of plague in a Gunnison's prairie dog colony complex from New Mexico. *Journal of Wildlife Diseases* **33**:706–719.

Cully, J. F., Jr., S. K. Collinge, C. Ray, D. Conlin, B. Holmes, W. C. Johnson, T. Johnson *et al.* (*Manuscript in preparation*). Small mammal communities associated with black-tailed prairie dogs.

Daszak, P., A. A. Cunningham, and A. D. Hyatt. (2000). Emerging infectious diseases of wildlife—threats to biodiversity and human health. *Science* **287**:443–449.

Dobson, A. P. (2004). Population dynamics of pathogens with multiple host species. *American Naturalist* **164**(Suppl.):S64–S78.

Enscore, R. E., B. J. Biggerstaff, T. L. Brown, R. F. Fulgham, P. J. Reynolds *et al.* (2002). Modeling relationships between climate and the frequency of human plague cases in the southwestern United States, 1960–1997. *American Journal of Tropical Medicine and Hygiene* **66**:186–196.

Gage, K. L. and M. Y. Kosoy. (2005). Natural history of plague: perspectives from more than a century of research. *Annual Review of Entomology* **50**:505–528.

Gage, K. L., R. S. Ostfeld, and J. G. Olson. (1995). Nonviral vector-borne zoonoses associated with mammals in the United States. *Journal of Mammalogy* **76**:695–715.

Gese, E. M., R. D. Schultz, M. R. Johnson, E. S. Williams, R. L. Crabtree, and R. L. Ruff. (1997). Serological survey for diseases in free-ranging coyotes (*Canis latrans*) in Yellowstone National Park, Wyoming. *Journal of Wildlife Diseases* **33**:47–56.

Girard, J. M., D. M. Wagner, A. J. Vogler, C. Keys, C. J. Allender *et al.* (2004). Differential plague-transmission dynamics determine *Yersinia pestis* population genetic structure on local, regional, and global scales. *Proceedings of the National Academy of Sciences, USA* **101**:8408–8413.

Grover, J. P. (1997). *Resource Competition.* Chapman and Hall, London.

Henke, S. E. and F. C. Bryant. (1999). Effects of coyote removal on the faunal community in western Texas. *Journal of Wildlife Management* **63**:1066–1081.

Hinnebusch, B. J., A. E. Rudolph, P. Cherepanov, J. E. Dixon, T. G. Schwan, and A. Forsberg. (2002). Role of Yersinia murine toxin in survival of *Yersinia pestis* in the midgut of the flea vector. *Science* **296**:733–735.

Hoar, B. R., B. B. Chomel, D. L. Rolfe, C. C. Chang, C. L. Fritz, B. N. Sacks, and T. E. Carpenter. (2003). Spatial analysis of *Yersinia pestis* and *Bartonella vinsonii* subsp. *berkhoffii* seroprevalence in California coyotes (*Canis latrans*). *Preventive Veterinary Medicine* **56**:299–311.

Holt, R. D., A. P. Dobson, M. Begon, R. G. Bowers, and E. Schauber. (2003). Parasive establishment and persistence in multi-host systems. *Ecology Letters* **6**:837–842.

Hoogland, J. L. (1995). *The Black-Tailed Prairie Dog: Social Life of a Burrowing Mammal.* University of Chicago Press, Chicago, IL.

Keeling, M. J. and C. A. Gilligan. (2000). Metapopulation dynamics of bubonic plague. *Nature* **407**:903–906.

Kotler, B. P. and J. S. Brown. (1999). Mechanisms of coexistence of optimal foragers as determinants of local abundances and distributions of desert granivores. *Journal of Mammalogy* **80**:361–374.

Kotliar, N. B., B. W. Baker, A. D. Whicker, and G. Plumb. (1999). A critical review of assumptions about the prairie dog as a keystone species. *Environmental Management* **24**:177–192.

Lomolino, M. V. and G. A. Smith. (2003). Terrestrial vertebrate communities at black-tailed prairie dog (*Cynomys ludovicianus*) towns. *Biological Conservation* **115**:89–100.

Maddon, M. B., J. C. Hitchcock, R. M. Davis, C. M. Myers, C. R. Smith, *et al.* (1997). An overview of plague in the United States and a report of investigations of two human cases in Kern County, California, 1995. *Journal of Vector Ecology* **22**:77–82.

McCallum, H. and A. P. Dobson. (1995). Detecting disease and parasite threats to endangered species and ecosystems. *Trends in Ecology and Evolution* **10**:190–193.

Mellink, E. and H. Madrigal. (1993). Ecology of Mexican prairie dogs, *Cynomys mexicanus*, in El Manantial, northeastern Mexico. *Journal of Mammalogy* **74**:631–635.

O'Meilia, M. E., F. L. Knopf and J. C. Lewis. (1982). Some consequences of competition between prairie dogs and beef cattle. *Journal of Range Management* **35**:580–585.

Parkhill, J., B. W. Wren, N. R. Thomson, R. W. Titball, M. T. G. Holden, M. B. Prentice *et al.* (2001). Genome sequence of *Yersinia pestis*, the causative agent of plague. *Nature* **413**:523–527.

Parmenter, R. R., E. P. Yadav, C. A. Parmenter, P. Ettestad and K. L. Gage. (1999). Incidence of plague associated with increased winter-spring precipitation in New Mexico, USA. *American Journal of Tropical Medicine and Hygiene* **61**:814–821.

Perry, R. D. and J. D. Fetherston. (1997). *Yersinia pestis*— etiologic agent of plague. *Clinical Microbiology Reviews* **10**:35–66.

Poland, J. D. and A. M. Barnes. (1979). Plague. In J. F. Steele, ed. *CRC Handbook Series in Zoonoses. Section A: Bacterial Rickettsial, and Mycotic Diseases 1* pp. 515–597. CRC Press, Boca Raton, FL.

Pollitzer, R. (1954). Plague. *World Health Organization Monograph* **22**:1–698.

Pollitzer, R. and K. F. Meyer. (1961). The ecology of plague. In J. M. May, ed. *Studies in Disease Ecology*, pp. 433–590. Hafner Publishing Company, Inc, New York.

Roach, J. L., B. Van Horne, P. Stapp, and M. F. Antolin, (2001). Genetic structure of a black-tailed prairie dog metapopulation. *Journal of Mammalogy* **82**:946–959.

Silverman, J. and M. K. Rust. (1981). Influence of temperature and humidity on the survival and development of the cat flea, *Ctenocephalides felis* (Siphonaptera: Pulicidae). *Journal of Medical Entomology* **18**:78–83.

Silverman, J. and M. K. Rust. (1983). Some abiotic factors affecting the survival of the cat flea, *Ctenocephalides felis* (Siphonaptera: Pulicidae). *Environmental Entomology* **12**:490–495.

Stapp, P., M. F. Antolin, and M. Ball. (2004). Patterns of extinction in prairie-dog metapopulations: plague outbreaks follow El Niño events. *Frontiers in Ecology and the Environment* **2**:235–240.

Thomas, R. E. (1996). Fleas and the agents they transmit. In B. J. Beaty and W. C. Marquardt, eds. *The Biology of Disease Vectors*, pp. 146–159. University of Colorado Press, Niwot.

Tilman, D. (1982). *Resource Competition and Community Structure*. Princeton University Press, Princeton, NJ.

Tompkins, D. M., J. V. Greenman, P. A. Robertson, and P. J. Hudson. (2000). The role of shared parasites in the exclusion of wildlife hosts: *Heterakis gallinarum* in the ring-necked pheasant and the grey partridge. *Journal of Animal Ecology* **69**:829–840.

US Fish and Wildlife Service. (2000). Endangered and threatened wildlife and plants; 12-month finding for a petition to list the black-tailed prairie dog as threatened. *Federal Register* **65**:5476–5488.

Index

Note: page numbers in **bold** refer to material in boxes.